WELLNESS
AGAINST ALL ODDS

Sherry A. Rogers, M.D.

1994

 Prestige Publishing
Box 3068 3500 Brewerton Rd.
Syracuse, NY 13220

i

Copyright © 1994

Prestige Publishing
P.O. Box 3068
3500 Brewerton Road
Syracuse, NY 13220

For information address Prestige Publishers, Box 3068, 3500 Brewerton Rd., Syracuse, NY 13220.

Library of Congress Card Catalog Number: 94-065045

ISBN: 0-9618821-5-8

Printed in the United States

Dedication

Whom else, but to LUSCIOUS.

But when I read Elizabeth Barrett Browning's words,

"How do I love thee,
let me count the ways.....
I love thee to the breadth and height my soul can reach",

I asked myself, whom else could she have been talking about but Luscious?...I guess they must have had an affair sometime.

Anyway, not to be out done (after all, I do have the advantage of 25 years with him); To Luscious. . . . . .

We've slept in our Caribbean treehouse, and the cornfield by the pond,
In the milkhouse at the barn, and French castles, of which we're fond.

From Rome to that floor in Shanghai . . . . sometimes we didn't have a bed.
From Melbourne to the Ganges; each place I've laid my head,

Each one has become my favorite night, with which none can e'er compare.
The reason is plain and simple; it's because **you** were always there.

DISCLAIMER

This book is not intended for self-treatment. It is intended to be a source of information that will lead one to seek out the appropriate type of physician to help one implement the ideas this book has to offer.

In Loving Memory

K B

ACKNOWLEDGEMENT

Thanks to Mr. Dan Grigoriew for
his expertise, caring, and patience
with my endless corrections.

FOREWARD

Dr. Sherry Rogers is truly one of those remarkable health practitioners who has survived the traditional medical education route, only to retain her sensibility, vision, and perspective about what being a doctor is all about: serving people with the best, lowest-technology means possible.

I have known Dr. Rogers for more than ten years, and I have always been amazed by her ability to couple the scientific underpinnings of medicine and all its technicalities with a high degree of skill in communication and humanness in the way she delivers her message to the patient. She has found a remarkable system, whereby these two, sometimes disparate, world views become a cohesive, almost seamless end product which results in improved outcome, health, and healing in her patients.

As one of the acknowledged world experts in environmental medicine, which is a rapidly advancing field, Dr. Rogers has broken new ground in understanding the relative relationship of the environment to health and disease processes, and how nutrition and other lifestyle principles play a role in ameliorating and helping to defend against toxic insults from the environment.

In her most recent book, *Wellness Against All Odds*, I find another, very creative link between basic science, anatomy, physiology, and mechanistic understanding of disease, and how people really live. This takes up where her book, *The E.I. Syndrome*, left off. I believe it is a user-friendly guide to implementing the concepts that she also describes in her book, *Tired or Toxic?* By using a case-study style, along with liberal examples from her own clinical experiences, with an underpin ning of science to support her assumptions, she is able to develop a great lesson plan for the reader on how a disease might be produced by lack of attention to the details of lifestyle and nutrition, and what to do about it.

There are many "sensible," easily applied concepts included in this book that fly in the face of what many of us learned in our traditional schools of health sciences, nutrition, or medicine; however, these are presented in such a way that the reader recognizes there are whole new approaches at the cutting edge toward the improvement of health and vitality in individuals who have had a series of chronic health problems or are at risk for serious disease.

The book has an extensive series of referrals and other information that can be used to help the reader find answers to questions that may have been on their minds for some time, yet they were unaware of where to look for solutions to their concerns. It also contains a significant amount of nutrition and dietary information which can be applied directly by the reader in areas of specific health concern. I found this to be a book with a wealth of information that would be difficult to locate in standard reference sources, and even more difficult to consolidate into one readable manuscript.

There are an extraordinary number of health books published every year, but it appears to me that this book does a unique job of putting together clinical information which has been tested and proven to be successful; individual case histories which are anecdotal, but which come from one of the most respected leaders in environmental medicine as authentic; basic emergence of the science of nutrition, immunology, and environmental health; and consumer information that can be utilized directly in a personal health improvement program. This is quite a handful, and very difficult for any author to get into one book, but believe Dr. Rogers has accomplished that goal in this very interesting distillation of her years of clinical experience.

I would recommend *Wellness Against All Odds* to any individual looking for a cogent, articulate discussion of where and how medicine is advancing, and how that applies to individuals taking charge of their own health and finding the path toward health enhancement that works best for them.

Jeffrey S. Bland, Ph.D,
C.E.O.
HealthComm Inc.
Gig Harbor WA
January, 1994

TABLE OF CONTENTS

Title page   i

Copyright   ii

Dedication   iii

Disclaimer   iv

In Loving Memory   v

Acknowledgement   vi

Forward   vii

Chapter 1 - In the Beginning or How this book came about   1

Chapter 2 - Give us this day our daily bread   11

    What diverse Cancer Therapies Have In Common   11

    The Metabolic Cross   14

    General Guidelines For Transitional Vegetarian   21
    and Carnivore Diets

    General Dietary Guidelines: Transitional Vegetarian   30

    General Dietary Guidelines: Transitional Carnivore   37

    Case Story: Severe Chemical Sensitivity   46

    Lessons from the Carnivore Switch   47

    The Basis In Biochemistry   50

    Damaged Cell Membranes Leak Calcium   54

    High Potassium Is Critical To Healing   57

    Steaming Preserves Potassium   59

    The Silent Sick   60

    Down With Guilt!   61

What Diet Should I Start On? 63

Many Need an Unbalanced Diet To Begin With 64

The More Serious The Condition, The More
Dangerous Are "Subtle" Differences In Diet. 66

Leukemia As An Example 69

Opposites Attract 73

The Bottom Line 73

Resources 74

Chapter 3 - Purification 81

"The Coffee Break" 81

History Of Coffee Enemas 82

How Does The Coffee Enema Work? 90

Would This Help The Common Cold? 91

The Lethal Retinoic Acid Syndrome 92

Steady As She Goes 92

Questions about coffee enemas: 93

Procedure For Coffee Enemas 95

Procedure For Making The Enema 96

Scientific Evidence 98

A Hot Date With Juan Valdez 103

For The Dying Patient Who Cannot Eat:
Cachexia And Hydrazine Sulfate 105

References   107

Chapter 4 - Man Does Not Live By Bread Alone: 110
    Enzymes, Juicing, Cleansing, Flushing And Brushing

    Enzymes   110

    How It Was Discovered That Enzymes Destroy Cancers 113

    What Can Cause Enzyme Deficiencies?   116

    What Type Of Enzyme Should I Use?   117

    Other Conditions That Enzymes Help   119

    Juicing   121

    Immaculate Intestines: 123
    Gut Grooming Or Cleansing

    Colon Cleanse Protocol   124

    Alternative Directions: 125

    Procedure: 125

    Flushing   126

    Materials & Procedure: 129

    The Purge   131

    Brushing   132

    Additional Detoxification Routines   133

    Candida And Leaky Gut Syndrome   134

    Resources   141

Chapter 5 - Atoning For The Biochemical Sins Of The 21st Century   145

Fixing What's Broken 145

Dispelling Another Myth: 147
Nutrient Deficiencies Are Rare In The U.S.

How Do We Get Nutrient Deficient? 148

Copper Deficiency As An Example 150

The Nutrient Connection 154

If You Fail To Identify And Correct Nutrient 160
Deficiencies, The Sick Get Sicker, Quicker

Chromium Deficiency Causes 167
The Craving Cycle And Hypoglycemia

The Vicious Chromium Cycle: 169

The Magnesium Cycle Of Disease 169

References

Why Leukemics Need High Calcium Prescriptions 173

Potassium And It's Relation To Healing 179

References 181

Vitamin A Cures Some Cancers 184

Cancer Patients Are Cheated 186

References 187

How The Sick Get Sicker, Quicker, 193
By Following Current Medical Protocol

Magnesium Leads The Way As An Example 196

Is There A Conspiracy Of Ignorance And Arrogance? 202

Beware of Crooked Science 205

"If You Eat A Balanced Diet, You Can't Get Deficient" 206

References 211

Books Of Interest 220

Help! I'm Being Magnesiumed To Death! 221

Chapter 6 - The Ecologic Trinity: 223
    Clean Air, Food And Water

The Total Load 223

What You Can Do Today? 225

Create A Bedroom In Which You Can Heal 225

Start A Diet With Which You Can Heal: 226

Start With A body Which Can Heal: 227

Start With A Mind That Is Ready To Heal: 227

What Is Wrong with Chlorinated Water? 228

An Environmental Medicine Approach 231
To Chronic Back Pain

Resources 237

Heavy Metal Toxicity 239

How To Diagnose Heavy Metal Toxicity 244

Parkinson's Disease As An Example 245
Of Heavy Metal Toxicity Disease

Never Underestimate The Importance 248
Of A Tincture Of Time

Food Allergy And Gluten-Sensitivity Can Mimic 249
Many "Undiagnosable And Incurable Diseases

D-xylose Test 254

Silent Pesticide Poisoning   256
Can Ruin Your Life In A Day

Should I Take Hormones?   259

Thyroid   259

Adrenal Hormones   260

Testosterone   261

Estrogen   262

Melatonin   264

What's Your Passion?   265

The Candida Solution   266

Total Load Checklist   271

How To Avoid Dying In The Hospital   276

Resources: 281

Chapter 7 - The Faith Factor   284

Spirituality   284

For God's Sake Don't Mention Religion In Your Book!   291

Facilitated Healing   295

Spirituality And E.I. Have Much In Common   296

The Corrosion And Collapse Of Character   301

Drug To "Prevent" Breast Cancer   306
Can Cause Leukemia And Blindness

What Do We Call This Program?   311

Resources   316

Chapter 8 - Humble Healing   321

How Not To Die From Labelitis   321

Case Example   322

The Most Common Blunders Of Medicine   328

No One Has More Power Over Your Health   331
Than The Person Who Prepares Your Food

Alcoholism As A Multi-Faceted Disease   333

How Do I Start?   334

The Seven Trade-Offs   335

Humble Healing Program   345

Notes On The Individual Aspects Of The Program   345

"I'm Overwhelmed!"   351

Resources   355

Scientific Publications of Sherry A. Rogers , M.D.   358
in Peer Reviewed Medical Journals

Scientific Articles By Sherry A. Rogers In   359
Proceedings of International Symposia

Books By Sherry A. Rogers, M.D.   361

Chapter 1

In The Beginning
or
How this book came about

In the beginning, I was a simple country doctor at heart with specialty boards in family practice and additional certification in allergy. I was happy practicing medicine just like my colleagues. It wasn't until I started to develop an endless array of diseases and symptoms that nobody in medicine could cure, that I started straying from the pack.

My husband and I literally roamed the United States, even going to hypnosis courses in Washington D.C., trying to find a cause and a cure for my multiple maladies. At night I would go to bed in tears after having spent hours laboring over my medical books, crying "Why isn't what I have in here?". But all these diseases and symptoms were one of God's many gifts to me, because I was then shown that they had causes that could be corrected. From that point on, we departed from the point of view that current medicine still embraces, namely that "a headache is a Darvon deficiency".

We departed from the world of drugs to enter the world of environmental medicine and nutritional biochemistry where the cause of symptoms can be found and real cures brought about. Not only did we learn how to do nearly **drug free** medicine, but we also learned an important rule of modern medicine, and that is, that the **patient is the keeper of the keys to wellness.** After I had devoured every book on the subject, only to find that we had a great deal of information that was not to be found in any other books, I felt compelled to share it with those who were suffering as I had.

So even though I had never dreamed of writing a book, had no talent for such an endeavor, and still had some brain fog of my own, we wrote **THE E.I. SYNDROME**. It spelled out how to diagnose food, chemical, mold, and Candida sensitivities as well as nutrient deficiencies, and much more. In Fact, to this day it has multiple facts the chemically sensitive person needs to know that just are not in print anywhere else. So I thought we had accomplished our goal. I thought we were done.

In spite of learning how to clear so many of my maladies, new ones kept cropping up and challenging us. My asthma, migraines, chronic sinusitis and eczema were cleared with mold and food injections. I had identified multiple vitamin and mineral deficiencies which had contributed to my chronic fatigue and periodic, unexplained depressions. Multiple chemical sensitivities were identified that caused the brain fog, chronic back pain and a multiple of other symptoms.

Then I started to develop bloody colitis; next a chronic shoulder problem that nobody could figure out, way out of proportion to anything I could have subjected the shoulder to. I felt I had started the disease-of-the-month-club. But the chemical sensitivities at that point were the worst problems because they limited my freedom. There were lots of places I could not go without suffering brain fog for days as a result of "normal" chemical exposures like perfumes, natural gas or new carpets. I kept looking at every possible way that people had made themselves well and kept being drawn back to macrobiotics. There were multiple people who had cleared their very cancers with that diet and I kept thinking that if they could do that, then my problems had to be a piece of cake; and indeed hundreds of us lost our chemical sensitivities or drastically reduced them with the macrobiotic diet.

So, we wrote **You Are What You Ate** to teach our patients about the diet and the special modifications of it that are necessary for allergic people. Then, I thought we had accomplished our task. I thought we were done. However, I was still wrong because people would come to our office from all over the country and go home to their family doctors exuberant and say, "Doctor, I thought you would like to know how I got myself well. You've worked so hard to try to help me and when nothing worked, I went to see a specialist in environmental medicine. Now, I know the causes for my symptoms and I'm starting to get well. One of the things that I'm doing is the macrobiotic diet"

Numerous patients told us that their doctors looked down at them declaring, "There's no evidence for that stuff, you know". It was then that I decided that they were going to have evidence that was irrefutable and so we wrote **Tired Or Toxic?** which gives over 33 biochemical mechanisms of why macrobiotics is so healing. It also gives over 8 mechanisms of how Candida can cause the baffling symptoms that it does. It also goes into a tremendous amount of nutritional biochemistry, showing not only the biochemical explanation for chemical sensitivity, but showing how undiagnosed mold, food, and chemical sensitivities as well as hidden vitamin and mineral deficiencies can masquerade as just about any symptom, including the terrible brain fog that had plagued us all.

It provides the diagnosis and treatment for all of this, plus the scientific evidence. In fact, it is the first book to do this and simultaneously be written for both the physician and the patient. I felt this was the only way of protecting the patient against doubting Thomases who really had not the faintest glimmer of knowledge about the subject. And THEN I thought that we were done.

But again, I was wrong. We had written three books in less than five years with a full-time private practice in addition to lecturing and teaching around the world sandwiched in. I thought we we were peddling just as fast as we could, but people showed us another urgent need.

As it turned out, since **You Are What You Ate** got people started on the macrobiotic diet, I figured the scores of other macrobiotic books with recipes and menus would guide them further. But not one single book actually spelled out in detail what it was that all those people with cancers did day to day in order to clear their cancers with the macrobiotic diet. There were numerous autobiographies by people who had cleared their cancers with the diet, some of whom were physicians themselves. But none actually spelled out in detail what it was they did day to day. Every time I read of how someone had miraculously recovered totally from an end- stage incurable cancer, I was left asking, "But what was it exactly that they did day to day?" The only way I could think of to find out was to go to the top.

So, I flew to Boston every month for half a year to work with the leading living authority in macrobiotics, Mr. Michio Kushi. He was wonderfully gracious and allowed me to sit for days on end with him as long as I needed, as he went through scores of patients from around the world. I watched as they cleared numerous "incurable" conditions. Being a very fast writer, I wrote everything that he told each person and when finally I found myself writing what he would tell them to do, before he even said it, for three days straight, I knew I had it. Then we wrote **The Cure Is In The Kitchen.** Then I thought we had accomplished our goal. I thought we were done. And for the fourth time, I was wrong.

This time it was because we saw that many people were starting on the diet for their own special needs, but the rest of the family turned up their noses and said "Yuk! I'm not eating that stuff." So, we had to figure out recipes and menus for the rest of the

4

family, while utilizing the grains, greens and beans that the sick person has to have so that the cook would not be doing double duty. That's when **Macro Mellow** was born through the marvelous talents and loving efforts of Mrs. Shirley Gallinger. Then I thought surely we were done and that we needn't write any more books. After all, I'm not a writer, I'm a physician. For the 5th time, I thought we were done. And for the fifth time, I was wrong. Because then the most startling thing of all happened, and I knew once again it was up to us to make this very important message available to those who would need it. It never ceases to amaze me that there is such a hard working, underground network of people desperately trying to survive against all odds and making it. They will not sit back and take a life sentence pronounced by a doctor, just because they have a certain cancer or other illness. Instead, they start looking to find what it is the doctor doesn't even know and how they can make themselves well, against all odds.

It all began in the summer of 1989, when an adorable, young attorney presented to my office with acute myelogenous leukemia. She said half a year ago she had been given a 5% chance of living one year by three major medical centers. She had been recommended three courses of chemotherapy and a bone marrow transplant all of which would amount to about $200,000.00.

For this price, she had a one in three chance of dying from the treatment, but if she lived it would buy her most likely two years. The quality of those two years however, was questionable. So she herself, decided that she wanted to go on the macrobiotic diet, analyze her nutrient levels and try to heal her body against all odds. Her story you have read in **The Cure Is In The Kitchen**, how her leukemia cleared while on the diet.

However, just after the book was published, she went off the

5

diet; and as you know, cancer victims who go off the macrobiotic diet, especially before seven years, usually end up with their cancers coming back with a viciousness and so it did with my friend. In fact, it was so bad that the oncologist called me in the middle of my office hours and told me she had exactly 48 hours to live and no longer; that there was nothing more that could be done by anyone, anywhere to save her.   I'll tell you it was one of my worst days, trying to practice with a broken heart!

The next morning she showed up in my kitchen.   She had gotten her transfusion, signed out AMA (against medical advise) and had come to say "Good-bye". She said she knew she was dying and had about 24 hours left and said that she felt worse now than she had in the beginning when her leukemia was first diagnosed. My heart dropped to my knees as I thought of all the fun times we had had together and that I was not ready to part with my friend. "Wait a minute!", I said, "Macro isn't the only way people have beat cancer, let's try another way."

For years I have been studying alternative forms of cancer therapy, merely because I thought there were some lessons to be learned by people who had conquered it, that might be useful for my patients with chemical sensitivities.   I was familiar with the very good track record of the Gerson therapy. The only reason I had never explored it for my E.I. (environmental illness, chemical sensitivity) patients was that it's too time-consuming for someone who works.

I immediately went right into my home study, got out my Gerson book and we hot-footed it down the street to the health food store and pharmacy and got all of the things that we needed. I even had a Gerson juicer already, so she was ready to start out at that moment.

6

A month later she was still alive and rallying, actually looking better and feeling better. It was at that point that we realized that she couldn't stay on the Gerson treatment. It's so time-consuming that all you have time for in life is cleaning out your juicer. With hourly fresh juices as part of the involved therapy, by the time you're all cleaned up, it's time to start peeling and preparing the vegetables for the next juicing. And being a type A personality, she was still actively practicing office and courtroom law as well as being a mother to two gorgeous children. So at that point, I introduced her to another idea hoping that she would agree, and she bit —— hook, line and sinker.

It was the Kelley Program, started by a dentist in the late 60's in Dallas who cleared his own cancer of the pancreas and is still alive at this writing. This program promised to be a bit more compatible with being a full-time practicing attorney and mother of two beautiful children. And so, she embarked on the third program which cleared her cancer the second time around, against all odds.

Seeing the remarkable results of this program led me to a massive night and day exploration of every aspect of both of these programs. I was driven. I wanted to extract from them anything and everything that might be of use to my friend as well as my patients from all over the world with all sorts of "undiagnosable" and "untreatable" conditions. And through my explorations, I encountered a whole silent underground of people who have done the impossible. But they do not speak out for fear of being thought of as "weird" or crazy. For we have all been brain-washed to believe that it would be impossible to do what they have done, and if it were true, why is it that the whole world is not aware of these startling findings?

As a result of this intensive search, there has been an avalanche of information that we have uncovered in the last few years. It turns out that there are a number of natural and inexpensive programs with which people have done the impossible. It was screaming to me that there was a bigger message here for anyone who was willing to take the time to study all these methods and determine, first why they worked at all, and then to see what they had in common. And, last but far from least, it seemed to be screaming to me to explain how this information could be useful for those who were still suffering from "undiagnosable" or "untreatable" conditions.

And as you can guess, especially if you have followed the previous 5 books, it not only opens up a whole new world of medical possibilities, but changes all the rules of medicine. And, most importantly, it empowers the person with the illness - - - it puts the control in his hands, where it ought to be. Physicians are merely his consultants; **the patient is the one who plays the major role in determining whether or not the patient gets well.**

Couple all that with what I have learned from my continual research into the biochemistry and medical journals, as well as from all the courses I attend and teach in and from my wonderful and loving patients, and you can appreciate why I thought it actually criminal not to write this book and make this knowledge available to anyone who would like to explore these concepts with the help of their physician.

As you will see, some of the things initially will sound really far out, but when it comes right down to it, everything is God given, very inexpensive compared with prescription medications, chemotherapy, radiation and surgery, and is very natural. On the contrary, these techniques do not poison, burn or mutilate the body tissues. They do just the reverse. They allow the body to get so healthy that it can reverse or heal disease.

8

Furthermore, for many cancers, for example, there are no chemotherapy programs that have a proven track record to justify using them. But nonetheless, they are used out of desperation. And of course, **all chemotherapy can cause cancer eventually.** In fact the nurses and pharmacists who even handle it are at risk (McDevitt JL, Lees PSJ, McDiarmid MA, Exposure of hospital pharmacists and nurses to antineoplastic agents, JOM, 35:1, 57-60, 1993).

And the techniques in this book do not make the assumption that a headache is a Darvon deficiency. Arthritis is not a Motrin deficiency, high cholesterol is not a Lopid or Mevocor deficiency, **cancer is not a chemotherapy deficiency.** These techniques do not make the victim rely solely on drugs to mask symptoms, only to eventually allow another symptom to arise in the same or a different target organ. But instead, these techniques merely allow the body to get so bloody healthy that it eventually heals itself.

The irony is that some of these techniques have been around for over 90 years, and some for over 2,000! But with the advent of the pharmaceutical era, they have been ignored, save for a silent minority of physician sleuths. We've been very fortunate in receiving hundreds of fan letters from people who have read the other five books, telling us how much they have helped them diagnose and treat their own problems. For anyone utilizing the therapies in this book, I would strongly recommend that you read all five of the previous books, because there is a great deal that the patient must know in order to bring about wellness that is contained in those volumes and cannot be repeated here. Actually, the books represent stages of necessary growth, and this volume will build on that knowledge.

The patient dedicated to wellness against all odds, actually has to go to medical school, so to speak. And too often someone (whether it be a patient of mine or a non-patient who has written to me or scheduled a phone consultation with me to brain-storm) will relate that in finally addressing one of the recommendations from one of the other books, they had turned a corner and were now on the road to wellness. The problem is, no one knows what factors will change the course of illness for you. So I would recommend fervently that you read all the preceding five books to develop **the total load concept** and to garner all the facts you can.

Because the concepts in the preceding books are useful regardless of whichever program in this book a person follows, for brevity, I will have to assume that you possess that knowledge so that we can proceed to higher levels of wellness in this volume. But suffice it to say, that if someone merely reads this book and does not find improvement, I would like to caution that it is most likely because he is not addressing the total load.

And so, there are concepts in this volume applicable not only to those who follow the macrobiotic program, but for those who hate it, and for those who simply cannot do it because it makes them worse, and especially for people who are trying to get **well, against all odds.** I'm not into selling books. That is not how I make my living. Heavens! If I were, I would have hired a ghost writer and gone with some big, fancy publisher and gotten a lot of publicity. Instead, we don't advertise, we don't market, but merely rely on word of mouth amongst people who are just plain interested in getting themselves as healthy as possible.

Likewise, we do not write for the "average" person. Our readers are advanced physicians and lay people who know more about health than the average physician. They read and search for **wellness, against all odds.** I hope this work makes that possible now for you.

Chapter 2

GIVE US THIS DAY OUR DAILY BREAD

What Diverse Cancer Therapies Have In Common

It is fascinating to me that there are many diverse therapies with which people have cleared cancers. Let's concentrate on only a few that I have verification of and see what they may have in common. The Gerson program comes to mind, because many have succeeded with this and several have written their stories. The now deceased Dr. Max Gerson was very sincere in his efforts to popularize this and expended great effort to enable others to follow the program and share in his astonishment of what the healthy body can heal.

Interestingly, though, I know off several people who went to the Gerson clinic with E.I. (environmental illness, chemical sensitivity) and had no improvement. They told me that when they entered, they looked the healthiest, while everyone else was brought in in wheelchairs and stretchers, cachectic (wasted), and near death. As the weeks rolled by, however, the cancer people started to rally and looked progressively better, while the chemically sensitive got worse. I still do not know the answer to this, unless they were just not, as you will learn, on the correct metabolic diet for them, or having reached a specific stage, did not then re-adapt the program accordingly.

Basically, the **Gerson program** includes a diet of multiple fruit and vegetable juices as well as raw liver juice throughout the day, in fact totalling 13 times throughout the day. As well, there are digestive enzymes, potassium, iodine, thyroid, vitamins, vitamin injections, and coffee enemas and caster oil treatments.

11

One can go to the Gerson Institute in Mexico or do the therapy on their own with their physician.

Essentially, it reminds me of hydroponics. **Hydroponics** is a method of greenhouse farming where no soil is used. Instead, an irrigation system maintains a steady flow of fresh water which carries in vital nutrients and flushes out the wastes. The reason why the Gerson Treatment reminds me of hydroponics is because in that program the body is literally flooded with nutritional juices from fruits, vegetables, and raw liver; then coffee enemas stimulate the liver to flush out the toxic wastes, speeding up the detoxification procedure. It is just like the greenhouse plant grown without soil, flooded constantly with life-giving nutrients and simultaneously being unburdened of metabolic wastes. This most likely has a great deal to do with why this treatment has worked with many impossible cancers, as you will read.

There is another program which also has a good track record with impossible cancers. The **Kelley program** merely borrows extensively from Gerson's program, while recognizing that there are different metabolic types, some of whom could not tolerate the Gerson program. And so it escalates to yet another level. Dr. Kelley appreciated the fact that many people have cleared cancers with juices, but on the other hand, many have cleared cancers with macrobiotics.

And when both of these failed, Dr. Kelley discovered that some people could clear their cancers with high meat and fat diets. And as with Gerson, the Kelley program simultaneously relies heavily on supplements, coffee enemas, enzymes, and juicing as well. But this appears to be the first time that someone recognized that we might have differing metabolic requirements from one another in terms of food.

12

Most of you are aware of the macrobiotic program with which many have also totally cleared end-stage "incurable cancers" and subsequently written their books about the experience. **Macrobiotics**, in contrast to the above programs, consists of all cooked foods, no meat, no fruits, no raw foods, no juicing, no enemas, no enzymes, no fat or oil, and no supplements. Instead, it relies on many vegetables to include highly nutrient-dense sea vegetables, plus whole grains, greens, and beans. This strictness, however, is temporary, as this program, more than any other that I know of, recognizes that with healing, the diet needs to broaden with the eventual inclusion of any and all of these items that might be needed.

And even macrobiotics is not so far removed from any of the other programs. The high iodine prescribed in the Gerson program to support the thyroid can be obtained from the sea vegetables of macro. Likewise, the potassium prescribed in the Gerson program is more than made up for with all the vegetables of macro. And, the emphasis on chewing over a hundred times per mouthful in the strict phase of macro most likely substitutes for the enzymes.

All the programs stress **whole organic foods** as much as possible. The sick body cannot rally if it is busy detoxifying pesticides and other chemicals. And one of the many benefits for the cooking of foods with the macrobiotic program is that it improves digestion and lowers the antigenicity of foods, making an allergic reaction to them less likely. So despite their outward differences, they all have a good track record for accomplishing the impossible, and concentrate on flooding the body with so much high density food and/or nutrients that it is able to heal itself. And probably it is of equal importance to know what all the diets have in common in terms of what they disallow, as it is for what they do allow.

13

For many will rally, regardless of diet chosen I suspect, once they are off white flour, sugar, cigarettes, alcohol, soft drinks, processed foods, pesticided foods, etc. Getting off chlorinated city water, meats and fowl loaded with antibiotic and hormone residues, and packaged foods loaded with chemicalized salt, hydrogenated oils, and bleached sugar are probably major ways of unloading for many.

THE METABOLIC CROSS

As it turns out, there are different metabolic types of people. These metabolic types stem from our genetics and land of origin. Eskimos live on a diet high in fat and over 40% of it is cold water fish and mammal (whale) blubber. And yet in spite of an extremely high fat diet, they have a very low rate of heart attack. But bring them to the United States to eat the American diet and they enjoy the same high rate of heart attack that we have here.

Likewise, a Caribbean native would not do very well on an all meat diet and in fact, many Caribbean islands now have escalating levels of cancer, diabetes and hypertension, in part because they are copying the U.S. diet of processed foods high in salt, fat, sugar, alcohol, processed foods loaded with chemicals, and red meat.

Likewise, Japanese women have a higher rate of breast cancer once they move here and adopt our diet high in dairy, chocolate, and fat. Studies show that many cultures suffer an increased incidence of disease once they veer from their native diets. An example is that Africans develop bowel cancers when they leave their high roughage diet and eat American processed foods.

It would be fairly easy to figure out what a person should eat

14

based on his ancestors' native land, if it were not for the fact that most of us are now such a hodge-podge of ethnic groups. There are very few remaining people who are "pure". This complicates the job of deciding which diet is best for you at a particular point in time.

To make matters more complicated, a person's metabolic type is not fixed, but can vary with environment and state of health. So unlike the lion who must have meat and the horse who must have grain, people can and do switch metabolic needs, often in mid-stream as they are healing and reaching a new plateau of wellness. To make the switch at the right time is the trick.

In determining the type of diet suitable for a particular person at a specific time, the diet needs can be thought of as falling on two axes, a horizontal axis and a vertical axis. With time, I'm sure this will become more sophisticated, as it turns out that there is a whole spectrum of needs depending upon one's heredity, constitution, diet and environment. The problem is that these needs are not static, but change over time and are under the influence of various overloads, least of which is serious disease.

Let's look first at the horizontal axis. On the far left is the person who needs an **alkalinizing diet** in order to heal and therefore does very well with **macrobiotics**. The strict phase is the diet with which so many end-stage "incurable" cancers have been totally reversed.

Elaine Nussbaum is a splendid example. As a New Jersey housewife in her 30's, she developed cancer of the ovaries. She had surgery, but it spread anyway to the liver and lungs. She had chemotherapy and irradiation, and still it spread, this time to the backbones. And as they were eaten away by the vicious cancer, they collapsed, crushing the delicate spinal nerves .

15

This left her painfully bed-ridden, at which point she developed pneumonia.

But at 78 pounds, bald and bed-ridden from he two year fight with metastatic cancer, her physicians did not dare give her an antibiotic. With less than a month to live, they feared she was too weak to tolerate any more medicine. It was at this point, yes, when all hope was lost, that she decided to go on a macrobiotic diet.

That was over 9 years ago. The happy part is that I was lecturing with her last year in Miami. She had just come in from jogging. She is an exuberant picture of health, and wrote her story in **Recovery**. I would recommend this book to everyone. For whenever someone asks me, "Do you think macrobiotics could help me clear my problem ?" I just think of what Elaine has accomplished.

But back to our metabolic cross. On the opposite side from macrobiotics, on the far right is the highly **acid-loving metabolizer.** He is what we call the **carnivore,** or the person who requires a **high meat and fat diet**, at least temporarily. He is also often the person with chronic Candidiasis who can only eat meat, and triggers symptoms if the slightest amount of grain or fruit and even other carbohydrates like root vegetables are ingested.

As people normalize they tend to shift toward midline because a truly healthy person should be able to eat a little of everything. But most do not make rapid shifts, but gradually swing toward the midline as they heal, broadening and expanding their diets with caution. If they get worse, it may be a sign to slow down and hold back. The body is not ready yet.

On the vertical axis we have at the bottom, are cooked foods.

Many people are so ill that they have to have everything cooked for them for a while in order to best assimilate or digest and incorporate the nutrients. Macrobiotics is a nearly fully cooked diet. And some are so ill in terminal stages of cancer that they can only eat brown rice, fish, sea vegetables, and other vegetables that have been twice cooked with double the amount of water. It is like a very soft, extremely digestible baby porridge.

At the top of the vertical axis is the all raw foods diet. These are the people who go to the Ann Wigmore Clinics and other **raw food** programs and do well for a while. This also includes the **juicing** fasts. The problem is that people eating on the extreme ends, either all cooked or all raw, often need to do so only temporarily while they are healing. For once they are healed, the dynamics of assimilation and metabolism are changed. They now have different requirements.

It is logical that healing bodies have very different requirements from healed bodies, for they are bodies in a different metabolic balance. So once they are healed, they come more toward the midline of both axes. For the midline allows us to obtain the best from all diets. **If they fail to evolve as they heal** (fail to change the diet as they change), **they often start to decline and can't figure out why they did so well for a while** and are now deteriorating.

Dr. Kelley, who has retired, stumbled onto the need for a high meat and fat diet when he got stuck with a patient who was on an alkaline macrobiotic diet who was not doing well. He then wisely thought, if they are not doing well on this, let's go to the opposite extreme and see if the person could rally doing an all meat and fat diet. Happily surprised, that's exactly what happened.

The left hand side of the metabolic cross has been described in our three books on macrobiotics, and constitute the Macro Almanac. (1) **You Are What You Ate** will tell you **how to get started** in the macrobiotic diet and lifestyle. (2) **The Cure Is In The Kitchen**, will then go further and detail exactly how it's done, day to day, and give the **details of the strict macrobiotic diet** that lies to the far left of the horizontal axis. This is the diet that people like Elaine Nussbaum used. It is also **the diet that the majority of people heal on.** The reasons are many; one of which is that most enzyme systems in the body function best when the body is slightly alkaline. In fact when the body is very sick or going through a reaction, it is usually acid. (**Tired Or Toxic?** gives over 33 biochemical reasons why it heals).

Basically, macrobiotics is a diet of "grains, greens, and beans, seeds and weeds, roots and fruits". The sea vegetables or seaweeds, for example are so extremely rich in minerals, that it is one of the few diets that has not also required large amounts of supplements. However, because of the modern polluted world, this is even changing. We are the first generation ever exposed to such an unprecedented level of chemicals in our daily life. But the work of detoxifying the 21st century environment uses up nutrients. So **even people with excellent diets can become nutrient deficient.** We have seen many people who were macrobiotic counselors and ate a wonderful diet. But when we identified hidden nutrient deficiencies, they cleared conditions they had been unable to with diet alone.

(3) As one gets more well, or if one is not as severely affected to begin with, then he can come more toward the midline and eat from **Macro Mellow**. This is the **transitional vegetarian diet,** and it is outlined below. On the opposite end of the horizontal axis is a transitional carnivore diet. That likewise is outlined. The transitional diets are so named, because they are merely a temporary stopping point until greater wellness can be attained, and thus a broader diet as well. They are also a

transition from the really strict ends to middle-of-the-road wellness, and the most appropriate for the majority of people.

In terms of what diet you need, that will be a difficult decision between you and your doctor. For example, I know of two people who have ten year survivals with leukemia on the macrobiotic program. I also know people who have reversed it with Gerson and with a carnivore diet. Therefore, there is tremendous biochemical individuality.

If a person does not have cancer, deciding which diet to use is easy. It's much akin to the provocation-neutralization skin testing that we use for food and chemical sensitivity. You go in one direction and if the patient gets worse, you go in the opposite direction. It is very simple. The same thing with the diet plan. Since the majority of people heal with macrobiotics, the odds are in your favor that that is the diet to start with. If you become worse, or intolerant of some of its fundamental foods, like grains, that is a good sign to switch gears and employ the transitional carnivore diet.

However, there is more to the decision than that. For example, you want to first rule out other possibilities for wanting to abandon macrobiotics. These include not cooking it well, not learning to cook foods that you like, eating out of balance as in not having enough oil, or not enough higher quality protein. But by far, **the most common reason we see for people going off the macrobiotic diet is being overwhelmed by cravings. And the most common cause for these cravings has been hidden vitamin, mineral, amino acid, essential fatty acid, or hormonal deficiencies.** For as you will learn, chromium and manganese deficiencies are extrememly common in the American diet, and a major cause of uncontrollable hypoglycemia and irristable cravings. There are many other causes, too, like carnitine deficiency, as well as chemical and food sensitivities,

19

but all that later.

The only problem is that with cancers, we can't afford the luxury of making people worse. More specialized diagnostic work needs to be done before deciding on that, with a physician who has an unquenchable thirst for this type of information; but some general ground rules will be given later, after more background.

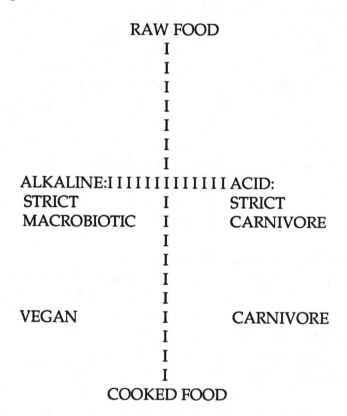

THE METABOLIC CROSS

GENERAL GUIDELINES FOR TRANSITIONAL
VEGETARIAN AND CARNIVORE DIETS

On these diets, we encourage the use of primarily organically grown produce, as well as organic sources of animal protein. Organic fruits, grains, nuts, seeds and vegetables are grown without synthetic chemicals, fertilizers, or pesticides. They are picked when ripe and not artificially ripened; they are stored and shipped also without the use of fumigants, pesticides, and other carcinogenic chemicals. Likewise, organic chickens and cattle are raised without the use of hormones, growth stimulants, and antibiotics.

A growing body of evidence indicates that **organic** food sources are the cleanest, and certainly tend to be the most nutritious, having often 2 1/2 times the nutrient value, as studies from Rutgers University (J APP NUTR, Smith R, 45:1, 1993 study available from Doctor's Data, Inc., Lisle, Illinois) have shown, as example. And you can be sure that if the measured nutrients are 2 1/2 times greater, that there are most likely additional nutrients present in the organic foods that are not in the chemicalized foods grown on depleted soils. In other words, they did not just happen to measure those nutrients that were higher.

Other words you want to look for as well as organic are **bio-dynamic**, meaning that the animals are not fed chemicals; their manure is used to fertilize the crops, which also are grown with minimal chemicals, and are fed back to the animals. In other words, it is done as in olden days, using a God-given recycling program with minimal reliance on unnatural store-bought synthetic, incomplete chemicals.

Most towns and cities have at least one good health food store or co-op, that provides good quality organic food at reasonable prices. In some areas of the country, such food may still be difficult to find, so create a demand and start to find some sources. Check with local farmers and support groups. Join forces with local HEAL, macrobiotic, or Candida support groups and make your clout felt.

Right now, however, there are some **caveats** that bear mentioning. For example, if you have any **skin condition** such as eczema, acne, atopic dermatitis, all citrus and usually including pineapple needs to be avoided. This means you have to be careful with vitamin supplements containing citrus- derived antigens, like bioflavenoids, as an example, as these can keep the skin flared, in spite of all your dietary efforts.

With **diabetes**, you probably will need to avoid all fruit juice and dried fruits. And you will have to be careful with vegetable juices and check your sugars carefully. Canned, frozen, processed and sweetened fruits are completely unacceptable.

In terms of **cooking techniques**, vegetables can be gently steamed, baked, or stir-fried. Never boil a vegetable. When you do, many valuable nutrients leech out into the water, and then are lost. Always save the liquid, either to drink or for soups or bean dishes. Although there is no perfect way to cook, steaming does preserve most of the nutritional content of vegetables. You can purchase a stainless steel steamer at any appliance store.

Vegetables and Vegetable Products:

There is **no limit** on the amount or the number of servings of vegetables you can eat each day. Basically, eat as much from this category of foods as you wish. The diets emphasize raw vegetables, but some people have a gut that is not yet healthy enough, and requires more cooked food for best assimilation. The following list contains vegetables that are generally easy to find, and which are acceptable on either diet. Use them as you wish:

Avocado

Cruciferous vegetables, or the Brassacea Family: Broccoli, Brussels sprouts, cabbage, cauliflower, kale, collards.

Green Leafy Vegetables: Beet tops, Swiss chard, and spinach, carrot tops, escarole, dark lettuce, and 2 more Cruciferous, kale and collards.

Legumes (Bean Family): Black beans, chickpeas, green beans, kidney beans, lentils, lima beans, pinto beans. You should, however, avoid peanuts and their products (peanut butter) which can harbor a mold that produces a very carcinogenic chemical, a mycotoxin called aflatoxin. You should also avoid soybeans and their products (miso) for now, because they can, depending upon source and cooking technique, contain a potent enzyme inhibitor.

Mushroom Family: All edible varieties.

Nightshade Family: eggplant, peppers (green, yellow, red, and pimento), tomatos, potatoes. **Important note:** Do not touch this family which also includes cayenne, chili, paprika, and tobacco if you have **arthritis**. In 74% of people with any form of arthritis (degenerative, traumatic, rheumatoid, lupus, osteoarthritis, etc.), this family of foods is a common hidden and unsuspected cause of arthritis. And once the food is eaten, the arthritis can last for as much as three months after the LAST ingestion of even the tiniest amount of any member of this family. Paprika, for example, is often hidden in the generic ingredients of "spices"and "curry". Also hidden in the term "spices" can be cayenne or chili, especially in sausages, sauces and soups. Another way the antigen is hidden is in many commercial soups and breads which contain potato water or modified food starch.

Onion Family: Garlic, leeks, onions, asparagus. Root Vegetables: Beets, carrots, radishes, yams and sweet potatoes (not related to the nightshade family which contains white and red potatoes above), turnips.

Squash: All varieties, including zucchini, cucumber.

Vegetable Juices: Freshly made raw vegetable juice is important to the success of these nutritional programs. Raw juices are concentrated sources of many essential vitamins, minerals and enzymes, and are more easily digested than the whole, raw vegetable itself. Carrot juice, rich in beta- carotene, must nevertheless be restricted because of its high sugar content.

Juices must be made fresh, as many of the important nutritional substances deteriorate within hours. It is best to drink your juice slowly, being sure to mix it well with saliva, within 20 minutes of having made it. The use of a straw helps many prolong the mixing with saliva, which is very important for getting the maximal nutrition from the juice. Do not make the whole day's worth at once, or carry it to work. It must be drunk when made for maximum effectiveness.

You should make, and drink, at least a total of one pint of juice each day, spread throughout the day in small (freshly made) amounts, rather than being consumed all at once. You are not limited to carrot. **Additions** to your vegetable juice could be celery, beet, cabbage, cucumber, endive, lettuce, parsley, Kale, potato, spinach, apple (in small amounts), and turnip.

Always make your juices from vegetables that are at room temperature. Cold juice inhibits digestive juices.

The addition of a clove of **garlic** is a good anti-fungal for the gut. As well, it **decreases** the ability of the blood to **coagulate** (a problem that leads to a heart attack or the laying down of lipid [cholesterol] deposits on blood vessel walls, called **arteriosclerosis**). This then can lead to high blood pressure, stroke, or heart attack). Do not use garlic if you have a bleeding problem, low platelets or leukemia.

There are a number of good juicers available on the market, such as the Omega and Champion juicers. There are many others of good quality as well, and as with air cleaners, all have their good and bad points. The extreme example is the Gerson model. It keeps the food clearest of electromagnetic and centrifugal destruction, but is the most cumbersome to use and clean. Do avoid juicers, however that require the addition of ice or other liquids, as this dilutes your efforts. Likewise, avoid those models where the pulp is still in the juice, as this causes diarrhea and therefore limits the amount of juice one can tolerate.

Sea Vegetables: Don't laugh! Sea vegetables (seaweeds) are a wonderful source of precious minerals. You can learn to disguise them in food, such as blending them into soups. Read **MACRO MELLOW** for details.

Grains: This category of plant product includes alfalfa, barley, buckwheat, corn, flax, rice, millet, oats, rye, wheat. Normally, grain products are eaten cooked, such as in breads, cereals and pasta. We prefer the grains raw, to provide the maximum nutritional benefit. However, grains cannot be eaten straight off the stalk: first of all, they're too hard, and second, they contain enzyme blockers which must first be neutralized. They also contain phytates that inhibit the absorption of nutrients and can promote toxins in the gut to be absorbed that can act like any chemical in damaging specific enzymes.

Sprouting, is an excellent way to prepare **edible raw grains.** Sprouted alfalfa and wheat berries, if made fresh, are actually quite tasty, even sweet: don't confuse freshly made sprouts with those commonly available in your supermarket, which may be moldy, days old, and taste like it. Essene bread from health food stores is nutritious and is made entirely from sprouted grain.

In addition to sprouted grains, we recommend you eat at least 3-4 tablespoons of **seven to fourteen grain cereal.** The fourteen grain cereal consists of fourteen different beans, grains, nuts and seeds: alfalfa, almonds, barley, buckwheat, brown rice, corn, flaxseed, lentils, millet, mung beans, oat groats, rye, sesame, and wheat berries. This cereal was designed so that a human could literally live on it, and eat nothing else: it provides virtually all the nutrients, even the protein, we need for sustenance (but read celiac section).

You can purchase from Arrowhead Mills a 7 grain cereal and add to it with the various ingredients to make the fourteen grain cereal. You could make it up once a month or buy the cereal already mixed from ARG Patient Services (1 800-number in Resources), which provides the cereal in one pound bags. Each evening, merely grind 3-4 tablespoons in a blender. Grind the mix into a fine powder, place in a bowl, add apple juice or other fruit juice. Let soak overnight at room temperature. The following morning, you can add blackstrap molasses, honey, maple syrup, or yogurt or cream, and eat without cooking.

Many patients find the cereal tasty: others refer to it as bird food. Regardless, you should eat it for the first six months of your program, as it provides good nutritional insurance. It is obviously great for travel; just grind up a batch and go. You can order mineral water or juice the night before.

These diets allow breads as long as they are made from 100% whole grains, such as whole wheat, whole oatmeal, sprouted wheat, whole rye, etc. Such breads should be made without synthetic chemicals, hydrogenated oils, additives, preservatives or sugar. Some nutrients will be destroyed during the baking process, but whole grain breads do add variety to the diet and also provide protein, complex carbohydrates and dietary fiber, as well as the B vitamins, minerals such as magnesium and zinc, and chromium. You can have whole grain breads each day.

Cooked **brown rice** is excellent if you tolerate grains, but some need to restrict to small portions because of the high carbohydrate load. With beans, rice makes a complete protein and in this combination can substitute for animal products. As with bread, the cooking process will destroy some of the nutritional value, but cooked brown rice still provides many valuable nutrients.

You must **avoid all refined grain products,** such as white flour, white spaghetti, white bread, and white rice. These foods have been stripped of most of their nutrients, and should never be eaten during a healing phase. For example, during the refining process, 22 essential nutrients, including fiber, are removed from wheat: 3-4 nutrients are then replaced, so that the bakers can label this depleted food as "enriched". White rice, like white wheat flour, is also nutritionally inferior, and as we have stated elsewhere, Schroeder's 1969 studies show that white flours contain only about 1/5 th of the original minerals.

Nuts: Nuts of all types, including almonds, Brazil nuts, cashews, filberts, pecans and walnuts, are excellent sources of vitamins, minerals, fatty acids and good quality protein. Nuts should be eaten raw, unroasted, without salt or sugar. On these diets, we specifically request that you eat a small handful (10-20 almonds) of almonds for breakfast and again for lunch. Almonds, of all the nuts, are a superb source of protein, and have the fewest nooks and crannies to harbor mold and carcinogenic mycotoxins. Avoid peanuts.

Should you have difficulty chewing almonds, you can soak them overnight, or boil them 20 minutes, squeeze them, and pop them out of their skins. As a last resort, two tablespoons of almond butter can substitute for the whole raw almonds. Note that almonds, and other nuts, can also be sprouted, providing that they are still living and organic. If they will not sprout, I would investigate the source.

Beverages: No coffee, tea (except macrobiotic), alcohol, or soft drinks. And no carbonated beverages, even water. For these become carbonic acid in the blood and deplete or use up precious buffers (like calcium) in order to be neutralized.

Allergies: Never eat a food that you suspect or know you are sensitive to or that produces any adverse reaction. Likewise, do not eat any food that you suspect worsens any dysbiosis(abnormal bugs), such as intestinal yeast, like Candida. Always begin a program using your safest foods first. Once you are stable and starting to heal, you will have plenty of time to eventually reintroduce unknown foods to see if you now tolerate them. Remember, as you get healthier, you tend to lose a number of sensitivities, and tolerate things that you have not tolerated in years. If you do not tolerate many foods, it would be best to rotate foods **(THE E.I. SYNDROME)** in order to delay the development of further food allergies.

But if you have a **serious reaction to any food** such as anaphylactic throat swelling, asthma, loss of voice, loss of consciousness, etc., do not test these. If you are really determined to test them, they should be eaten in the physician's office who is trained in the treatment of serious anaphylactic reactions. I always feel the safest place for you to test anything of that nature is right in front of me, with all the emergency tools at my disposal.

Mycotoxins are chemicals that molds make. These toxins are numerous and some of the most potent causes of cancer known to man. They can be prevalent on moldy foods, especially moldy grains, beans, seeds and nuts. There is no perfect way to test for them, plus they are usually invisible, tasteless, and odorless. The best way to protect against them is to be sure that these foods are stored in dry, cool places. Also having minimal light in the storage pantry decreases the deterioration that occurs with light and time..

Avoid the microwave: Microwaves are high-frequency electromagnetic waves that cause a vibration of food molecules up to 2.5 billion times per second to create friction and the resultant heat. In the process, nutrients are damaged, and some are changed into carcinogens and other chemicals damaging to body chemistry. Studies show it really deteriorates mother's milk that has been briefly warmed in the microwave. The IgA antibodies are destroyed 98% and 96% of liposomal activity is lost as well (J PEDIATRICS, Apr 1992).

Other studies show higher cholesterol levels after eating diets of "waved" foods. This most likely because some of the altered or damaged nutrients are the very same ones needed to properly metabolize the cholesterol. Furthermore, carcinogenic plasticizers in plastic and styrofoam containers can migrate into the food (Bishop CS, Dye A: Microwave heating enhances the migration of plasticizers out of plastics, J ENV HLTH, 44:231-235, 1982. Microwaves. INT J BIOSOCIAL & MED RESEARCH, 1993; Spec Subj. Vol 14:224- 228 [commentary on a review article, "Microwaves: Scientific proof of dangers", from J FRANZ WEBER 1992:193-10]. Yoshida H, et al, Effects of microwave cooking on the molecular species of pumpkin seed triacylglycerols, NUTR REPORTS INT, 1988;37(2):259-268).

General Dietary Guidelines:

Transitional Vegetarian

If you have been prescribed a Transitional Vegetarian diet, it is to determine if you thrive on a diet consisting of at least **60% raw foods** such as raw vegetables, fruits, grains, nuts, and seeds. For optimal functioning, most will require a certain amount of lean animal protein chosen from eggs, cheeses, fish, poultry and occasional servings of red meat. **Organic** is the key to healing however.

Salads: Eat at least one salad a day, and more if you like. Use as many different vegetables as you like: carrots, parsley, cucumber, broccoli, cauliflower, leafy greens, peppers, tomatos, onions and sprouts.

Fruit and Fruit Juices: Fruit provides many vitamins, enzymes and minerals, as well as good quality fiber. We suggest you include 2-3 pieces of fruit daily, taken after the meals to avoid fluctuations in your blood sugar. Do not juice fruit, since it is high in sugar.

On this diet all fruits are acceptable: apples, bananas, berries, citrus (oranges, grapefruit, lemons, limes, tangerines), kiwi, melons, nectarines, pears, peaches, plums, and tropical fruit such as mango, papaya, and pineapple. You should have at least three servings of fresh whole fruit a day, and more if desired. But try to keep a sensible balance with other foods. We don't want this to become a fruit diet, unless you are craving this. Then we should explore what this means. More about this later.

Seeds: Raw seeds, such as pumpkin, sunflower, flax, and sesame are rich in protein, vitamins, minerals, certain trace minerals and essential fatty acids. Seeds should be refrigerated or frozen, to prevent the fatty acids from turning rancid. Learn to taste and smell rancid seeds and nuts, for this means the oils have become oxidized (aged) to become chemicals that now are damaging to the body chemistry.

Remember grocery store oils do not become rancid, because the portion that could become rancid has been chemically changed by hydrogenation to delay or inhibit it. But the same process that does this also forms trans fatty acids and removes many of the beneficial nutrients like vitamins A, C, and E. These are crucial in preventing the development of nearly every disease, including arteriosclerosis and cancer, the number one and two causes of death in the U.S.

Sprouts: Freshly made sprouts are a particularly nutritious food that makes an excellent addition to salads, especially in winter. You can have sprouts as often as you like, and as much as you like. Virtually any bean, grain, nut, or seed can be sprouted. Anything that sprouts is still alive and contains the

31

life force to make a whole plant.

Such foods are valuable for a number of reasons. First, certain foods, such as beans, which cannot normally be eaten raw, can be eaten uncooked when sprouted. Sprouting also increases the nutritional content of many seed type foods; during the sprouting process, the cells begin manufacturing useful substances such as chlorophyll. Finally, raw beans, grains, nuts, and seeds contain powerful enzyme blockers which are destroyed during the sprouting process. These enzyme blockers can be harmful if eaten in the active form.

Sprouting should not be a time-consuming affair. When preparing sprouts, remember to use active seeds uncontaminated with fungicides or other toxic chemicals. Seeds for sprouting are generally available at health food stores. A company called The Herb and Spice Collection provides a wide variety of organically produced seeds for sprouting. You can obtain their catalogue by calling the company at 1-800-365-4372.

Beans: Beans are an excellent food, rich in fiber, proteins, minerals, trace elements and vitamins. In addition to raw sprouted beans, also use cooked beans, several times a week.

Animal Protein: For optimal nutrition, plan at least 5-6 servings of fish, poultry or cheese main dishes each week, supplemented with occasional red meat, if you feel like it, especially the following:

Eggs: Despite bad publicity because of their cholesterol content, eggs are a complete food, containing high quality protein, essential fatty acids, vitamins and important trace elements. Transitional Vegetarian Metabolizers can easily handle the cholesterol, so such concerns are not important for you.

And whenever there is doubt, merely have your 12-hour fasting cholesterol, triglycerides, HDL, VLDL, and apo-lipoproteins A1 & B checked. Then you will know exactly where you stand. You may have at least one egg each day, perhaps taken along with your fourteen grain cereal. You may poach or soft boil the eggs, as this form of cooking least disrupts the protein content Buy fertile, range-fed, organic eggs.

Dairy Products: Providing you do not have a lactase deficiency (lack of an intestinal enzyme to metabolize milk, leading to intestinal gas, cramps, diarrhea, constipation and pain) you may have butter, yogurt and cheeses. Raw cheeses, available in most health food stores, are more suitable than pasteurized and processed milk and cheese products. Often the bacteria in cheese and yogurt have digested the milk sugar lactose enough that a person with a deficiency of the enzyme, lactase, will be able to tolerate this form of dairy product without symptoms. You should **avoid milk** itself, since many patients are allergic to it. It also causes mucous, especially increased nasal congestion, sinus pressure and infection, and asthma in many. You should also avoid bright yellow and orange cheeses, which are usually colored with synthetic chemicals. As well, avoid highly processed cheeses, such as American cheese and cheese spreads, which tend to be filled with additives and preservatives.

Don't force dairy products; eat only as much as you actually crave. If you like it, use yogurt a few times a week to restore the bowel flora to normal. Be sure the package says it contains live acidophilus cultures.

Vegan types tend to **store calcium** very efficiently, so you don't need much in your diet. And remember that millions of Chinese, for example, never have milk or cheese and do not have the high rate of osteoporosis that we have. That is because the many vegetables they eat contain not only the calcium (2 cups of green have about as much calcium as a glass of milk), but also the trace minerals necessary to put the calcium in the bones. Also they are not eating all the sweets and meat that we do. These acid foods require buffering of the body so that it does not become too acid itself. **Calcium is the buffer** the body uses up to compensate for these extremely acid foods. By avoiding sweets and meats, the calcium buffers are spared or saved and stored.

Compare this to the American who has multiple trace mineral deficiencies from eating lots of sweets, fat, alcohol, and processed foods. When eaters of this type of food ingest extra calcium, the trace minerals that allow it to be put into bone are not sufficient. So instead, the calcium becomes toxic, and is therefore placed in the toxic waste sites of the body, namely the blood vessel walls (arteriosclerosis).

So the **person who takes calcium supplements** without eating correctly and without knowing if the nutrient levels in their body are good, **is accelerating the development of arteriosclerosis** (which leads to high blood pressure, heart disease, senility, strokes) by accelerating the deposition of calcium in the blood vessels.

Seafood: You should include lean white seafoods (cod, flounder, haddock, halibut, perch, sole, trout, whitefish) twice each week, as well as the fatty fishes such as bluefish, mackerel, salmon, swordfish and tuna; also crab, lobster, scallops, and shrimp.

Because of serious problems with bacterial contamination, try to avoid all raw shellfish; the risks of illness are too great. Also, avoid farmed fish, as they have the wrong fatty acids. Remember, real fish eat seaweeds and other fish, high in omega 3 oils. Farmed fish eat pelletized commercial animal food high in omega 6 oils.

And do not forget that when you have a good piece of organic **fish** (or any organic flesh with bones for that matter), to be sure to render all the precious minerals by making a soup. For fish, the addition of carrots, onions, squash and non- bitter greens plus ginger, as an example, can make a sweet and pungent fish tea or soup. This is where you get a lot of your minerals (besides from the sea vegetables).

Sea Vegetables: Make Kombu tea or cook Kombu into soups to add to the mineral content of your diet. Or make nori rolls to carry to work. But if this stage is not for you, omit it for now. Excellent source: Maine Coast Sea Vegetables, Dept. M, Franklin ME, 04634. Also most health food stores carry sea vegetables.

Poultry: Poultry, particularly the leaner varieties such as chicken, turkey, and Cornish hen, are excellent sources of animal protein for you. Lean poultry can be eaten 1-2 times each week. Because commercially grown poultry is so over-loaded with carcinogenic hormones plus antibiotics and pesticides, you must use only organically raised fowl.

Red Meat: Many Transitional Vegetarian Metabolizers do well with 1-2 servings of lean red meat a week. Beef such as calves' liver and veal, and lean lamb make suitable choices. Try to include your servings of red meat with the lunch meal. If you can get game, such as venison, so much the better, as these have superior levels of beneficial essential fatty acids over commercially raised meats. It is best to have the meat at the noon meal, as it is better digested then.

If you do have an occasional urge for a more fatty meat like bacon, boil it for a couple of minutes first before frying it. This can considerably reduce the fat and salt content.

For cancer patients, one of the mainstays of the Gerson diet was **raw calves' liver**. If it is prescribed for you, buy organic only, cut it up into tablespoon sized pieces, and freeze. Each day, you should blenderize from 3-6 tablespoons, and add the blenderized concoction to a glass of carrot or freshly made tomato juice. The juice should cover the taste. You may not like the liver, but it can temporarily be a vitally important part of the program. Of course, fresh is best, but very difficult to obtain.

Desserts: In addition to fruits, you may tolerate daily portions of honey and maple syrup, in small amounts only as a sweetener. Also permitted are limited use of jams and jellies as long as they contain only whole fruit and fruit juice as a sweetener, and no refined white sugar or synthetic chemicals.

Herbal teas may be used if you absolutely feel you need them. But on the whole, you want to make sure that every food is of the highest nutrient density possible, and there is not that much to be gained, unless you need the liquid or feel you specifically benefit from some particular herbs. You must avoid alcohol, as it overloads the detox system and in many, can set back your progress actual weeks and months. And never use Nutra-Sweet, Equal or other synthetic sweeteners.

Oils: This diet allows small quantities, 1-2 tablespoons a day, of oil. Oils with omega-3 oil include flaxseed, canola, hempseed and walnut oil. However, these would be best used in a blender to make salad dressing (add lemon, lime, apple cider vinegar, herbs, garlic, parsley, other oils, etc., as individually tolerated. If you add anchovies, be sure to wash the salt off). Do not heat these oils, but use extra virgin olive oil for cooking.

Never buy oils that simultaneously are clear and come in non-opaque clear glass bottles. Clear, colorless and odorless oils(typical of what you see in the grocery store) are stripped of nutrients. The clear bottles reflect the fact that the manufacturer knows he has stripped the nutrients, so there is no point in protecting the oil from light that further hastens its deterioration. Eat seeds as often as you like, at any time of the day, as they are the unadulterated source of the oil. But remember to chew them well.

Use MACRO MELLOW for your guide to menus and recipes. And make liberal use of sea vegetables, high in minerals. And put your heart, intellect and instincts into your cooking. For it is one of the pivotal instruments of wellness. But most importantly, keep a balance where at least 50% of the diet is organic vegetables

****

General Dietary Guidelines:
Transitional Carnivore

For the Transitional Carnivore diet despite the considerable media antagonism to animal fats and red meat in general, some metabolic types thrive, at least for a while (and others indefinitely) if they include fatty red meat and other animal proteins in their diet. This is because this is the optimum "fuel" for this body type or enzyme-type, or metabolic-type. Remember our old analogy of the automobile engine. Some people are just plain diesel engines, and you cannot expect them to run on gasoline.

If you have ever put the wrong fuel in a car, as I have, it will be indelibly imprinted in your memory how bad the wrong fuel is. There is a sudden slowing and lurching, bumping, and grinding of the engine, as you become engulfed in smoke and the whole engine dies. And it really is not too dissimilar to what a person eating the wrong type of diet for him at that particular point in his life feels like. Remember, whenever the guilt of eating this high cholesterol diet starts gnawing at you, merely get your fasting lipid levels drawn and check it out. The other thing to remember is that it is often temporary while the person rebuilds tissue. Then he can begin to migrate more toward the midline of the metabolic cross with a healthier reduction in meat and fat.

This diet also emphasizes **root vegetables**, such as potatoes and carrots, but restricts certain vegetable foods, such as leafy greens and fruits, which are generally not suitable for this metabolic type. Actually, if you read Ms Jean Auel's wonderful series of books, beginning with THE CLAN OF THE CAVE BEAR, it is a diet much like they ate. There are several ways in which this diet differs from the standard American high cholesterol diet that is so deadly in the U.S.

Let's take a look at just a few examples: (1) When your nutrient levels are normal, the body is able to more properly metabolize cholesterol. Consequently, the use of organic meats provides many benefits including higher nutrient levels. (2) Also, what you are not getting may be just as important as what you are getting. Organic meats are raised without pesticides, herbicides, and hormones. These compete for and use up nutrients that are necessary for proper metabolism of cholesterol.

(3) By avoiding sugars, processed foods, white flour products, and hydrogenated oils, you are getting a higher nutrient density diet with which to better metabolize cholesterol. Just look at the grocery store hydrogenated oils: they have had vitamins B6 and E removed and been exposed to exorbitant heat to form trans fatty acids that actually promote arterioscle-

rosis.

So there is not the concern about high cholesterol with this diet as there should be with the "regular" standard American high cholesterol diet as eaten by unknowledgeable people. For their diets are higher in chemicals that can compete for nutrients that are necessary for the proper metabolism of cholesterol. And when in doubt, you can always check your levels to verify this.

(4) Furthermore, cave dwellers ate whole foods, and when it came to animals, they did not waste any of it. They made soups from the bones and ate the mineral-rich organs. In this way they procured many of the trace minerals that are necessary for metabolism of fat and meat. This represents just a smattering of the biochemical blunders that have invaded our food system and make it so radically different from original meat diets.

Specifically, you should plan your meals to include the following:

Red Meat: Despite the widespread prejudice against animal fats in general and red meat in particular, Transitional Carnivore Metabolizers function most efficiently if they include at least 5-7 servings of fatty red meat such as beef, lamb and pork in their diet each week. Often the best tolerated are beef and lamb, but occasional servings of pork such as pork sausages and bacon (without preservatives) are also recommended. The more rare you like your beef, the better, but of course, this then means all the more care must be taken to be sure it is of good organic quality and free of bacterial contamination.

In addition, occasional servings, according to your taste, of **organ meats** such as calves' liver, heart, kidney or brains are recommended, as these contain much more minerals and vitamins than muscle meat. There is no limitation on serving size; if you want a pound of red meat at a sitting, then eat it. In general, an average serving size of from 8-14 ounces. But should you put on undesirable or unneeded weight, check back with your physician for a diet reassessment.

If you find yourself craving red meat every day, then you should consume it every day. You should also eat as much fat as you wish. For you, a prime rib with the fat is an ideal food. Of course, don't force yourself: adjust portion size, frequency of servings and fat intake to suit your taste and appetite. If your body does well with animal fats and animal proteins, you will know in a few weeks as you begin to feel better. And you can check your lipids to be sure that it is biochemically a good diet for you. This includes cholesterol, triglycerides, HDL, LDL, and apo-lipoproteins A1 & B.

And remember, you have not finished your organic meat until you have made use of the **bones.** Do not discard the bones. Make a soup with vegetables and bones, and add a little organic apple cider vinegar to the pot to help in extracting the calcium form the bones. Boil on lowest temperature to maintain a gentle rumbling for 1-2 hours. You can then add your root vegetables or beans, etc., in the last 20 minutes so they are not overcooked. One of the many mistakes we make these days is in not using the whole animal, if we are going to be carnivores. The high calcium from making soup from the bones, for example, replenishes the calcium lost by the body in its attempt to buffer the high acidity from eating the amino acids of meat.

Poultry: In addition to red meat, you should consume poultry products at least 2-3 times a week. You will actually do well with fatty birds such as duck, but chicken and turkey are excellent choices. Don't hesitate to eat the skin or the fat at the bottom of your roasting pan; your body needs such fats to work effectively, and repair damaged cell membranes, at least initially. You can make excellent tasting gravies with a roux of 1 tbs of whole wheat flour and 1 tbs of heavy cream. Add this to the meat drippings, cooking until thickened.

Chicken or turkey sandwiches make an excellent lunch. You should choose the serving size and the frequency of serving of these products according to your appetite and taste.

Seafood: Several servings (2-3) a week of fatty fish such as bluefish, haddock, halibut, mackerel, salmon, swordfish, and tuna. Herring and sardines are also excellent choices, and include shellfish, such as crab, lobster, scallops, and shrimp in your diet.

Avoid the leaner white fishes such as sole and flounder, which will not satisfy your appetite or your body's physiological needs. And, because of serious problems with bacterial contamination, avoid all raw shellfish; the risks of illness are simply too great.

Eggs: For Transitional Carnivores, eggs are not a particularly good food. However, if you like eggs, you might tolerate 3-4 eggs each week. You can cook the eggs any way you like; poaching and soft boiling are particularly good ways to cook eggs, because the proteins are least disrupted, but omelets and hard boiled eggs are acceptable.

Diary Products: Transitional Carnivores tend to do well with whole milk yogurt and butter. **Never use margarines,** as they contain as much as 35% trans fatty acids which are damaging to cell membranes and promote arteriosclerosis. You can have a cup of whole milk yogurt daily, and as much butter as you wish, keeping in mind that butter is loaded with calories. Be sure that all yogurt says it contains live acidophilus cultures. To be sure, make some of your own yogurt from it. If it does not make good yogurt of similar taste, get another source. Usually the grocery store yogurts are of poor quality and you will need to go to a health food store. Unless otherwise instructed you should avoid milk, cheese and other dairy products initially.

Grains: Specifically, you can have whole grain breads each day. You can have brown or wild rice as often as you like. But if you have Candida problems, you are best advised to omit grains entirely for a few weeks, then add them back to evaluate the effect. Some people can get away with grains as long as they keep them under 30% of the diet. Essene bread from health food stores is nutritious and is made entirely from sprouted grain, with no yeast.

Whole grain cereals such as oatmeal make excellent breakfast foods. Although **this diet forbids milk,** you can have cooked and other cereals with yogurt, butter or a tiny amount of heavy cream.

Pasta as a main dish is acceptable, again, as long as it is **100% whole grain.** However, because you do need frequent servings of animal protein, we suggest pasta be served with meat sauce. Ideally, if you have the energy and like to cook, home made whole grain products, for example, home made whole wheat bread, would not only taste the best, but would be the freshest and most nutritious.

For cancer patients, one of the mainstays of the Gerson diet was **raw calves' liver.** If it is prescribed for you, buy organic, cut it up into tablespoon sized pieces, and freeze. Each day, you should blenderize from 3-6 tablespoons, and add the blenderized concoction to a glass of carrot or freshly made tomato juice. The juice should cover the taste. You may not like the liver, but it can temporarily be a vitally important part of the program. Of course, fresh is best, and organic is mandatory.

Vegetables and Vegetable Products: There is no limit on the amount or the number of servings of vegetables you can eat each day. Basically, eat as much from this category of foods as you wish.

In general, you will do best with root vegetables such as beets, carrots, potatoes, sweet potatoes, turnips and yams. Also recommended are asparagus, avocado, broccoli, Brussel sprouts, cabbage, cauliflower, celery, and peas. You can eat these vegetables as frequently as you wish. Organic pickled vegetables, such as pickles, sauerkraut, and relish are also highly recommended. Use relishes according to your own tastes and preferences.

However, you should avoid most leafy green vegetables, with the exception of spinach. Many of this metabolic type simply cannot utilize these particular plant products, in fact they will be seen in the stool undigested. **So for you, a leafy green salad is not a "healthy" food.** If you want a salad, make coleslaw slaw or a bean salad, which for you are excellent choices. A daily salad of raw freshly shredded cabbage, onion, celery, carrot and radish would be excellent for you. So get familiar with root vegetables, as these are more suitable for this diet type.

Beans (legumes): are a high protein vegetable: this group includes black beans, chickpeas, green beans, kidney beans, lentils, navy beans, pinto beans and all other beans; a daily serving, if you wish, would be excellent.

Beans are an excellent food, rich in fiber, proteins, minerals, trace elements and vitamins. Beans also contain certain nutrients (like molybdenum) that help with detoxification.

Vegetable Juices: Freshly made raw vegetable juice is absolutely critical to the success of your nutritional program. You should drink, one half to one quart of carrot juice each day. The use of a straw is good if it allows you to hold the juice in your mouth a little longer and mix it with your saliva. This promotes better digestion. In addition, you should have the juice of other vegetables, such as celery, cabbage, or beet. You might make your own vegetable mix: additional vegetables for your punch include cucumber, endive, potato, spinach, kale, and turnip.

Fruits: For you, we recommend certain fruits such as apples, bananas, berries, melons, nectarines, peaches, pears, and plums. However, you must **avoid most other fruits**, particularly citrus fruits (grapefruit, lemon, lime, orange, tangerine), as they tend to slow down your metabolism. And, you should limit quantities, even of the allowed fruits; one piece a day is the limit.

Fruit juice is not a good food for you, even if it comes from the health food store. It is merely concentrated sugar with dead enzymes that have been sterilized to kill bacteria and mold, thereby destroying the vitamin C. However, the mold antigens still persist and can trigger symptoms. Because of the destruction of vitamins, a smattering of artificial vitamins is added back and bragged about on the label.

Desserts: For your type, we recommend an occasional fatty dessert such as cheesecake, perhaps once a week at most. Otherwise, you should avoid all refined sugars, but could have small amounts of honey, maple syrup and molasses as sweeteners; but in general, this body type does not metabolize sugars well, even natural sugars efficiently.

Never use Nutra-Sweet or other synthetic sweeteners.

Oils: The best oils are flaxseed, olive, and canola (in that order). Use as much olive oil as you want in cooking and on foods. Do

44

not cook or heat flax oil.

Hempseed oil (Sorry, even though this is the marijuana seed, the oil is free of tetrahydrocannabinol or THC; the part that is responsible for the drugged effect of marijuana. Therefore, it is legal, and is a great source of omega 3 oil. It is 19% alpha linolenic or omega 3; 57% linoleic or omega 6, and 12 % oleic or omega 9. It is available from The Ohio Hempery, Inc., 14 N court ST, #300, Athens, OH 45701, phone (614) 593-5828, but very expensive. However, it is a temporary alternative for allergic people. Do not heat this oil, just as you would not heat flax or cod liver oils.

Beverages: Pure water is the best beverage, along with the vegetable juice. Herbal teas are acceptable, but remember, no lemon.

For all diet types, no coffee, tea (except macrobiotic), alcohol, or soft drinks while you are attempting to heal. And no carbonated beverages, not even carbonated spring waters. For these become carbonic acid in the blood and deplete or use up precious buffers (like calcium) in order to be neutralized.

Don't be afraid to put your heart, intellect and instinct into your cooking. Your very health hinges on how well you do. And make liberal use of sea vegetables **(see MACRO MELLOW),** as these are high in important minerals. Use reputable, less contaminated sources, like Maine Coast sea vegetables.

CASE STORY: SEVERE CHEMICAL SENSITIVITY

M.S. was a 48 year old highly chemically sensitive teacher. She had consulted many medical specialists, including allergists and ecologists with minimal improvement. One of our most important discoveries was that she was highly magnesium deficient. In spite of this and other parts of the total load program helping her to reduce her symptoms and increase her tolerances, she was not totally well. The macrobiotic diet helped her come up a few more rungs on the ladder of wellness. Suddenly she became intolerant of all grains, having symptoms of the brain fog every time she ate them.

When I suggested the carnivore diet, like everyone else we have suggested it too, she at first thought I was nuts. Here was the author of four books on macrobiotics, including three firsts: (1) the first book to ever give over 33 biochemical explanations of why macrobiotics is so healing and why it could possibly reverse end-stage cancers, and (2) the first book to ever explain in detail the strict phase healing diet that so many wrote their autobiographies on of how they had cleared their end-stage cancers, and (3) the first macrobiotic book to address the special needs of the allergic, chemically sensitive, and the Candida victim, telling here to eat a carnivore diet of meat and fat.

But as we were to find out later, many rallied on such a diet change, for a number of reasonsthat will be explained. And, as expected, there was predictably a small core of the people who could not handle the thought of the carnivore diet for ethical reasons, others for philosophical or religious reasons.

Anyway, she too, took the leap of faith and was ecstatic with the results. "I can't believe I feel so much better, in such a short time, and with nothing more than a diet change!"

LESSONS FROM THE CARNIVORE SWITCH

There are several lessons to be learned from this, foremost being that people can change metabolic types in mid-stream. In other words, **a person can change their metabolic requirements at any point in time.** I heard one physician argue that they were never on the correct diet for themselves to begin with. He argues that, as an example, if a person started out on a macrobiotic diet and did well for a while, that it was because it was such a wrong diet for him that he was actually digesting his own tissues, which are hypoallergenic, and hence he had reduced symptoms, albeit marked weight loss.

Although I could see some evidence for this in some individuals, I think caution should be reserved before jumping to that conclusion for everyone who eventually drifts more toward the carnivore side, since many have done extremely well for much too long a period of time on a macrobiotic diet to have it be the wrong type for their metabolism. Some thrived on it for years before needing a change.

Furthermore, even if a radical change to carnivore diet is needed, it is often temporary, and then they eventually drift toward the middle of the metabolic cross. It is almost like a temporary over-compensation in the opposite direction before a more healthful swing to the midline. In observing people who eventually drift more toward the midline after having been macrobiotic for several years and having made remarkable restorations in their health, I think it is merely the natural progression of things. For part of healing is to be able to eat (and to require) a broader diet.

I suspect that most of us should fall in the middle once we are healthy, and should enjoy foods from all realms, acid, alkaline, raw and cooked. After all, isn't that a sign of a truly healthy person, one who can eat anything once in while? It is what we eat day to day that determines our overall health, but a varied diet provides the opportunity to get a wide source of nutrients. And we should not be on such a delicate balance that one dietary indiscretion blows us away for days, as it did with many of us when we were very ill with multiple food and chemical sensitivities.

For example, before macro, just a whiff of wine gave me a headache. A sip produced chest phlegm, hoarse voice, and asthma. A mouthful would leave me with facial eczema for a couple of weeks. Now that I am well, I can have a whole bottle of wine with no problem. But of course, if I made that a part of my daily diet, in a short while I would lose all the tolerance I had gained. (I had fun finding this out, though.)

Nowadays I feel best on a modified vegan with occasional meat (for the **work of detoxifying the environment uses up proteins, especially glutathione)**, as well as indiscretions as mentioned. It sure makes life in the real world a lot easier, too. But I would go through the 3-4 years of macro a thousand times again, for it restored my health to a point I never dreamed possible. Then after a while I, too, needed meat.

It is great that people like John Robbins (A DIET FOR A NEW AMERICA) and Michio Kushi (THE CANCER PREVENTION DIET, DIET FOR A STRONG HEART) have shown us the problems of a meat diet, not only on personal but global levels. But remember, you can't fight genetics, and more importantly, this era has so radically changed our needs, that all bets are off, and many rules have had to be broken. **The work of detoxifying the environment uses up proteins.** Remember, the work of detoxifying the environment throws away proteins.

For you will recall from **TIRED OR TOXIC?** THAT WE ARE

THE FIRST GENERATION TO EVER BE EXPOSED TO SUCH AN UNPRECEDENTED NUMBER OF DAILY CHEMICALS in our air, food and water. The body has to detoxify this stuff, or we get ill. But the work of detoxification uses up, wastes, looses forever, many priceless nutrients. One of these is the **tri-peptide, glutathione. For every molecule of a chemical you detoxify, you throw away forever a molecule of glutathione.** That in itself should alter your protein requirements, at least until you reduce your environmental total load of chemical stressors. Even if you do not perceive any odor, every time you walk into a grocery and detoxify just one molecule of pesticide, you throw away one molecule of glutathione forever. Your body used amino acids and energy to make this. So **our 21st century environments are using up our nutrient stores at an accelerated rate.**

Remember the woman above who had done so well with macro for so long and then did even better when she switched to carnivore? Part of the reason is that she lives in an indusatrial river valley which is socked in with a high level of industrial pollutants. Some individuals will never heal as long as they live there, for their bodies can never catch up or get ahead. They are always loosing specific detox nutrients (which include proteins that form glutathione) faster than they can assimilate them.

Still another physician felt the switch in metabolic types is often due to the development of grain sensitivities from either not following a rotated diet, or from a diet too high in grains. Although this is always a possibility, there is more to the problem than mere grain intolerance, for the removal of grain does not bring the wellness that the full carnivore switch does.

THE BASIS IN BIOCHEMISTRY

The basis for the metabolic types lies partly in the chemistry of energy synthesis. Entry into the **citric acid cycle** in the body chemistry, where **energy** is made, can occur via **two pathways**. One pathway to enter the citric acid cycle chemistry to make energy is through pyruvate metabolism; and carbohydrates (grains, greens and beans or vegan food) are the fuels the body uses to make energy via this path. The other way to enter the energy path is via acetyl coenzyme A, and fats and proteins (the carnivore diet) are the fuels for this. This is standard elementary human chemistry. Thus we have a biochemical explanation for the different metabolic types.

How a person changes metabolic types in mid-stream can depend on multiple factors. As an example, they may have used up certain nutrients in the work of continual detox, as described above, and need a temporary carnivore switch so they can make more detoxifying glutathione. Or they could have a gut full of Candida from a recent sugar binge or antibiotic and this can change requirements. For example, some species of Candida make thiaminase, an enzyme that destroys thiamine (vitamin B1) before it is even absorbed. Since thiamine is necessary for the pyruvate cycle, it could push metabolic requirements to a path that does not need as much.

Likewise, recall how as we all got sicker with chemical sensitivity, we suddenly could not tolerate chemicals that prior were tolerable? Then as we got well, we started being able to tolerate some chemicals, and not others? Well just as certain detox enzymes and whole pathways can be out of commission for a while, so can parts of the metabolic pathways.

But the determination of which routes your body needs at a particular point in time is usually always multi-factorial and far from simple. It depends on many factors, to include your genetics or hereditary predisposition, your current overload in terms of disease, hormones, enzymes, nutrient levels, diet, climate and temperature, symptoms, chemical overload, harbored toxins and heavy metals that may be poisoning some regulatory enzymes, and other factors. So you see it is not a simple thing that can be easily taught, and to complicate matters, it changes as these parameters change.

There are some **simple clues** for easier cases, however, as to when a switch might be needed. Some who may need **to be carnivores** can

(1) have been macro for a while, then it stopped working
(2) they stopped feeling good, or
(3) they were overcome with cravings, or
(4) lost too much weight,
(5) developed a loathing for greens, or
(6) an intolerance for grains.

Sometimes deciding if the program is right for you is compounded by the fact that some really sick individuals get more toxic for a few days to weeks as the body tears down tissues to rebuild. Usually this is right in the beginning of the program, unless the person is so sick that the body has to get to a certain state of readiness before it is prepared with enough reserve to start to heal. So **feeling worse does not always mean a diet switch is due.**

Once on the carnivore diet, when cravings occur for greens and salads, then this may be a sign to widen and swing back toward midline. But cravings for sweets (alcohol craving should be treated as sugar craving) often mean that not enough energy can be extracted from the food as eaten. Again there are a number of reasons, like they may need cooked versus raw food,

51

or may need some protein and fat, or have a gut full of Candida, or have digestive enzyme deficiencies or nutrient deficiencies like chromium or manganese that inhibit proper metabolism of carbohydrates, or have diabetes, thyroiditis, etc.

The more **raw** the diet, the better. But as discussed, some have such weak digestive systems, that the all-cooked strict macro is optimal at that point in time, as proven by numerous cases. **Raw foods** have **three factors** going for them. (1) First, there is less loss of nutrients without cooking. (2) Second there are live enzymes which are beneficial in many ways to the body. (3)Third, when foods are cooked with high heat so that there is a browning, as in charcoal grilled steaks, the chemistry of the **browning** is called the **maillard reaction**, which forms polycyclic hydrocarbons which can be a cause of cancer and accelerated aging (Monnier VM, Nonenzymatic glycosylation, the maillard reaction and the aging process, J GERONTOL: BIOLOG SCI, 45:4, Bl05-111, 1990).

Ah, would the world be so simple that we would only have to wonder if we were macro or carnivore. But as you know, there are people for whom neither diet is adequate. Some are such inefficient metabolizers that they need concentrated sugars until they can get their nutrient levels, chemical overload, etc. under control. Some have so little life force remaining, that they need nearly everything raw.

Others are so inefficient in digestion, that raw would go right through them. And still others need to give the gut a rest on a synthetic nutrient formula designed to aid detoxification (Ultra Clear or Sustain, available at N.E.E.D.S.). Others are so extreme, like the extreme carnivore, that they can only tolerate meat or intravenous amino acids.

Some are so severe that we send them to **Dr. William Rea's**

Environmental Health Center in Dallas for special **hyperalimentation** and an unparalleled total load program. "Hyperal" involves giving the gut a rest, just as you would rest a broken leg. Instead nourishment is given intravenously or in the vein for a while. Suffice it to say, trials are fine, but the sicker you are, the more the need for medical supervision.

Fortunately, mainstream drug-oriented medicine is just beginning to appreciate how important the acid-alkali knowledge is. For example, a severe allergic reaction was inhibited by sodium bicarbonate and reported in a medical journal. The irony is that this has been recommended and used by ecologists for years and is in **THE E.I. SYNDROME** for patients. But most doctors don't know about it, and a decade later it is reported as a new finding. I wonder how long it will be before they discover buffered C and the other related treatments (Katsunuma T, et al, Wheat-dependent exercise- induced anaphylaxis: inhibition by sodium bicarbonate, ANN ALLERG, 68:184-188, 1992).

Regardless of metabolic type, **sugar is one of the most damaging foods.** As with everything, there are exceptions. For some have such damaged intestines or metabolisms, that the only fuel they can utilize is sugar. So when you find that, you need to correct the leaky gut and nutrient and hormone deficiencies that cause it. For the damages caused by sugar can cause not only arteriosclerosis but cumulative and irreversible damages in other organs (Brownlee M, Cerami A, Vlassara H, Advanced glycosylation end products in tissues, the biochemical basis of diabetic complications, NEW ENGL J MED, 318:20, 1315-1321, May 19, 1988; and Smith D, The atherogenic effects of hyperinsulinism, PRIMARY CARDIOLOGY, 17:3, 65-67, Mar 1991).

DAMAGED CELL MEMBRANES LEAK CALCIUM

With this in mind, and because we have explained so much of how the alkaline diet works in TIRED OR TOXIC?, let's look at the **carnivore or acid-loving** person. Often they have damaged cell membranes (nutrient deficiencies, years of hydrogenated oils from French fries, chemical exposures that were not entirely detoxified, etc.) or leaky membranes. One of the things these membranes leak is calcium (that is why calcium channel blockers are a leading prescription medication for everything from angina, hypertension, and arrhythmia to migraines).

When the calcium is not on the correct side of the membrane, many other things go wrong as a result. For one, the cell loses vasoactive peptides (proteins that can control body swelling) and the person starts reacting to everything. These are the people who get edema or swelling frequently and can hardly tolerate a thing, even water. As well, the neurons (nerve cells) cannot fire as they should, so the person is a slow starter, depressed, fatigued, and gains weight easily on low calorie diets.

Anyway, LEAKY CELL MEMBRANES, from years of processed foods, for one, allow calcium to leak back into the cell in too large an amount, where it damages and can prematurely kill the cell. But when the system is acid, known as acidosis, this can blunt the influx of calcium into the cell (Kitakaze MH, Weisfeldt ML, Marban E, Acidosis during early reperfusion prevents myocardial stunning in perfused ferret hearts, J CLIN INVEST 82:920, 1988). Thus a slightly acid system keeps more of the calcium on the outside of the cell where it will not damage the cell interior.

So when these people who need to be carnivores are tested, it can appear that they have too much calcium inside the cell, but not enough calcium if the assay used looks at calcium outside the cell in the serum. If an intracellular assay only is looked at, it might show excessive calcium.

But it is not that these people do not need calcium, on the contrary, they need lots of it, but on the proper side of the cell (Herman B, et al, Calcium and pH in anoxic and toxic injury, TOXICOLOGY, 21, 2:127-148, 1990). And acidosis helps to do that, and eating an acid or carnivore diet fills the bill. This does not mean that everyone who has been prescribed a calcium channel blocker should be a carnivore; it is much more complicated than that, for many rally superbly on macro.

The treatment for the acid requiring type is the carnivore as described above, emphasizing red meat (raw as possible), root vegetables (potatoes, beets, Jerulsalem artichokes, turnips, carrots, onions, cassava, etc.), organic fat, cruciferous vegetables (raw cabbage salad, brussel sprouts, broccoli, cauliflower), beans, vinegar, sauerkraut, cider, honey, yogurt, etc. Also they usually need to avoid greens, citrus, and magnesium for a while. And they usually need much additional calcium and much potassium. The potassium requirement comes from the fresh vegetable juices and cabbage salads and other vegetables.

And for those still obsessed with the dangers of eating high cholesterol diets like the carnivore, remember it is usually transitory; just as lions and Eskimos do it with no problem, because it suits their chemistry, many have rallied through the impossible with a carnivore diet. And you can check your lipids any time; but remember when the body has a proper amount of complementary nutrients, cholesterol is actually a free radical scavenger, or natural anti-oxidant of the body.

And even drug-oriented medicine is beginning to realize now

that cholesterol is not the main cause of coronary heart disease. It would be great if it were that simple! But look at the people with high levels in their 80's with no signs of disease, and young men with normal cholesterol who die suddenly in their 40's. Indeed, "Lowering serum cholesterol concentrations does not reduce mortality and is unlikely to prevent coronary heart disease" (Raunskov U, Cholesterol lowering trials in coronary heart disease: frequency of citation and outcome, BRITISH MEDICAL JOURNAL 305:15-19, July 4, 1992).

Whereas, by contrast, the **alkaline-loving vegan or macro** generally has tight cell membranes, with nutrient deficiencies that subsequently do not correct very easily. And they need a preponderance of magnesium and potassium, versus the calcium and potassium of the carnivore. And when they do need calcium, it is of a different source than that which helps the carnivores: Cal amo (a calcium chloride with extra hydrochloric acid to aid ionization and assimilation) or calcium phosphate or calcium citrate for the carnivores, versus calcium gluconate or calcium lactate or calcium carbonate for the macros.

But the macros, remember, can extract calcium rather efficiently from collards and other greens as well as grains, soy products, and sea vegetables. So they do not need as much. As you recall, **arteriosclerosis is a disease of excess calcium in vessel walls** (Landauer JA, The cause and prevention of coronary heart disease, J ADV MED, 5,4:233-245, 1992). These victims usually need a high magnesium and low fat diet to dissolve the calcium (and enzymes as you will learn).

So now you understand why the macrobiotic diet has been so successful in reversing arteriosclerosis in people for whom vascular surgery and drugs had failed. For within one year of a modified macrobiotic diet, they had documented reversal of their arteriosclerosis by PET scan (Ornish D, DR. DEAN ORNISH'S PROGRAM FOR REVERSING HEART DISEASE, Random House, NY, 1990, and Ornish D, et al, Can life-style changes reverse coronary heart disease?, LANCET, 336:129-133, 1990).

Now you can more readily understand why calcium would not be indicated for this type; they already have too much, and in fact need diets high in magnesium and potassium to off-set the excess calcium. Is it starting to make sense?. But once they have obtained their health objective, many can swing back toward the midline where they can enjoy an occasional old favorite steak, etc.

HIGH POTASSIUM IS CRITICAL TO HEALING

These damaged or leaky cells also leak other important minerals, one of the most crucial being POTASSIUM. The potassium pump (which is in the cell membrane) is often damaged, for example, from years of hydrogenated oils (grocery store oils, French fries, etc.). But it is rarely diagnosed since the serum potassium is the most commonly assayed form, and it is necessary that a more sensitive assay, the RBC (red blood cell) potassium test be done to find this defect.

The macrobiotic and Gerson diets have a high potassium ratio in common, as one of their healing factors. This is accomplished in part with the high amount of vegetables and vegetable juices. Other researchers support this, as do the U.S. government and National Cancer Institute dietary recommendations of more vegetables and fruits. But the successful cancer programs push the potassium to a higher level, out of necessity.

An interesting fact for me was that in 1978 the United States government Office of Naval Research supported research that

57

explained that high potassium is one of the important reasons that the Gerson therapy has such a good track record in healing incurable cancers. A high potassium diet is one with a preponderance of vegetables and fruits; and raw carrot juice makes it even higher.

But it has only been in the last few years that we have heard of these recommendations for more vegetables. It is also distressing that they failed to make the reasons why more vegetables are helpful understandable to physicians, and that they neglected to recommend juicing, an even faster way to raise the potassium. It took 15 years to decide to get the message out to the average person. (Cope F, A medical application of the Ling association-induction hypothesis: the high potassium, low sodium diet of the Gerson cancer therapy. PHYSIOL CHEM PHYS. 10:465-4687, 1978)

At a recent meeting, Indian physicians presented a study that showed that men recovering from a heart attack have four times a **reduction in death** or complications when fed a **diet high in anti-oxidant foods with raw fruits and vegetables** (Niaz MA, et al, Effect on mortality and reinfarction of adding anti-oxidant rich foods to a prudent diet in the Indian experiment of infarct survival, Center on Nutrition Research, Medical hospital and Research Center, Moradabad-10, UP—24001 India). This information should be used in feeding recovering heart attack patients in place of the notoriously poor but standard hospital diet.

Right now there is a drug receiving a great deal of attention because it helps turn around multiple sclerosis and even restores conduction in demyelinated nerves. The drug, 4-aminopyridine, is a potassium channel blocker. In other words, it compensates for a damaged potassium pump. But by not fixing what's broken the users of it have found that the benefit dwindles with time, as you would expect. Whereas those, for example, who have turned their MS around with the healing phase of the macrobiotic diet and nutrient corrections, tend to steadily improve, because they are repairing part of the fundamental defect (Davis FA, Stefoski D, Rush J, Orally administered 4-aminopyridine improves clinical signs in multiple sclerosis, ANN NEROL, 27:2, 186- 192, 1990. van Dieman HA, Polman CH, van Dongen TM, van Loenen AC, Nauta JJ, Taphoorn MJ, van Walbeek HK, Koetsier JC, The effect of 4-aminopyridine on clinical signs in multiple sclerosis: a randomized, placebo-controlled, double- blind, cross-over study. ANN NEUROL, 34:2.123-130, 1992).

Anyway, when it is known that one of the important parts of all cancer therapies is to get a high level of potassium, it becomes evident why the macrobiotic diet with its soups, sea vegetables, sweet vegetable drink, and high amount of vegetables is so healing. Every one of these is high in potassium.

And in terms of assessing your potassium, do not let anyone waste your money by checking a serum potassium. It is far too insensitive. **Insist on an rbc (red blood cell) potassium** at least.

STEAMING PRESERVES POTASSIUM

Other work is just now appearing to prove that the way in which foods are cooked also has an important bearing on how much potassium is available. A paper from the M.D. Anderson Cancer Center tells us that processing of foods (the processed foods in grocery stores make up the majority of food for sale) loses about 45 % of the potassium and the way we cook it can lose another 45%.

For example, a raw potato has a potassium to sodium ratio of 104. If you boil that potato in 1% salt water, the ratio drops to an abysmal 0.7, which is counterproductive to healing. If, however, you steam the potato, the ratio is 100, promoting healing.

Now you can appreciate why the recommendation to steam as many vegetables as possible is so important. At first glance, many unknowledgeable about these facts might be inclined to say, a food is a food, and it matters little how you cook it. But how wrong they are, for it totally changes its worth.

The moral of the story is to eat at least 1/2 of the day's food in vegetables, steam all that you must cook, drink the liquid, and reduce the salt. (Jansson B, Dietary, total body and intracellular potassium-to-sodium ratios and their influence on cancer. CANCER DETECTION AND PREVENTION, 14:563-565, 1990). And when foods brown with cooking, this chemistry of browning foods with high heat forms **nitrosamines** which are polycyclic amines and are carcinogenic and mutagenic; another reason to steam. That is why for the cooked food of macro, it is not recommended to exceed 140 degrees Centigrade, and foods should be steamed, low-heat sauteed, or baked.

THE SILENT SICK

I'm not trying to confuse you with too much information, nor withhold information, as I know much of this science is difficult for many. I've tried to keep references and chemistry to a minimum, as well, to make it more "user-friendly". But I feel it is important for those who need it to have available some of this information, since it is not available anywhere else at this point, much less collated with all the other material that is present here. So if parts of this seem too much for you, just continue to plough through, for you will be amazed at how much you have learned by the end.

I never cease to have an ever-increasing respect and love for that silent underground of ill, who against all odds are determined to get well. They have ferreted out information and learned things that I don't think I could have learned without all the science background that I have. But these unscientifically trained people have decided that their health depends on how well they educate themselves, and they have done an unbelievably admirable job.

And I know of many people, who without any training in science, will understand and use the information I present. Likewise, when my writings seem to stray too far from a point, or get disproportionately too technical in some areas, it is because I am talking to someone I have in mind. They may think that with all my patients I could not possibly be thinking of them, but I am gifted with a peculiar memory.

DOWN WITH GUILT !

This brings us to a very important point of GUILT. We should ditch it completely ! If a person cheats, there must be a reason. Either he has

(1) **nutrient deficiencies** (like chromium, manganese, or carnitine deficiencies causing sweet cravings and hypoglycemia, as an example), or

(2) an **overload** in the external environment like too heavy a **chemical** exposure causing uncontrolled cravings, or

(3) an overload in the internal environment abnormal metabolism like a thyroid deficiency, diabetes or cancer or intestinal parasites like Candida, heavy metal toxicity, chronic pesticide poisoning, too much stress, or

(4) he is on the **wrong diet** for his present metabolic needs.

(5) Another cause of cravings is that the individual is not on any program and is way **off balance**, eating a diet of processed foods, coffee, alcohol, or much sugar, etc., which also are powerful causes of cravings.

(6) One last cause can be unresolved anxiety, anger, boredom, sadness, guilt, and other **unhealthy emotions**, which can drive one to eat either on a psychological basis, or a biochemical one. For excess worry, for example, can cause adverse changes in the pH (balance between acidity and alkalinity) and cause cravings by that mode. Or by stimulating the sympathetic nervous system, diminish the activities of glands, digestion, and other parasympathetic mechanisms that promote more satiety.

I have observed that our **metabolic types** are not always cast in stone, but **can shift with time** in some people, and are dependent upon many seemingly unrelated factors. These could range from nutrient status to stress level, to activities in the body like cancer or major healing, and much more. Since guilt is certainly a negative in terms of healing and serves no real useful purpose when people are eating the "wrong" things, it should be abandoned.

The preferred tack would be to try to determine why you are craving, and what can be learned from the craving that would teach us more about you. I cannot stress enough that cravings are like any other God-given symptom; they are a golden opportunity to determine what is wrong with the system before it gets worse, and fix it.

It is analogous to the red oil light of your car going on. You can either smash it with a hammer so that it goes out (analogous to taking medications for symptoms), or you can figure out what the car needs and get some good quality oil into it. And if you should chose to merely mask the symptoms, you know the damage to the system is magnified many times over by the time the next warning symptom presents itself.

The only difference is that with the car, we expect that there will be a major catastrophe with the engine without oil. Whereas with the body, we somehow have been brain-washed into thinking that a headache is a Darvon deficiency (Darvon propoxyphene, for those youngsters in the group, was a very popular prescription pain medication in the 1960's and 1970's).

Many actually believe that to suppress symptoms is a healthy and a smart thing to do, and that no harm should result. If they do worry, it seems to be misdirected toward wondering what side effects could come from the medication. They seem to have totally overlooked the fact that the chronic degenerative diseases of "old age" (which are occurring at younger ages nowadays) take years of ignoring or covering up of symptoms to produce.

WHAT DIET SHOULD I START ON?

For the vast majority of people, if they have no idea of where to start, and want to merely ease into a healthier diet and get rid of their cravings, the best diet would be the **transitional vegetarian**. It also is the diet recommended by Harvard Medical School, the American Heart Association, the American Cancer Society, and the United States Government health departments, as it is heavier in whole grains, vegetables, and beans, which form the base of the food pyramid. At the top of the food pyramid, there is fish and fowl, and even red meat for those who need it.

Since public health recommendations historically lag behind

available information, it has taken far too many years to evolve the currently recommended diet. Since it is evolving directly toward what macrobiotics has recommended for decades, it would seem prudent to not wait another 20 years to discover and recommend the highly nutritious sea vegetables (which can be so skillfully hidden in foods that you will not know of their presence) and the other advantages of the macrobiotic diet. For example, sea vegetables are a very potent yet inexpensive source of minerals that have been stripped from the average diet, the deficiencies of which are responsible for a vast amount of chronic disease and undiagnosable symptoms.

The **best cookbook** at this time **for the transitional vegetarian** diet would be Shirley Gallinger's **MACRO MELLOW**. It will teach you how to make high density nutritious foods of whole grains, vegetables (including sea vegetables), and beans and still make them taste like "regular food". It also provides menus as well as gardening ideas. It is a great start for the family that wants to improve their health, but cannot handle a drastic program. It enables you to ease into more healthful cooking, before seeing the doctor for a prescribed diet.

MANY NEED AN UNBALANCED DIET TO BEGIN WITH

Since the vast majority of people heal fastest with the **alkaline** diet, it is statistically **the best diet for the most**. However, the more off base you are and the more severe your health problems, the more unbalanced your initial diet may need to be. It is quite analogous to the correction of nutrient deficiencies. You recall that when a person has several serious vitamin and mineral deficiencies, we have to write a program to correct these deficiencies.

In doing so, the nutrients that were found to be deficient on blood and urine tests must be corrected. In order to do so, the

64

prescribed dose of nutrients to correct specific deficiencies must be abnormally high and therefore out of normal balance. Remember, you need an unbalanced prescription to correct the imbalance of severe deficiencies. The schedule we could end up writing would look very strange to a biochemically trained physician if he did not know that we were correcting several severe defects. For he would look at it and say that it was way too high in certain elements and was bound to create a problem. And he is correct.

The trick is to correct the problem and then stop this prescription regimen before the imbalance appears. That is why we warn right on the prescription that it must be taken only for the few months as prescribed. For to take it longer, would be to risk getting other deficiencies as these high levels inhibit the uptake of other precious nutrients.

For example, a copper deficiency is very common (in about 80% of the population in the U.S.) and can cause fatigue, chemical sensitivity, high cholesterol, premature aging, depression, thyroid conversion defect, and much more. Copper is also very difficult to correct. If it is not carefully monitored and the dose of copper lowered when the correction has taken place, the excess copper can now inhibit the absorption of molybdenum, chromium, iron, etc., thereby creating new deficiencies and new symptoms.

A similar situation occurs with diet changes. For a while a specific diet, like very alkaline strict macro, can produce wonders, and then slowly not be enough. This is where there must be a compensation for the metabolic swing. A macrobiotic or alkaline type may feel hungry all the time and need more high quality protein, for example. Or he may start to crave nuts or chips signaling the possible need for more fats and oils. So if cravings develop, they may be a sign of the need for a change, not the need to smother the already ailing person in health-robbing guilt. And this craving can be a good sign. For a swing toward the more liberal midline, and away from strict macro, can be a sign of improved health.

THE MORE SERIOUS THE CONDITION, THE MORE DANGEROUS ARE "SUBTLE" DIFFERENCES IN DIET.

On the other hand, very small changes in the diet can mean the difference between success and failure. This is progressively more true in proportion to the condition of the person's health. As an example, there are many reasons why **the strict alkaline or macrobiotic diet**, spelled out in detail in THE CURE IS IN THE KITCHEN, has been so successful in helping many people not only stop but totally reverse and lose "incurable" end-stage cancers and other diseases. And although over 33 of these mechanisms explaining how this can happen (complete with their scientific references), are in TIRED OR TOXIC ?, there are over 2 dozen more that have been found since writing that.

For example, there is another reason why solid tumors are usually best treated with a macrobiotic diet. The metabolic products of meat digestion include substances like putrescene and spermidine, that once absorbed from the gut into the bloodstream may act as toxins. But radio-active labelling of these polyamines reveals that although they are necessary for normal body metabolism, they trigger solid tumors to grow. The body's copper-requiring enzyme, polyamine oxidase helps to limit the absorption of these substances from meat that promote tumor growth. And, of course, just plain not eating meat while healing a solid tumor would be the optimum choice (Bardocz S, et al, Polyamines in food—implications for growth and health, J NUTR BIOCHEM, 4:66-71, Feb 1993).

As another example, burdock root is used in the strict healing phase. Yes, the root comes from the same weed that grows wild, but can also be purchased in health food stores if you want to avoid the back-breaking job of digging your own. Many groups of researchers have shown that the root of the burdock weed (Arctium lappa) has anti-tumor activity. (Morita K, et al, A desmutagenic factor isolated from burdock (Arctium lappa Linne). MUTAT RES, 129:25-31, 1984, and Foldeak S, Dombradi G, Tumor-growth inhibiting substances of plant origin. I. Isolation of the active principle of Arctium lappa. ACTA PHYS CHEM, 10:91-98, 1964, and Dombradi C, Foldeak S, Screening report on the anti-tumor activity of purified Arctium lappa extracts, TUMORI 52:173, 1966)

According to the World Health Organization, burdock has also proven to have an "inhibitory activity against HIV (AIDS) virus (WHO, In vitro screening of traditional medicines for anti-HIV activity: Memorandum from a WHO meeting. BULL WHO [Switzerland] 67:613-618, 1989).

Or look at the USA TODAY and NEWSWEEK articles November 1, 1993 about kudzu. It is a part of the macrobiotic diet, and has been known as a harmless white root with medicinal properties for 2000 years. Finally a Harvard researcher began looking into all this and the fact that it makes alcoholics reduce their cravings by 50% within weeks of regular use. When it made front page news, the government said it would have to do animal studies and make it into a drug! I wonder how long it will be before they find out it has been used for years, or when they will "rediscover" its other properties like healing leaky gut syndrome.

Once you are aware of special medicinal properties of certain foods, it becomes evident where some of the older remedies came from. For example, there was a man named Hoxsey who put an old dying horse out to pasture because he couldn't bear putting him down. When the horse improved, Mr. Hoxsey started to observe that the horse selected only certain weeds and grasses to eat, leaving others alone. So another sick horse was put in the same pasture and also improved. Eventually a mixture was made of these selected weeds and sold as a treatment for humans. Some claim to have had success with it. One of the ingredients was burdock. Burdock is also an ingredient in another controversial Canadian herbal cancer treatment, Essiac.

But as you know, just as a headache is not a darvon deficiency, one herb, one vitamin, one food, etc. is not going to turn around many diseases, much less cancer. It is a **total load problem**. And the more serious the problem, the more precarious the balance. And the more successful the program, the more it seems to concentrate on flooding the system with high density nutrients in as many forms as possible.

Likewise, **sea vegetables**, in addition to their high mineral content, have other polysaccharide moeties that are strongly **anti-cancer.** For example one type caused complete remission of advanced leukemia (Furusawa E, Furasawa S, Effect of pretazettine and viva-natural, a dietary seaweed extract, on spontaneous AKR leukemia in comparison with standard drugs. ONCOLOGY 45:180-186, 1988). Other sea vegetables have had anti-cancer effects and caused regression of cancers, including leukemias (Schwartz J, Shklar G, Regression of experimental hamster cancer by beta carotene and algae extracts, J ORAL MAXILLOFAC SURG, 45:510-515, 1987, and Miyazawa Y, et al, Immunomodulation by a unicellular green algae (Chlorella pyrenoidosa) in tumor-bearing mice, J ETHNOPHARMACOL, 23;135-146, 1988).

But as with anything, there must always be a **balance.** Plus all modalities in life seem to have a bell-shaped curve in terms of effect. This means there is one particular range for a dose that is beneficial for a particular person, and as you extend further and further in either direction from that dose, there is diminishment of the effect and/or even toxicity and death. And so it is with sea vegetables. People who have overdosed on them have gotten iodine-induced hyperthyroidism, thyrotoxicosis (Ishizuki Y, et al, [Transient thyrotoxicosis induced by Japanese kombu}, NIPPON NAIBUNPI GAKKAI ZASSHI, 65:91-98, 1989). Everything has a fine balance.

LEUKEMIA AS AN EXAMPLE

But now let's take a look at an example of a serious life-threatening condition like leukemia. There are different forms of it, with different prognoses (expected outcomes) and standard recommended treatments. Some forms are not considered treatable (well, you can treat anything, but the bottom line is how many survive, and at what expense, and with what quality life). Anyway, some leukemics (and other related cancers of blood forming tissues like lymphomas) cannot and should not do an alkaline diet.

Instead, many need a transitional and sometimes even strict carnivore diet, full of animal fat and meat. They probably need the red meat and fat, as these are the substances that could most rapidly repair what is missing from the diseased bone marrow. But also they need high calcium supplementation, as well. This is in part because calcium is so integral in the blood-clotting mechanisms. Interestingly, calcium also can block the toxicity of the high amount of fats needed for this metabolic type (Buset M, et al, Injury- induced by fatty acids or bile acid in isolated human colonocytes prevented by calcium, CANCER LETT, 50: 221-226, 1990).

Since dairy and meat are high in calcium, you might think that these are the only benefits. But **butter** (remember the transitional carnivore as prescribed is a diet high in fat as well as meat) contains **butyric acid**. This substance of itself can make mouse leukemia cells differentiate in a test tube; that means they start to become normal cells and stop being cancer cells (Nordenberg J, et al, Biochemical and ultrastructural alterations accompany the antiproliferative effect of butyrate on melanoma cells, BR J CANCER, 55: 493- 497, 1987). Russian scientists found the same effect on a child in relapse with acute myelogenous leukemia who was already resistant to all conventional therapy (Novogrodshy A. et al, Effect of polar organic compounds on leukemic cells. Butyrate-induced partial remission of acute myelogenous leukemia in a child. CANCER, 51: 9-14, 1983).

Everyone knows that you need vitamin D to make calcium work, and if a leukemic has special need for calcium, he most likely will need more **vitamin D**. But this vitamin also has **anti-cancer properties** of its own, and especially anti- leukemic, rendering cells benign (again, transformed into normal cells) after treatment (Tanaka H, et al, 1(alpha),25-dihydroxycholecalciferol and a human myeloid leukaemia cell line (HL-60). The presence of a cytosol receptor and induction of differentiation. BIOCHEM J, 204: 713-719, 1982; and Honma Y, et al, 1(alpha),25-dihydroxyvitamin D3 and 1(alpha)-hydroxyvitamin D3 prolong survival time of mice inoculated with myeloid leukemia cells, PROC NATL ACAD SCI USA, 80:201-204,1983).

Likewise, **the more serious the condition, the more attention that must be paid to each detail.** For example, **garlic** (Allium sativum) is an herb of the Lily family (asparagus, onions, leeks, scallions, shallots). Aside from **lowering cholesterol and blood pressure and blood sugar**, it contains high amounts of sulfur which are good for the detox system (Nair SC, et al,

Differential induction of glutathione transferase isoenzymes of mice stomach by diallyl sulfide, a naturally occurring anti-carcinogen, CANCER LETT, 57:121-129, 1990).

And in addition to being anti-fungal for patients with dysbioses (unwanted organisms growing in the gut) like Candida, **garlic** also has **anti-cancer** properties. In fact UCLA scientists said it appeared to be as good as or better than more toxic and expensive drugs (Hoon S, et al, Modulation of cancer antigens and growth of human melanoma by aged garlic extract, FIRST WORLD CONFERENCE ON HEALTH SIGNIFICANCE OF GARLIC AND GARLIC CONSTITUENTS, Washington, DC, 1990)

BUT, REMEMBER GARLIC STOPS THE CLUMPING OF PLATELETS (Foster S, Garlic "Allium Sativum" (Ist ed.) Austin TX: American Botanical Council, 1991:7 (AB Council, Botanical Series; vol. 311). So it would be most deleterious to administer it to someone with leukemia, head trauma or other recent injury, or on blood thinners (anti-coagulants). I tell you these tidbits, not to make you experts in leukemia, or any other cancer, but to give you a feel of how careful one must be as the seriousness of the disease state increases. **Hippocrates said, "Let thy food be thy medicine."** And now you can appreciate just how potent it can be, and that there is 21st century evidence and explanation for this wisdom that is thousands of years old.

And, **garlic** is not the only herb or spice that is **strongly anti-clotting. Cumin,** the spice of chili con carne, and turmeric, the yellow color of **curry** and , are both anti-platelet (Srivastava KC, Extracts from two frequently consumed spices —cumin (Cuminum cyminum) and turmeric (Curcuma longa) — inhibit platelet aggregation and alter eicosanoid biosynthesis in human blood platelets, PROSTAGLANDINS LEUKOT ESSENT FATTY ACIDS, 37:57-64, 1989)

And since the integrity of the clotting system is so important for the leukemic, they need extra **vitamin K.** But even more importantly, vitamin K has some anti-cancer (and anti-leukemic in particular) effects of its own. I love it how there are so many dual roles for items that are beneficial (Chlebowski RT, et al, Vitamin K in the treatment of cancer, CANCER TREAT REV, 12:49-63, 1985, and Chlebowski RT, et a;, Vitamin K3 inhibition of malignant murine cell growth and human tumor colony formation, CANCER TREAT REV, 69:527-532, 1985.

And because **vitamin K is manufactured in the intestine,** it is crucial to have good intestinal flora. That is an additional reason for daily yogurt (containing live acidophilus) in the carnivore leukemic. Good food sources of vitamin K include alfalfa, green leafy vegetables, and kelp (a sea vegetable).

And as with nearly every nutrient, vitamin K has a strong connection to the detox system. As a small example, you already know that one of the most important roles of vitamin K (especially for the leukemic) is in blood clotting. It works by carboxylating **glutamic acid** to form prothrombin. (Anderson SA, Effects of certain vitamins and minerals on calcium and phosphorus homeostasis, p23, FDA, Wash DC,Sept 1982, Life Sciences Research Office, 9650 Rockville Pike, Bethesda MD 20814).

But remember, that **glutamic acid** is one of the three peptides that go into making **glutathione, a major conjugator or detoxifier for control of chemical exposures.** But recall that glutathione is thrown away with the chemical that is being detoxified. In other words, it is **used up, and lost forever.** So if the person trying to overcome a serious disease is not aware of the principles of environmental medicine and does not exercise good environmental controls and keep chemical expo-

72

sures to a minimum, he is in essence negating any benefit accrued from supplementing his nutrient deficiencies.

OPPOSITES ATTRACT

Opposites attract, yin and yang, male and female. Most couples are indeed opposites. We complement each other's inadequacies and revel in each others accomplishments. So don't let the next logical extension of this foul up your life. And that is, that usually a macro is married to a carnivore; an alkaline type is married to an acid-loving. Once you acknowledge and appreciate each other's metabolic type, you can reduce mealtime strife. Never try to cram someone else into your metabolic type.

THE BOTTOM LINE

The metabolic cross reveals a spectrum of requirements between acid and alkaline, as well as raw to cooked. So as not to complicate, we have omitted other axes at this point. But suffice it to say, there are other axes and this can get a great deal more complicated. For our purposes here, however, these two basic directions will take you a long way. For the vast majority, irrespective of the degree of unwellness, the **alkaline** side is the most healing.

For the neophyte, just getting off sugar, white flour, coffee, alcohol, sodas, cigarettes, and processed foods starts unloading them. Then the addition of nutrient-rich whole grains, greens and beans really starts to liven them up.

But as with all of life, there are the exceptions and outlyers, who do not fall into the average range. In fact some of the treatments could make them worse. An example is given for the leukemic who is a carnivore. He needs a diet high in fat and red meat for a while, with much more calcium (and other things like vitamin A as you will see), while simultaneously avoiding such seemingly harmless foods as garlic, which has anti-clotting properties and is in effect, anti-platelet.

So while the vast majority can evaluate which diet makes them feel the best, those with more serious conditions definitely need more specialized help. And should you find that at least for a while, you are a carnivore, remember to have a physician knowledgeable in lipids (essential fatty acids) help you factor and monitor these in your program. And remember that your needs can change.

RESOURCES

Nussbaum E, RECOVERY, Japan Publ., 1986, all Japan Publ can be obtained through Kushi Institute, Box 7, Becket, MA 01223
or N.E.E.D.S., 1-800-634-1380 (this is **the best autobiography I can recommend** about healing utterly impossible end-stage metastatic cancer, when given 3 weeks to live by doctors)

Faulkner H, PHYSICIAN HEAL THYSELF, Kushi Inst., ibid, 1992 (autobiography of British medical doctor who cleared his own "incurable" cancer of the pancreas at 74......I had dinner with him 5 years later and received a letter this year)

Satillaro AJ, RECALLED BY LIFE, Avon Books, NY, Kushi Inst., ibid, 1984 (another medical doctor who cleared his own metastatic prostate cancer with macrobiotics)

Eastwest Foundation with Ann Fawcett and Cynthia Smith,

CANCER FREE; THIRTY WHO TRIUMPHED OVER CANCER NATURALLY, Japan Publications Inc., 1991, and Kushi Institute, ibid

Kushi M, THE MACROBIOTIC APPROACH TO CANCER, Avery Publishing, Garden City Park NY 1991, and Kushi Inst., ibid

Gerson M, A CANCER THERAPY, RESULTS OF 50 CASES, Gerson Institute, PO Box 430, Bonita CA 92002

Gerson M, THE CURE OF ADVANCED CANCER BY DIET THERAPY, A SUMMARY OF 30 YEARS OF CLINICAL EXPERIMENTATION, ibid

Gerson M, The cure of advanced cancer by diet therapy: A summary of 30 years of clinical experimentation, PHYSIOL CHEM & PHYSICS, 10:449-464, 1978

Bishop B, MY TRIUMPH OVER CANCER, available through the Gerson Inst., P.O.Box 430, Bonita CA 92002

Haught SJ, CENSURED FOR CURING CANCER, The Gerson Institute, POB 430, Bonita CA 92002, 1962

Mae E, HOW I CONQUERED CANCER NATURALLY, Harvest House Publishers, 17895 Skypark Circle, Irvine CA 92714.

Brandt J, HOW TO CONQUER CANCER, NATURALLY, Treelife Publications, 255 N. El Col Cielo Rd., #126, Palm Springs CA 92262.

Rohe F, DR. KELLEY'S ANSWER TO CANCER, 1969, Wedgestone Press, POB 175, Winfield KS 67156

Eyre R, I FOUGHT LEUKEMIA AND WON, Hawkes Publ, 3775 S. 500 West, Box 15711, Salt Lake City UT 84115, 1982

Valentine, Tom & Carol, MEDICINE'S MISSING LINK. METABOLIC TYPING AND YOUR PERSONAL FOOD PLAN Thorsons Publishers, Inc, 1 Park Street, Rochester VT 05767, 1987.

Kelley WD, ONE ANSWER TO CANCER Wedgestone Press, Box 175, Winfield KS 67157, 1969.

Wigmore, Ann, THE HEALING POWER WITHIN, Avery Publinshing, Wayne NJ, 1983.

Tilden, JH, TOXEMIA EXPLAINED. Frank J. Wolf Publ, Denver CO. 1926. Keats Publ., 36 Grove St (Box 876), New Canaan CT 06840. Revised 1981.

Rohe F, METABOLIC ECOLOGY Wedgestone Press, ibid, 1969.

Bieler HG, FOOD IS YOUR BEST MEDICINE, Ballentyne Books, Random House NY, 1982.

Airola P, CANCER: CAUSES, PREVENTION, AND TREATMENT. THE TOTAL APPROACH, Health Plus Publishers, PO Box 10027, Sherwood OR 97140.

Ehret A, MUCUSLESS DIET HEALING SYSTEM , Ehret Literature Publ Co, Yonkers NY 10701-2714, 1989.

Bragg, Paul & Patricia, THE MIRACLE OF FASTING, Health Science, Box 7, Santa Barbara CA 93102, 1990.

Bragg, Paul & Patricia, TOXICLESS DIET. BODY PURIFICA-

TION AND HEALING SYSTEM, ibid

Shelton HM, FASTING CAN SAVE YOUR LIFE, American Natural Hygiene Society, Inc. P.O.Box 30630, Tampa FL 33630, 1991

Auel JM, THE CLAN OF THE CAVE BEAR, Bantam Books, Inc., 666 5th Ave., NY NY 10103, 1980

Shelton HM, Fry TC, Weger GS, HOW TO KEEP YOUR BODY PURE, Health Excellence Systems, 1108 Regal Row, Manchaca TX 78652- 0609

Walker NW, DIET AND SALAD SUGGESTIONS, FACT (Foundation for Advancement in Cancer Therapy), phone 215-642-4810.

Erasmus U, FATS AND OILS, Alive Books, P.O.Box 67333, Vancouver, B.C., Canada V5W 3T1, 1986

Bates C, ESSENTIAL FATTY ACIDS AND IMMUNITY IN MENTAL HEALTH, Life Sciences Press, P.O.Box 1174, Tacoma, WA 98401, 1987

Pique GG, OMEGA-3 THE FISH OIL FACTORS, Omega-3 Project, Inc., 10615-G Tierrasanta Blvd, Ste 347, San Diego CA 92124, 1986

Horrobin DF, CLINICAL USES OF FATTY ACIDS, Eden Press Inc., P.O.Box 51, St.Albans VT 05478, 1982

Nolfi K, THE MIRACLE OF LIVING FOODS AND THE CURSE OF COOKING, Health Excellence systems, 1108 Regal Row, Manchaca TX 78654-0609, 1991

Beasley VR, TRICHOTHECENE MYCOTOXICOSIS: PATHOPHYSIOLOGIC EFFECTS, VOL II, CRC Press, Boca Raton, FL, 1989

Books about natural ways to clear cancer also available from:

*   N.E.E.D.S.   1-800-634-1380
          527 Charles Ave
          Syracuse, NY 13209

*   Foundation for Advancement in Cancer Therapy
          Box 1242
          Old Chelsea Sta,
          NY,NY 10113
          phone 212-741-2790

*   Cancer Control Society
          2043 N Berendo St.
          Los Angeles CA 90027
          phone 213-663-7801

*   Kushi Institute   subscribe to ONE
          Box 7   PEACEFULL WORLD
          Becket MA 01223   for monthly cases of
          (413)623-5741   cancer cures

Other organizations of interest:

Committee for Freedom of Choice in Medicine, Inc.
1180 Walnut Ave.
Chula Vista CA 91911
American Biologics Mexico, S.A.
1-800-227-4258

Some sources for organic foods (others in MACRO MELLOW):

N.E.E.D.S.   1-800 634-1380
527 Charles Ave.
Syracuse, NY 13209

Gold Mine Natural Foods 1-800 475-FOOD
1047 30th ST
San Diego CA 82102

Mt. Ark Trading Co. 1-800 643-8909
120 S. East Ave.
Fayetteville AK 72701

Walnut Acres   (717) 837-0601
Penns Creek, PA 17862
The Ohio Hempery, Inc., 14 N court ST, #300, Athens, OH 45701,
phone (614) 593-5828 (hemp oil and products)

Scientific papers of interest:

Cope FW, A medical application of the Ling association-induction hypothesis: The high potassium, low sodium diet of the Gerson cancer therapy, PHYSIOL CHEM & PHYSICS, 10:465- 468, 1978

Jansson B, Geographic cancer risk and intracellular potassium/sodium ratios, CANCER DETECTION AND PREVENTION 9:171-194, 1986

Jansson B, Dietary, total body, and intracellular potassium- to-sodium ratios and their influence on cancer, CANCER DETECTION AND PREVENTION, 14:563-565, 1990

Zs-Nagy I, et al, Correlation of malignancy with the intracellular Na+:K: ratio in human thyroid tumors, CANCER RESEARCH 43:5395-5402, Nov 1983

Bishop B, Organic food in cancer therapy, NUTRITION AND HEALTH, 6,2:105-109, 1988

Smith B, Organic foods vs supermarket foods:Element levels, J APPL NUTR 45:1, 1993

Gerson M, Dietary considerations in malignant neoplastic diseases, REV GASTROENT 12:419-425, 1945

Anonymous, Diet changes may buy cancer patients time, SCIENCE NEWS, 142:324, 1992

Anderson KE, Dietary regulation of cytochrome P450, ANNU REV NUTR 11:141-167, 1991

As this book goes to press, I recently found a "must read autobiography" for those who still have doubts about healing themselves in spite of reading RECOVERY, RECALLED BY LIFE, and PHYSICIAN HEAL THYSELF: Frahm AE, A CANCER BATTLE PLAN, Pinon Press, Colorado Springs, 1992, available Successful Living Products, P.O. Box 832, Baldwinsville NY 13207-0832

Chapter 3

PURIFICATION

"THE COFFEE BREAK"

The coffee enema has saved many lives. A coffee what? An enema? With what? How gross! How weird! How sordid! You mean you stick it in your butt?? How disgusting! But on the contrary, how healing and how life saving. And for some it is the difference between life and death.

I thought we had reached the epitome of medical non- conformance when we started teaching about rotated diets, then the titrated new molds, then chemical sensitivity, food additives, trans fatty acids, free radicals, EMF (electromagnetic field) pollution, radon in basements, and then recommending macrobiotic diets. But coffee enemas sounded to me even more bizarre than anything I had ever heard of in medicine.

I recall coming home from lecturing over a decade ago and all enthused with what I had learned or was teaching. I remember saying to my husband, "There are chemicals in people's carpets that can cause chronic fatigue, arthritis, depression and just about any symptom, even cancer. But if I tell my patients, I'll be driven out of town as a quack".

But as time has passed, even the dullest of persons knows that there are some pretty nasty chemicals that we are all exposed to every day. They even showed the poor little mice in the jar with the carpet sample on T.V. The 4-PC emitted from the "normal" carpet backing left them dead as a door-nail by morn.

Then it was the discovery of the over 500 chemicals in the

drinking water, many of which can cause a host of diseases, including cancers. For years I dared not divulge this information except to my most intelligent patients. The rest of the world, including the medical profession, was just not ready or able to accept it, even with all the scientific backup. Now everyone knows it, and only the least medically sophisticated people are left drinking straight tap water. For even if you cannot afford glass-bottled spring water, you can boil out many of the volatile organic hydrocarbons from city water.

Then I remember saying, "There is an invisible radioactive gas in people's basements that can cause cancer, but if I tell them, they will think I'm nuts". Now everyone has heard of radon. Then it was electromagnetic fields from electric blankets and home wiring in the walls or overhead power lines that were capable of causing severe psychiatric problems, infertility, and even leukemia. And so it is always easy to recognize the pioneers in medicine. They are often thought of as the quacks, until the knowledge becomes commonplace. (They are also the ones with the arrows in their backs).

Anyway, when you put medical progress in perspective, it still boils down to the fact that coffee enemas sound outlandishly unscientific! But nothing could be further from the truth.

HISTORY OF COFFEE ENEMAS

Actually, coffee enemas have been around for scores of years in fact, they were in the **MERCK MANUAL** (a revered text in medicine) up until 1977; and then they were merely removed for lack of space because there were so many drugs on the market. In the 1920's before the drug era took over medicine, they were widely written about.

My first exposure to coffee enemas came from reading about

them as an important part of the Gerson program years ago. But frankly it sounded so peculiar, that I readily dismissed them (I did the same foolish thing when I first heard about macrobiotics. I wonder how many other wonderfully beneficial things I have over-looked in my life?).

The next time I was to encounter coffee enemas was in reading about Dr. Kelley, a dentist who had cleared his own cancer of the pancreas. He found that a highly nutritional diet and specific vitamins and minerals kept him alive when multiple medical physician experts all told him that he had only a matter of months to live. But when his cancer kept growing and he could feel rocky hard tumors in his liver, he knew he had to do something more.

He found that when he took pancreatic enzymes that the hardness and nodularity of the liver would go down (more about that in the enzyme chapter). In other words, it helped his cancer dissolve. But as the cancer was being broken down, he became so sick, dizzy, headachey and just plain toxic that he couldn't stand it and he would have to go off the enzymes. When he went off the enzymes however, the rocky, hard cancer nodules reappeared on the liver.

It wasn't until he discovered coffee enemas in the old medical literature, that he was able to detoxify his body. In other words, with coffee enemas he was able to get rid of the toxic waste that had accumulated from the rapid (enzyme-facilitated) break-down of the cancer. He was able to get rid of these wastes fast enough now, so that they would no longer back-log or accumulate and make him unbearably sicker.

And as I read through old medical books from the 1920's, I saw a recurring theme amongst the "natural hygiene" group. Their philosophy was that all disease was merely a question of

toxicity. It was the mere inability of the body to dispose of accumulated waste products, before they caused symptoms.

And in essence, all disease and every symptom is really a reflection of the **balance or imbalance** between the ability of the body to do its daily repairs and the **net accumulation of toxic wastes** that result from this process. If the toxins become too much, then we have **symptoms** in whatever organ or tissue the toxins accumulate in. If they accumulate in the joints we call it arthritis, if they accumulate in the bloodstream we call it fatigue or headache, flu or toxicity.

I became seriously impressed however, with coffee enemas when I watched their effects first-hand when my attorney girlfriend was clearing her leukemia with this program. As her cancer cells were being broken down she would become so toxic that her tongue and liver would visibly swell. She was often times barely able to speak clearly because of such marked tongue swelling. When she did a coffee enema, the tongue swelling, brain fog and liver swelling were reduced as well as the toxic, sick feeling. She made me promise to write about its effectiveness so that others might benefit.

Nevertheless, I was still leery of coffee enemas because I knew myself and many others were very allergic to coffee. I wouldn't drink a cup of coffee if you paid me $1000, because I would be wearing it on my face in the form of eczema for three weeks afterwards. I won't even taste my husband's coffee in the morning (on the rare occasion that I make it) to see if I've made it correctly, because just a sip will break me out. However, as you will learn, being allergic to coffee is not a contraindication for a coffee enema.

As fate would have it, I had another opportunity to test out the effectiveness of coffee enemas. As you know, the nightshades

84

are a botanical classification of foods which include potatoes, tomatos, green, red and yellow peppers, pimento, chili, cayenne, paprika, egg plant, and tobacco. The night shades and red meat happen to be very common causes of arthritis in many people. The reason people have had difficulty in ever figuring it out is that the arthritis usually does not occur for 48 hours and by then you have forgotten what you ate two days prior.

Even worse, once the arthritis is triggered by ingestion of nightshades, it does not usually go away for three months. This is because it is not a simple IgE mediated allergy like ragweed hayfever or dust allergy is. Instead, it is a different type of allergy where the body makes an IgG or IgM antibody to make immune complexes. These stay attached or glued to the cells much longer.

So, you can understand why someone with arthritis rarely figures out that nightshades are the cause. Just suppose someone loves potatoes or tomato sauce and goes without them for a couple of weeks; since his arthritis won't be one bit better in just a couple of weeks and now since he's on the "pitty pot", feeling sorry for himself that he has been denying himself his favorite foods for awhile, he'll usually go ahead and have them, proving to himself that it didn't make him any worse. Since it didn't make him any better either, it gives the poor arthritis victim the false notion that nightshades are not a part of the problem.

Anyway, I figured it out for myself the hard way years ago and because I'm not too smart, God always figures out a way to prove it to me so that I can stumble onto the connection. Within two days I get severe, dramatic swelling of my finger joints with the slightest amount of green pepper or potato. It happens like clockwork 48 hours after I have had it and the joints look and feel like somebody has just hit them with a hammer. It stays this way for about three months and then disappears suddenly one day. That must be the day that the antigen-antibody complexes are finally metabolized by the body and gotten rid of.

Anyway, I was foolish and tried to ignore my sensitivity because someone had gone to great lengths to prepare a special meal for me, and had hoped that it would not have anything in it that I couldn't eat. I ate the meal, carefully dissecting out the peppers. But this was stupid, for they had been cooked into the dish. So like clockwork, in 48 hours two finger joints were swollen, and this time (as in many other times) my lumbo-sacral back arthritis from the old ruptured disc 25 years earlier also flared up unmercifully.

I had torturous pain in the back every single moment, every single day. I was such a specter of doom and gloom with my chronic pain, it's a wonder anyone could stand to be around me (some couldn't). I did chiropractic adjustments 4 times a week, trials of bed rest, which for me is a real sacrifice, IV's of magnesium (which did simmer it down, but only for a few hours each time) and multiple other things to no avail.

Fortunately, because I was out of my mind with pain and at a loss for what else to do, I was doing the coffee enemas reli-giously every single day and in three weeks, suddenly one day, the back pain stopped as precipitously as it had come and was gone.

My analysis of the whole situation is that it is the coffee enemas that speeded up my healing time and helped the body metabo-lize the antigen-antibody complexes quicker, since the little scientist in me has repeated this several times over. I'm sure a lot of physicians and other people could argue with me, but they would have to be in this body to appreciate my analysis.

Never before in all the years of agonizing experimentation had it disappeared so precipitously and ahead of biological schedule! Especially in view of the fact that this was one of the more serious (high dose of nightshades) episodes.

If you think of the responsibilities of the human intestine, the gut has really two basic functions. One, is to remove the nutrition from the foods so that we can use it for energy, growth, repair and healing. The second function is to get rid of waste. And a major part of this waste elimination function occurs when the liver and gall bladder dump unwanted detoxified chemicals into the gut to be disposed of. Remember how the body hooks that big protein **glutathione** onto chemicals floating in the blood stream? From there they finish their pass through the liver and out into the gut.

So it's logical that when the body has an extra burden of waste, that there is a backlog of unmetabolized material in the rest of the body. This causes a **toxemia** which can manifest as any symptom or disease. It would be prudent to help the body unload this backlog by speeding the work of **detoxification**. The result would be more energy left for the work of repair or healing.

It's no different than lancing an abscess. We know if one has a huge boil or abscess that they get better much quicker and often times do not need antibiotics if we can lance the abscess and allow the infected waste products to drain off. We know if we don't lance a boil, this infection can be carried by the lymphatics into the system and effect other areas of the body. You could end up with a serious abscess in the brain or on a heart valve.

Also, if a boil is not lanced the infection may spread locally and antibiotics are required. But usually, once a boil is opened and drained, the burden or total load to the body is so reduced that it can heal itself without the aid of antibiotics. Sometimes soaking, salt compresses, or black drawing salve are other ways to help pull out infection and speed the work of healing by reducing the total load to the body.

And so, it should not be at all surprising that coffee enemas work by speeding up the emptying of the bowel. This in turn speeds up the emptying of the liver ducts which hold the detoxified materials taken from the blood and tissues. And this in turn speeds healing.

If you think about it, this should have excellent application in many other areas of everyday medicine. We know for example, when people have liver or kidney disease, in medicine we have to reduce the total load to the system by putting them on low protein diets to reduce the work of the ailing liver or kidney. Sometimes antibiotics are prescribed to kill the intestinal flora, because certain types of bugs in the intestine promote reabsorption of toxins and undesirable metabolic byproducts from the gut. Here is a common medical condition that could be helped significantly with a coffee enema.

It's really quite astounding that the old remedies of the 1920's have been forgotten when they could be so useful in these conditions. A coffee enema could save the day for these victims of overwhelming toxicity. As we have found, they are invaluable in numerous conditions, from post- operative healing, severe infections, severe and traumatic injuries, to speeding the recovery time from chemical exposures and cancers. Why just look at all the people suffering with gut-wrenching nausea and vomiting after their chemotherapy has dumped millions of poisoned cells into their blood stream. Coffee enemas could help attenuate this agony, not to mention save lives.

Tilden's 1920 book **TOXEMIA**, explores the notion that all disease is a matter of the body's inability to detoxify and clean itself out. There is an imbalance between the speed of accumulating wastes and the ability of the body to get rid of these wastes. This theory explains why fasting is so universally beneficial to so many diverse conditions. It merely unloads the diverse body of some of its daily work so that it can have more reserve for healing.

It is no different than if you were pushing to get several day's worth of gardening done in one day so that you could finish in time to ensure a long growing season. During that arduous day of work, you would not decide to do your daily fastidious housework and elaborate cooking as well. Likewise, if the body is busy with an inordinate amount of healing and detoxification, you don't make it digest a feast and run a marathon. Instead you concentrate on accelerating the detox.

In the ensuing decades after Tilden's work, medicine got roped into using drugs to mask or hide symptoms, postponing a golden opportunity to identify the cause of illness. So with time, as conditions treated with drugs worsened, the symptoms eventually expressed themselves in different target organs. But "specialists " in particular organ systems believed their part was done, once they had suppressed symptoms.

And to this day the specialist never dreams, for example, that the man who dies from sudden cardiac arrest might be because his orthopedic surgeon missed his magnesium deficiency as a cause of his chronic back pain, or his gastroenterologist missed a magnesium deficiency as the cause of his esophageal or stomach spasm. Instead they were treated with muscle relaxants and non-steroidal anti-inflammatory drugs, or antispasmodics or medication to suppress acid formation. Then when the magnesium deficiency escalated, causing spasm of the coronary blood vessels, it was all history. The patient was dead and no one knew why.

HOW DOES THE COFFEE ENEMA WORK?

The very last part of the colon is in an "S"-shape and because it is in an "S"-shape it's called the **sigmoid colon**. By the time stool gets to this part of the colon, most all of the good vitamins and minerals and other nutrients have been reabsorbed back into the bloodstream. Because the stool is so full of toxins and the products of putrefaction at this point, nature has made a special circulatory system between the sigmoid colon and the liver. There is a direct communication of veins called the **entero-hepatic circulation, or EHC.**

This enables the toxins to be sent directly to the liver for detoxication, rather than circulating them through the rest of the body and all of its vital organs including the brain and making the person sick. This system of veins carries sigmoid toxins directly to the liver so that it can detoxify these toxic materials and avoid making the person generally ill.

When a coffee enema is used, the caffeine from the coffee is preferentially absorbed into this **ENTEROHEPATIC** system and goes directly to the liver where it becomes a very strong detoxicant. It makes the liver dump out the toxins it has been accumulating in the bile ducts and unload so that then the rest of the toxic materials that have accumulated in the organs, tissues and bloodstream can begin to filter into the liver and be taken care of. This is why I do not break out when doing them, because the coffee does not go into the systemic circulation.

The caffeine contains some alkaloids that also stimulate the production of **glutathione-S-transferase**, an enzyme used by the liver to make the detox pathways run. It is pivotal in the formation of more **glutathione,** one of the **main conjugators of chemicals,** enabling them to be eliminated in the gut. So in other words, a coffee enema speeds up the detoxification process and minimizes backlog of yet-to-be detoxified substances.

WOULD THIS HELP THE COMMON COLD?

It seems likely that if you felt you were coming down with a cold that there are a number of things you could do to "rev up" the detox capabilities of the body. First, you would do a nasal saline lavage which would capitalize on the osmotic force of the sea salt solution to drain the sinuses (directions in THE E.I. SYNDROME).

You know how your finger tips wrinkle up when you are swimming in the ocean and how your sinuses feel so clear. You feel like you could drive a Mack truck through them. Well, the reason this is so is that the osmotic force of salt pulls water out of swollen and congested tissues that line the tiny pin point openings of the sinuses. Your fingers wrinkle in salt water, because the salt pulls water across skin cells, and out of the superficial tissues. The same happens to the swollen pin-point tubes that allow the sinuses to drain. Shrinking down the swollen cells in the passages allows the opening of the sinuses to enlarge and they can now drain.

Furthermore, the high osmotic force of the salt solution then pulls the infected material out of the sinuses as well. When you follow the directions in **THE E.I. SYNDROME** be sure to use sea salt and good, clean spring water.

Second, use a high dose of Buffered C throughout the day beginning with a teaspoon every hour to the point of bowel tolerance. You should back off as soon as you get diarrhea and that is the total cumulative dose for the day (the directions are in **TIRED OR TOXIC?**). Then raw, fresh carrot juice four times a day as well as coffee enemas twice a day should increase the anti-oxidant ability of the body as well as help clean out wastes quicker.

THE LETHAL RETINOIC ACID SYNDROME

There is even a lethal syndrome now that has been described in the scientific literature as a mysterious cause of death that could be abetted with the coffee purge. It is recognized that certain cancers, like certain leukemias, can be actually be reversed and cured with high medically supervised doses of retinoic acid, a derivative of vitamin A (more on this later).

The side effect of the treatment, which totally reverses the leukemia, is that some of the people die of a "strange" toxicity after the cancer has been cleared. It is called the "retinoic acid syndrome". What they report is that even though people were getting better and had remissions, they had all sorts of strange symptoms including fever, difficulty breathing, swelling of the legs, fluid in the lungs and heart sack, low blood pressure and some people died from these.

These, of course, are **clear indications for a coffee enema** because they are clearly toxic symptoms from the breakdown of the cancer and yet to this day to my knowledge, they do not have the faintest idea of this and in fact, would probably laugh if we told them about it. Happily, for someone, somewhere, this fact alone makes the price of this book a bargain, as it will prove pivotal to their survival.

STEADY AS SHE GOES

One of the things that impressed me in watching people

92

improve cancers, chemical sensitivity and other conditions with the coffee enemas is the steadiness with which it must be done. It must be a daily routine and for weeks on end there may be no improvement and then suddenly everything clicks in and improvement can be appreciated.

For some, it takes months before the body rallies. It is the steadiness however, that is so important and it is a steadiness of a total load program which includes the correct diet, enzymes, hormones, juicing, prescribed nutrients, periodic bowel cleanses and flushing, attention to one's spirituality, and environmental controls. These all constitute an important part of the total load whenever coffee enemas are used. They are not meant to be used in isolation or alone without a **total program**. And above all, they should be done with good **nutrient supplementation** and **periodic checking of nutrient levels**.

Questions about coffee enemas:

Q: Isn't a coffee enema harmful? Doesn't it flush out important minerals and electrolytes?

A: No, all the important vitamins, essential fatty acids, amino acids, and minerals including the electrolytes like potassium (which is really a mineral) have already been absorbed higher up in the colon. The coffee enema is only in the sigmoid portion of the bowel. It is **not a colonic** and it is **not a high enema**. Therefore it **does not wash out the protective IgA** nor the mucous covering of the bowel, either. But because we are the first generation to explore the effects of them in light of things that were not known earlier, **I would strongly urge that nutrient levels be periodically checked.** Minimum, I would suggest at 3 months and 9 months, and rbc zinc, rbc copper, rbc manganese, rbc chromium, and a magnesium loading test.

Q: Won't the coffee enema make my bowels dependant upon an enema?

A: On the contrary, after people have been doing coffee enemas, they often find they have better bowel movements once they stop because their body is healthier overall.

Q: Is the coffee bad for my heart?

A: Recent studies show there is "no association between coffee consumption and the occurrence of coronary heart disease". And as all of us with coffee allergy have shown, it is not absorbed into the systemic circulation (which it would have to be in order to affect the heart). However, there are no abolutes in life, nor medicine. If you experience any adverse symptoms, I would reccommend that you stop the enemas. And if you do get a reaction that most do not, such as cardiac stimulation, this suggests you need investigation for the leaky gut syndrome, or a hyperpermeable gut that allows absorption of toxins and antigens that most likely are contributing to your symptoms (more about that later). We measured the caffeine blood levels in the few people who felt stimulated by the enemas and it was undetectable.

Q: How long should I do a coffee enema for and how often?

A: I know people who have done coffee enemas everyday for 10 years. I myself tried them for over a year and a half with no adverse effects and in fact, was even healthier (and I thought that I couldn't get any healthier because I felt so well). The doctor will prescribe the dose and frequency for you. It can vary from once a week to once a day to several times a day. People with serious toxic conditions such as diagnosed end-stage cancers often need 6-10 enemas a day. But the higher the frequency, the closer should be the medical supervision, especially of nutrient levels.

A good rule of thumb would be once a day, three weeks out of every four. Then you can be sure of the effects. In over a hundred chemically sensitive people who have improved significantly with the enemas, there were less than half a dozen who did not feel well and discontinued them. And I have never heard of a permanent side effect from them.

PROCEDURE FOR COFFEE ENEMAS

You will need the following materials:

1. An enema bag, preferably one of clear plastic that you can see through (N.E.E.D.S.),
2. a special soft French catheter to fit over the hard plastic tip of the enema bag,
3. a large stainless steel cooking pot,
4. organic coffee or Folgers (red can) fully caffeinated, drip grind coffee,
5. a Pyrex one quart measuring cup with handle and pour spout,
6. unsulfured molasses, and
7. chemically less contaminated water; definitely do not use city tap water. If you have clean well water that's fine, or filtered water or glass bottled water (not in plastic bottles). The cheapest route is to use reverse osmosis on your house water or a faucet filter. If you must use city water, boil off the chlorine for 10 minutes.

The see-through enema bag is preferable, but there is nothing wrong with the old-fashioned type that doubles as a hot water bottle. If you want, you can buy a French or foley catheter, of very soft rubber. Because it is of softer rubber than the hard plastic tip of the enema bag, it is easier on your hemorroidal area. If you do get the extra catheter tip, be sure to cut the

95

bottom 2 inches off the enema bag's hard, plastic tip with scissors before attaching the soft red rubber catheter tip. Otherwise the soft catheter will cover only the end hole at the very tip, and coffee will run out the second hole that is on the side just above the tip.

PROCEDURE FOR MAKING THE ENEMA

Put 1 quart of clean water in a pan and bring it to a boil. Add 2 flat tablespoons of coffee (or the coffee amount that has been prescribed for you). Let it continue to boil for five minutes, then turn the stove off leaving the pan on the hot burner. Add one tablespoon of unsulfured molasses.

Allow it to cool down to a very comfortable, tepid temperature. Test with your finger. It should be the same temperature as a baby's bottle. It's better to have it too cold than too warm; never use it hot or steaming.

Next, carry your pan or pot and the Pyrex measuring cup into the bathroom and lay an old towel on the floor. If you don't use an old towel, you will shortly have many old towels since coffee stains permanently. Use another bunch of towels, if you want, as a pillow and bring along your BIBLE or some other appropriately relaxing literature. Pour the coffee from the pan into the measuring cup without getting the coffee grounds in the cup. Put your enema bag in the sink with the catheter clamped closed.

Then pour the coffee from the measuring cup into the enema bag. Loosen the clamp to allow the coffee to run out to the end of the catheter tip and re-clamp the bag when all the air has been removed from the enema tubing. Use a coat hanger to hang the enema bag at waist level. A door knob or towel rack is appropriate. Do not hang it high, as on a shower head, because it will be too forceful. It should flow very gently into the distal sigmoid colon only. It is not a high enema or colonic. It should only go into the distal rectum.

Lie down on the floor and gently insert the catheter. If you need lubrication, food grade vegetable oil such as olive oil would be fine. Avoid petroleum jellies like KY or Vaseline, etc. Gently insert the tube into the rectum a few inches and then release the clamp and let the first 1/2 of the quart (2 cups maximum) of coffee flow in. Clamp the tubing off as soon as there is the slightest amount of discomfort or fullness. Some prefer to roll to the right side, then the left and then back to the right and then the left again, staying a few minutes on each side and then lie flat and gently massage the abdomen.

Try to retain the enema for 10 minutes. Sometimes there will be an immediate urgency to get rid of it and that is fine. It helps to clean the stool out of the colon so that next time around you can hold more of the enema. Never force yourself to retain it if you feel that you can't. When you have clamped the tubing, remove the catheter tip and void when you have to. If you can hold it ten minutes each time, fine. After you have emptied the bowel, proceed with the remaining 1/2 quart and likewise hold that for 10 minutes, if able, then void.

The goal is to have two enemas, not exceeding 1/2 a quart (2 cups) each, that you are able to hold for 10 minutes each. Usually 2 or 3 times will use up all of the enema, but that is not your goal. Being able to hold it for 10 minutes is. During that time you will often feel or hear a gurgling or squirting out of liquid up under the right ribs. That may be your gallbladder discharging it's load into the bowel.

When you have finished your session, rinse out the bag and hang it up to dry. Periodically run boiling water, peroxide,or other comparable anti-microbial material through the empty bag just to discourage mold groth when it is not in use.

If you are hesitant to add the molasses, which serves to improve the efficiency of the enema, then omit it for the first few weeks, then see if you tolerate it.

If you feel "wired" or **hyper,** or have **palpitations** or irregular heartbeats after a coffee enema, you should reduce the amount of coffee, usually by half for a few days or weeks. Or consider that you really need organic coffee. And be sure the source of your water is good clean chemically less-contaminated spring, well, or filtered water. No chlorinated tap water for sure.

Usually you will hear or feel a squirting out and emptying of the bile duct. This occurs under the right rib cage, or sometimes more closely to the midline. If you hear or feel the release of the liver on the first or second enema, 2 is all you'll need. You can save the rest for the next time. If after a week of daily enemas you have never felt or heard the gall bladder release, you should consider making the coffee stronger, going up 1/2 tbs increments per qt., not exceeding 2 tbs. per cup. Or you may need a slightly larger volume, such as 3 cups at a time. Sometimes, 3 enemas (2 cups or less each) rather than two at a session are more beneficial for some.

Always discontinue the enemas if there is any adverse reaction whatsoever, and discuss it with the doctor at your next appointment. They are never meant to make you worse.

SCIENTIFIC EVIDENCE

In a scientific search of the medical literature through the American Academy of Family Practice, I was only able to find less than half a dozen articles reporting adverse effects with enemas, coffee or otherwise. These effects were electrolyte depletion. In other words, lowered potassium, magnesium, etc.. But there were loop-holes in the studies that would discredit them.

First of all, most assays in medicine today are inappropriate for potassium (i.e. most physicians order a serum potassium as opposed to the vastly more sensitive test, an intracellular rbc potassium) and magnesium assays are likewise inadequate (serum or rbc values are used instead of the more sensitive loading test). Couple this with the knowledge that the JOURNAL OF THE AMERICAN MEDICAL ASSOCIATION article (June 13, 1990) showed that 90% of physicians do not even check magnesium in sick and dying hospitalized patients with classical magnesium deficiency symptoms. This is inspite of the fact that U.S. Government surveys show that the average American diet provides only 40% of the magnesium a person needs in a day. And the same journal article showed that well over half the population is low in magnesium). Therefore, I cannot be impressed by the validity of these studies, since many of these subjects were most likely terribly low (yet undiagnosed) to begin with.

So in essence, most people unknowingly are so low or marginal in these minerals anyway, and sick people (who would be doing the enemas) are usually lower, that I fail to see how they could have been harmed by these, but suspect that their long overdue deficiencies became so blatantly obvious that they were finally diagnosed, even by the insensitive serum assays.

The coffee enema abuse most likely provided a scapegoat diagnosis for people who were probably already marginal or low: their deficiencies were blamed on the enemas, but none of the studies used the proper assessment of mineral status before the enemas were initiated. These enemas as I say, are not high enough to compromise the potassium. One would have to be on a slant board or elevate their hips and give the enema high up (either with pressure and/or a larger volume) in order to deplete these electrolytes. And most importantly, the appropriate tests were not done beforehand to see if these people were already marginal with their minerals. I personally do not recall anyone having or reporting serious electrolyte deficiencies with the coffee enemas. But be cautious, anyway.

In terms of the fact that caffeine has a stimulatory effect on the liver and makes it dump out its toxins, there are reports in the scientific literature to verify this and also that coffee actually increases the amount of glutathione-S-transferase which is necessary for the body to detoxify chemicals and toxins. As you recall, this enzyme is necessary to form the proteins that hook onto or conjugate nasty chemicals in the body. By attaching to them, they are then able to drag them out through the liver, bile ducts, gall bladder, and into the colon to get rid of them (detoxify) forever.

Caution should be taken that the **coffee enemas are never used alone. They must be part of a good strong supplement program** after assessing nutrient levels, usually hyposensitization injections, juicing, enzymes, periodic liver and colon cleanses, good environmental and dietary controls and much more. They are reserved for conditions that are severe and need the total load program.

Thus far we have had dozens of patients with a variety of problems from chronic fatigue to severe chemical sensitivities report that they are much improved by the enemas. Obviously they would be useful for a person who has an acute chemical exposure. They **reduce the recovery time**. Likewise, they speed the recovery from dietary indiscretions, injuries, and more.

I continued to survey the scientific literature to see if there were any legitimate reported problems with coffee enemas, and indeed, there were, but again I was unimpressed. And when you analyze them, you can see why. For example, one woman who died from them already had known achlorhydria (no stomach acid, which means she had serious uncorrected mineral deficiencies) and she was doing 12 a day (3 or 4 an hour!). Her admission electrolytes not compatible with life, as would be expected (Eisele JW, Reay DT, Deaths related to coffee enemas, JAMA, 244, 14:1608-1609, 1980).

As the guinea pig for most everything we recommend, it was logical that I try them first. I thought it would be futile since I'm no longer sick. With my lecture and practice schedule I have very little "free" time for myself. So I often overdo when I get a chance to do some of my other activities. One weekend I shoveled out the entire barn, then unloaded 2 roll-back truckloads of hay, and carried four 80 lb sacks of oats into the barn. Afterwards I worked with a horse and was thrown off, and worked in my organic garden. The next day I should have ached and hurt like crazy. I'm used to it.

But when I awoke at 5:30 a.m. I was amazed. I felt brand new, because of the coffee enemas. They rev up the detox system so there is **no backlog of unmetabolized muscle breakdown products.** With the clean-up system working more efficiently, there is no need to spend one or two achey days while the body plays "catch up". I have repeated this numerous times with the same predictable results. And if I forget to do the enema after abusing my body, I am quickly reminded of its benefits.

Likewise when we had the snow storm of 1993, I shoveled snow for 3 days. Some of the piles were actually 12 feet high. I never had so much as a solitary minute muscle ache. And yet with my back x-rays showing 2 missing discs (I never had surgery, but

101

ground them up and destroyed them myself) and extensive traumatic arthritis and having had no exercise like this since I had torn my shoulder apart a year prior, I should have been at least as sore as others who had done less physical labor than I had. But in fact, I'm the only person I know who did not hurt that weekend. It was a weird sensation. Here I was for hours throwing snow shovels full of snow over my head and shoulder so that they would miss a row of 9 feet high bushes, with not even the most minor hint of any muscle discomfort. The only thing I can attribute it to was the coffee enemas.

Likewise, if you go somewhere and become **chemically overloaded** and come home with **brain fog and headache**, do a coffee enema. Most of us were surprised that it alleviated the symptoms within minutes. If we had only known about this during the decade of suffering with our severe chemical sensitivities ! Or better yet, during our **macrobiotic discharges.** I'm sure my staff would have given anything for me to have done those instead of smelling like a dead rat for a few months.

Because we have the privilege of seeing some of the most sensitive patients from around the world, there were a few who were intolerant of the coffee. Although we haven't evaluated it as yet, I wonder if an equivalent dose of over-the-counter caffeine in the enema (as opposed to the coffee) would suffice? There is, on the flip side, something to be said for using whole natural products, unprocessed, and unrelated to medications or drugs. And indeed, real coffee contains other things that could also benefit. For example, every 100 grams of coffee contains 0.9 mg of niacin, or vitamin B3, which causes vasodilitation and is crucial in the liver's detoxication chemistry. It also contains 80 mg of potassium, which has multiple cellular benefits.

A HOT DATE WITH JUAN VALDEZ

In **summary**, coffee enemas have been used for over a hundred years, as a generalized detoxification procedure. Despite rumors to the contrary, coffee enemas are perfectly safe when taken as directed. Coffee enemas stimulate the liver and gallbladder to release stored toxins and wastes, and this enhances liver function, by relieving the backlog.

Unless otherwise specified, most people can take the enema each morning for a month to evaluate its effect. Simply prepare a quart of coffee, using 2 flat tablespoons of coffee per quart. The water should be purified with the reverse osmosis filtration unit; if you do not have such a unit, clean spring water will suffice. **Organically grown coffee is best** for this procedure: especially for the severely sick individual.

Most have been using Folgers in the red can, fully caffeinated, drip grind. Boy doesn't this provide a wealth of material for a clever comedian??? I can even think of a number, but they won't let me print them. With our most intimate friends we just explain that we have a hot date with Juan. But it sure brings new meaning to cafe' au lait (ole' !). One thing is for sure, they can no longer accuse us of being full of it.

A few reminders: The coffee should be made in a stainless steel or glass coffee-maker. **Aluminum is not recommended**, since aluminum is a toxic metal and can leach into the coffee while perking. You should add one tablespoon of unsulfered blackstrap molasses to each quart of coffee, while the coffee is hot: the molasses aids in retaining the enemas and also increases the efficiency of detoxification. It is acceptable to make the coffee the night before use; this allows the coffee to cool. The coffee is best used at body temperature. If it cools too much overnight, reheat slightly before using.

103

Again, use a natural lubricant, not the standard petrochemical derivatives, since everything put on the skin can be absorbed into the system. That is how nitroglycerine patches and estrogen patches deliver their medications, by dermal absorption.

Insert the colon tube slowly and gently, maximum 3-6 inches or less into the rectum; if it kinks, pull back and try again as kinking will block the flow of coffee. Release the stopper, and let about a pint of coffee slowly flow in, then reclamp. If the coffee won't flow, this usually means there is a kink in the tube, and you must withdraw the colon tube and reinsert. At first, it may be difficult to retain the enema, but try to hold the coffee about ten minutes, if able. At ten minutes, or sooner if nature demands, remove the tube and expel the enema. Some prefer to remove the tube as soon as the first 1/2 of the enema has been given, since the presence of the tube in some people can stimulate reflexes that make them less able to retain the enemas the full 10 minutes. Others leave the tube in until they are ready to expel the enema.

After expelling the first enema, repeat another 1/2 quart enema, holding for another ten minutes. One session consists of two 1/2 quart enemas, each held 10 minutes.

At first, you may feel slightly jittery, although most patients find the enemas relaxing. Usually, the jitteriness lessens after about the third enema. If the jitteriness continues, this means you are making the coffee too strong. If you never experience the feeling of a squirting out up under the right ribs, and you can hold 1/2 of the quart enema easily for 10 minutes, you may need a slightly stronger solution of coffee or larger volume.

If a person is too incapacitated, as with a bad back, and cannot get on the floor, the enema could be done in bed (with a bedpan and plenty of waterproof pads for easy clean-up). Or it could be done as the person is semi-squating or seated on the toilet. Merely insert the tube while seated and attempt to retain it 10 minutes for two times per session as above. In this natural position of elimination, however, it is usually more difficult to retain it for 10 minutes.

And remember that when it is known that **chlorine in city drinking water** has a positive association with a higher incidence of cancer of the rectum and bladder, for sure **you don't want it in your enema** (Morris RD, Audet AM, Angelillo IF, Chalmers TC, Mosteller F, Chlorination, chlorination by-products, and cancer: A meta-analysis, AMER J PUBL HEALTH, 82,7:955-963,1992)

In summary, remember how we likened the healing programs to **hydroponics?** Coffee enemas are merely a way of revving up the detox system, so that it can keep up with the wastes that must be excreted. For when they back up, they cause symptoms, can damage other areas of the body and even overwhelm the body and cause death. When you are flooding the system with high density nutritional food and vegetable juices, and breaking down old diseased and unwanted tissues, as well as detoxifying the daily overload of 21st century chemicals, it makes sense that we need to speed up the out-flow or clean-up phase. And the proof of the pudding is how you feel and the ultimate healing results.

FOR THE DYING PATIENT WHO CANNOT EAT:

CACHEXIA AND HYDRAZINE SULFATE

There is a special situation that merits mentioning here, and that is the dying patient who is just too plain toxic to eat. They are doing coffee enemas to speed the work of detoxication, but there is just not enough nutrition coming in. They have no appetite and loved ones painfully watch them shrink away day by day.

There is a non-toxic simple substance that has been unselfishly researched by a local physician, **Dr. Joseph Gold**, here in Syracuse for over 20 years. The reason you have never heard of it is that the chemical is so simple, that there is no patent for it: thus no money to be made. It is very cheap. However, it has inhibited the growth of leukemias, lymphomas, melanomas and other cancers.

But more importantly, it has also been studied for years, not only by Dr. Gold, but by Russian researchers and many others as an answer to the **wasting away (cachexia)** of the terminal cancer patient. And just as many have needlessly died because they did not know about coffee enemas to speed up detoxication, many have literally starved to death after they had cleared their cancers.

The dose has been 60 mg tablets three times a day for a month, then a rest for 2-4 weeks, and restart the cycle. Possibly with coffee enemas one might not need an off cycle, or the individual may be able to get off the hydrazine permanently and sooner.

Hydrazine sulfate is available from Ms. Donna Schuster, Great Lakes Metabolics, 1724 Hiawatha Ct, NE, Rochester MN 55904 (phone 507-288-2348).

REFERENCES

1. Sparnins VL, Lam LKT, Wallenberg LW, Effects of coffee on glutathione-S-Transferase (GST) activity & 7,12- dimethylbenz (A) anthracene (DMBA)-induced neoplasia. PROC AACR & ASCO. (AACR abstracts 1981) in CARCINOGENESIS, vol.22, abs #453, pg 114, 1981

2. Lam LKT, Sparnins VL, Wattenberg LW, Isolation & identification of Kahweol palmitate & cafestol palmitate as active constituents of green coffee beans that enhance glutathione-S-transferase activity in the mouse. CANCER RES, 42, 1193-1198, Apr. 1982

3. Myers MG, Basinski A., Coffee & Coronary heart disease. Arch Intern Med, 152: 1767-1772, Sept, 1992

4. Lyght CE, ed., The MERCK MANUAL OF DIAGNOSIS AND THERAPY, 10th Ed, p 1754-1755, Merck Sharp & Dohme Research Laboratories, Rathway, NJ, 1961

5. Lam LK, et al, Effects of derivatives of kahweol and cafestol on the activity of glutathione-S-transferase in mice, J MED CHEM, 30:1399-1403, 1987

6. Jansson B, Dietary, total body and intracellular potassium/sodium ratios. CANCER DETECTION AND PREVENTION 14:563-565, 1990

7. Lentner C, ed., GEIGY SCIENTIFIC TABLES, VOL I, UNITS OF MEASUREMENT, BODY FLUIDS, COMPOSITION OF THE BODY, NUTRITION, Ciba-Geigy Corp, West Caldwell, NJ 07006, 1981, pg 253

8. Awasthi YC, Msira G, Rassin DR, Srivastava SK, Detoxifica-

tion of xenobiotics by glutathione-S-tranferases in erythrocytes: The transport of the conjugate of glutathione and 1-chloro-2,4,-dinitrobenzene. BRIT J HAEMATOL 55:419-425, 1983.

9. Beutrel E, Gelbart T, Pegelow C, Erythrocyte glutathione synthetase deficiency leads not only to glutathione, but also to glutathione-S-transferase deficiency. J CLIN INVEST 77:38-41, 1986.

10. Gold J, Inhibition by hydrazine sulfate and various hydrazides of in vivo growth of Walker 256 intramuscular carcinoma, B-16 melanoma, Murphy-Sturm lymphosarcoma and L-1210 leukemia, ONCOLOGY, 27:69-80, 1973

11. Chlebowski RT, et al, Hydrazine sulfate in cancer patients with weight loss. A placebo-controlled clinical experience, CANCER, 59:406-410, 1987.

12. Tayek JA, et al, Effect of hydrazine sulphate on whole-body protein breakdown measured by 14C-lysine metabolism in lung cancer patients. LANCET, 2:241-244, 1987.

13. Chlebowski RT, et al, Hydrazine sulfate influence on nutritional status and survival in non-small-cell lung cancer, J CLIN ONCOL, 8:9-15, 1990

14. Filov V, et al, Results of clinical evaluation of hydrazine sulfate. VOPR ONKOL, 36:721-726, 1990.

15. Gold J, Hydrazine sulfate: a current perspective, NUTR CANCER, 9:59-66, 1987.

16. Chasseaud LF, The role of glutathione S-transferase in the metabolism of chemical carcinogens and other electrophilic

agents, ADV CANCER RES, 29:174-274, 1979

17. Sparnins VL, Wattenberg LW, Enhancement of glutathione S- transferase activity of the mouse forestomach by inhibitors of benzo(a)pyrene-induced neoplasia of forestomach, J NAT CANCER INST, 66:769-771, 1981

18. Sparnins VL, Effects of dietary constitiuents on glutathione-S-transferase (G-S-T-) activity, PROCEED AMER ASSOC CANCER RES & AMER SOC CLIN ONCOL, 21:80, abs 319

19. van Eys J, Nutrition and cancer: physiological interrelationships, ANN REV NUTR, 5:435-461, 1985

****

Supplies(like oraganic coffee) and nutrients listed available from:

N.E.E.D.S.   1-800 634-1380 or (315) 488-6300
527 Charles Ave.
Syracuse, NY 13209

ARG Patient Services, Nutricology
P.O.Box 489
400 Preda St.
San Leandro CA 94577-0489
1-800-545-9960 for information or 1-800-782-4274 to order

Chapter 4

MAN DOES NOT LIVE BY BREAD ALONE: ENZYMES, JUICING, CLEANSING, FLUSHING AND BRUSHING

Thus far you know that you need a diet appropriate for your current metabolic type, and coffee enemas to speed up the detoxification. But there is more to a total wellness program that can improve the chances of healing even more.

ENZYMES

Enzymes are proteins that facilitate or help other reactions to occur. There are many kinds of enzymes. The ones we are talking about are primarily used for digestion and breaking down material so that it can be more readily available to the body.

Enzymes improve assimilation and help to extract vitamins, minerals, amino acids and essential fatty acids from our food. If for no other reason, enzymes should be useful for the cancer patient to make sure that he extracts as much of the nourishment from his foods as possible, for you will remember from **TIRED OR TOXIC?**, that if you are zinc deficient, for example, then you don't have enough **carbonic anhydrase** and **carboxy peptidase.** If you are chromium deficient you don't have enough **trypsin,** etc. All these enzymes are necessary for digestion of our foods.

But there is another reason for enzyme utilization in severe conditions including cancers. Remember Dr. Kelley, the dentist with pancreatic cancer in the late 60's (whom at this writing is still alive) who found many foods that improved his body's ability to get strong enough to heal the cancer? Like myself, he was blessed with the ability to have a condition from which he could learn, and in turn help others. He could feel his swollen liver with the multiple rocky hard metastases from the pancreatic cancer.

He researched some old literature from a **Dr. John Beard** who reasoned that **the placenta is a lot like a cancer;** it is a tissue that **grows and invades the body.** It should be rejected by the body because it is **genetically incompatible.** For example, most mothers could not have a liver transplant or skin graft from their child, because they are genetically too dissimilar; half the child's genes are from the father and would usually be incompatible with the mother's tissues.

And yet in spite of these known facts, a placenta seems to break all the rules of nature. It not only allows a foreign tissue to grow inside a healthy woman, but the placental tissue, or **trophoblast** as it is called, is highly invasive and grows at a fast rate. Then all of a sudden at around three months of gestation, it magically stops growing and invading. It stops having properties of a cancer.

He was curious what would terminate this growth cycle because he thought that whatever terminated this growth cycle might also terminate a cancer. He found that at the very time the unborn baby or fetus's pancreas started growing and started making pancreatic tissue, that was the time at which the placenta stopped growing. And he found this repeatedly true for many species of animals, none of whom had the same gestation period.

So he did experiments to see if indeed large doses of enzymes would inhibit the growth of cancers or help them break down so they could be gotten rid of. Not only did he initiate work showing this, but others have carried it on, and some have

111

found that the enzymes can even dismantle antigen- antibody complexes, like the ones that can cause serious autoimmune diseases like arthritis and much more. But more about the other applications of this important yet little known phenomenon later.

When Dr. Kelley read of this, he started taking large doses of pancreatic enzymes and low and behold his liver got softer and the hard metastatic cancer nodules started to disappear. But as this happened, the release of all this toxic metabolic cancer waste material made him so sick and toxic that he had to stop. Then when he stopped the enzymes the liver swelled again, the rocky hard metastases appeared on it and he knew he had to take the enzymes again to control his cancer. He went back and forth with this until he discovered the coffee enemas as we have discussed.

There are several things to know about the enzymes. First, there are different types. The Kelley Program recommends **organic glandular pork pancreatic enzymes**. But there are people who can't take these, but could tolerate organic glandular lamb or beef. For others there are plant derived enzymes, but most of these are made from fungal antigens (Aspergillus oryzae). So it is a question of balancing the needs and allergic intolerances of each individual person.

Basically enzymes are taken with meals to help with assimilation of food. Then additional doses are taken between meals when there is no food competing for their use so they can actually penetrate tissues and break down cancers,antigen-antibody complexes, and arteriosclerosis. Now we were all taught in medical school that this is not possible, that enzymes are not absorbed, but they are destroyed in the gut, and they certainly do not go into the tissues.

However, I was surprised to find that there is plenty of evidence to the contrary and you will see the references to show that this is not a correct teaching. It is interesting how often the assumption is made also that orally administered enzymes are destroyed in the gut and never make it to the bloodstream and tissues, but numerous studies show that this is erroneous (Kabacoff BL, et al, Absorption of chymotrypsin from the intestinal tract, NATURE 4895,199:815, Aug 24, 1963).

For people with cancer, it is quite important also to be sure that there is one dose of enzymes in the middle of the night, because the body does the majority of its healing at that time. So it is important to set the alarm between 2 and 4 a.m. so they can be taken on an empty stomach when nothing else is happening or competing for their use. If you can fit in another time when the body is not busy digesting, like right before bed, so much the better.

Understand that people with severe conditions will need to have a coffee enema not only once a day, but morning and evening and sometimes even mid-day and mid-night if they feel toxic or sick enough from the breakdown of their tumors or other metabolic by-products. So if toxicity symptoms awaken you, it is no only a good time to do a coffee enema, but also to take more enzymes.

HOW IT WAS DISCOVERED
THAT ENZYMES DESTROY CANCERS

Because this is such an important point, and because current medical thought will try to denigrate these ideas, I'd like to give you more of the background and reiterate some of the points in more detail. Dr John Beard (1858-1924) was a highly respected comparative embryologist at the University of Edinburgh Medical School for over 30 years. As shown, he theorized that the development of the pancreas in the fetus was what stopped the trophoblast from further growth, the trophoblast being the placental tissue that allows this "foreign" tissue to grow unattacked in the uterus. He thought it resembled a cancer in that it enabled the embryo, containing 50% foreign genetic material, to borrow into the uterine wall.

For remember, the fetus is seen by the mother's body as totally foreign. Furthermore, if this tissue, the trophoblast of pregnancy grows unchecked, and does not stop growing, it becomes one of the most malignant of cancers, choriocarcinoma.

So here is this foreign tissue happily growing in the uterus of the mother, that if we tried to transplant into any other area of her body would most likely be rejected. But for some reason the body tolerates this cancerous-like process as it takes over and expands in the uterus, allowing the fetus to be nourished and grow. Then around 56 days, the trophoblast stops growing. It no longer enlarges and no longer continues to invade the uterine wall.

The baby continues to grow, but the trophoblast does not. Dr. Beard was very astute to wonder what turned this tissue off, this tissue that acts somewhat like a cancer. He decided it was the presence of the pancreatic tissue which matured at that same time as the trophoblast stopped growing, around the 56th day of gestation or pregnancy. Dr. Beard studied many species of animals, and in every case, the day the pancreas appears is the day the trophoblast stops growing.

Some of his original papers and references are in a 1978 book called LAETRILE, NUTRITIONAL CONTROL FOR CANCER WITH VITAMIN B-17, by Glenn Kittler (Nutri-Books Corp, Box 5793, Denver CO 80217, or Royal Publ, 790 W. Tennessee Ave., Denver CO 80223). But Dr. Beard published this in the well-respected medical journal, LANCET in 1902, and his own book (which I would love to find), THE ENZYME TREATMENT OF CANCER AND ITS SCIENTIFIC BASIS (Schatto & Windus, 1911).

This is one more example of how this type of knowledge makes you feel almost clairvoyant when you read articles describing the impossibility of controlling cancer because it is "self-contained and impervious to control" (Nicholson GL, Growth mechanisms and cancer progression, HOSPITAL PRACTICE, 43-53, Feb 15, 1993). I hope these authors and others in medicine will learn about pancreatic enzymes and become familiar with this research done 91 years ago.

Other more modern researchers have found that the addition of enzymes like **brinase** (from the mold, Aspergillus oryzae) and **streptokinase** could significantly increase T cells in cancer patients, thereby improving the immune system strength and even reversing **anergy** or the lowered reactivity that often accompanies cancer (Holcenberg JS, Enzyme therapy of cancer, future studies, CANCER TREAT REP, 4:61-65, 1981, and Holland PD, et al, The enhancing influence of proteolysis on E rosette forming lymphocytes (T cells) in vivo and in vitro, BR J CANCER, 31:64-69, 1974).

And other studies refuted other ideas we were taught to reject, such as the use of other glandulars. For example, radionucleotide studies of oral glandulars (thyroid, thymus, adrenal, ovary, pituitary, etc.) show that these are concentrated in the similar glands. This explains why they work for a while and are no longer needed. They apparently supply specific gland micronutrients that correct a deficiency and restore function,

(Warshaw AW, et al: Protein uptake by the intestine: evidence for absorption of intact macromolecules.

115

GASTRENTEROLOGY, 66:987-992,1974. Martin GJ, et al: Further in vivo observations with radioactice trypsin, AM J PHARM 129:386- 392, 1964. Leibow C, Rothman SS: Enteropancreatic circulation of digestive enzymes, SCIENCE 189:472- 474, 1975.)

It is fascinating when you study scattered works on enzymes in the current scientific literature. As mentioned, hydrolytic **enzymes have been reported to decouple immune complexes** and mobilize them so the body can get rid of them. This has great potential for auto-immune phenomenon, like rheumatoid arthritis, lupus, thyroiditis, etc. (Stauder G, et al, The use of hydrolytic enzymes as adjuvant therapy in AIDS/ARC/LAS patients, BIOMED & PHARMACOTHER, 42:31-34, 1988). And indeed, I have witnessed it speeding the improvement of some **autoimmune food-induced arthridites.**

These facts translate into the fact that there is enormous potential for healing to be derived from the collation of old, safe and inexpensive remedies as we are outlining in this book. And one of the most surprising things to me was that the modern day evidence exists to support them.

WHAT CAN CAUSE ENZYME DEFICIENCIES?

Now that we know that extra pancreatic enzymes can dissolve antigen-antibody complexes and cancers and arrest their invasive nature. But let's look at some of the factors that might decrease our own innate enzyme secretions.

First off, you know that **mineral deficiencies** like zinc as an example will decrease pancreatic secretions. Also overworking the pancreas as in eating a great deal of sugar or eating in between meals can deplete pancreatic secretions. In addition an overgrowth of unwanted intestinal organisms (as we will discuss in the intestinal dysbiosis and leaky gut syndrome section) can adversely impair pancreatic (amylase) secretions.

Many **pesticides and other chemicals** (one of the worst ones is ingested alcohol) can also preferentially damage the pancreas (Marsh, et al, Acute pancreatitis following cutaneous exposure to an organophosphate insecticide, AMERICAN JOURNAL OF GASTROENTEROLOGY, 83:1158-1160, 1988). And others also have shown that the pancreas is particularly susceptible to pesticide poisoning, and we know how ubiquitous that silent killer is (Parries GS, Hokin-Neaverson M, Inhibition of phosphatidylinositol synthases and other membrane-associated enzymes by stereoisomers of hexachlorocyclohexane, J BIOL CHEM, 260:2687-2693,1985).

And you guessed it, reports show that **stress** has an important effect in reducing pancreatic function (Holtmann G, et al, Differential effects of acute mental stress on interdigestive secretion of gastric acid, pancreatic enzymes, and gastroduodenal motility, DIGESTIVE DISEASES AND SCIENCES, 34, 11:1701-1707, Nov 1989).

But by far the commonest cause is probably a **diet** high in **fats and sugars,** since it demands more enzymes.

WHAT TYPE OF ENZYME SHOULD I USE?

Bacillus cereus is supposedly a contaminant of most pancreas sources available (according to personal communication with Dr. Kelley, 1992). The New York State Department of Health lists this organism as the 4th commonest bacterial pathogen for food-borne illness from 1980-1989 (EPIDEMIOLOGY NOTES, 6,6: June 1991, NYS Dept of Health, Albany NY 12237-0608). But the organic sources are reportedly free of this (see Resources). Dr. Kelley was adamant in recommending only

117

organic glandular pancreatin, preferably pork (available from ARG and Klaire Labs: both carried by N.E.E.D.S.)

But there are always exceptional patients who are allergic to so many things. Some may prefer plant enzymes (Tyler's Similase or some of the enzymatic formulations by NESS Company are examples), which seem comparable for conditions other than cancer, and are less expensive (Griffin SM et al, Acid resistant lipase as replacement therapy in chronic exocrine insufficiency: a study in dogs. GUT, 30: 1012-1015, 1989)

If the patient fears having trouble using an enzyme based on fungal antigens, we can often cover that with (temporary) hyposensitization injections to the mold and other fungi that cross react with it.

In rare cases (which I have never seen) where pancreatic enzymes were used in very high doses, it supposedly caused an elevated uric acid (Stapleton FB: Hyperuricosuria due to high dose pancreatic extract therapy in cystic fibrosis, NEJM 295:246-251,1976). So whenever we enter unchartered waters, it is logical to use medical monitors, just as is done with any disease, anyway. **Never forget basic good medicine.**

In **summary**, it looks like **pancreatic enzymes** have the potential to **stop the growth of cancers and facilitate their breakdown.** They can also do the same with **arteriosclerosis and autoimmune complexes,** as in reducing arthritis pain and its duration. It looks as though something very important has been ignored for years. I tell you I would not have been this impressed if I had not witnessed it with my own eyes.

The dose should be worked out for you with your physician in concordance with your total program, since there is such great individual variation. Some people are initially too sick to use

118

enzymes. Others have such a rampant cancer that they can go through a bottle of 60 capsules in one or two days. That produces a lot of toxic wastes. And, of course, they should never be done without the total program of organic foods, vegetable juices, enemas, and nutrient corrections.

OTHER CONDITIONS THAT ENZYMES HELP

O.K., so enzymes eat cancers, you say, but are they of any help in other conditions? As we showed, they can dissolve antigen-antibody complexes, which covers a broad range of symptoms and diseases. But as with all the other techniques in this book, they are used for healing, generally without regard to label or diagnosis. For healing is what cures, not drugs. The bottom line is always what does it take to get this particular system at this time healthy enough so that it can heal itself?

Enzymes have been used in a number of conditions or diseases to improve healing. They have helped some cases of **lactase deficiency** where gas, bloating, pain, diarrhea, and malabsorption have resulted from ingestion of milk. The problem was that these people did not have enough lactase, an enzyme in the gut wall to digest milk sugars, so milk became an irritant to the system and produced symptoms (Solomons NW et al, The relative contribution of exogenous beta- galactosidase to intraluminal lactose digestion in lactase- deficient individuals, AM J CLIN NUTR, 1988).

Enzymes have been used to **dissolve arterial obstructions** as well. So you can see why I think it would be an exciting addition, for example, to the macrobiotic program to reverse coronary artery obstructions (Ornish, Lancet, 1990). In these cases, as in cancers, we have a definite time crunch to work against, so anything that facilitates the desired outcome is welcomed. (Verhaege R et al: Clinical trial of brinase and anticoagulants as a method of treatment for advanced limb ischemia, EUR J CLIN PHARMACOL 16;1650170, 1979).

And later you will read about another hidden source of suffering, **celiac disease** or **gluten enteropathy.** But it turns out that enzymes can help this, too. So you can literally have your cake and eat it too (Phelan JJ, et al, Coeliac disease: the abolition of gliadin toxicity by enzymes from Aspergillus niger. CLIN SCI MOLEC MED 53: 35-43, 1977).

As my last example of some of the innovative ways that enzymes can be used to heal, let's look at probably one of the worst diseases in medicine. A disease worse than cancer or AIDS. Worse, because only one set of physicians deals with it, and they mainly use drugs. These people are the true lepers of the 21st century, because there are not even any environmental units in the world that will take these victims. The disease is **schizophrenia.**

Fortunately there are just as many causes and cures as for other diseases. But because the target organ is the brain, you end up with an adult who needs a 24 hour baby sitter when they are in their worst stages. And to save money and nurse-power, when they are having a flare-up that is bad enough to require hospitalization, they are drugged rather than being chaperoned and worked up for environmental triggers and biochemical defects.

But research shows us that many of these victims have severe wheat sensitivity, celiac antibodies, and increased intestinal permeability. You will read more about these causes as we move on. I cannot recall one who did not have numerous sensitivities as well as many nutrient deficiencies and other biochemical glitches. And every time we discover new findings, it makes me wonder who we might have helped in the past. (I hesitate to digress but must state there is a wonderful network of orthomolecular psychiatrists who actually do look for the biochemical causes in schizophrenia).

The point of this is that **the same pathologies or causes of disease can manifest in countless ways. It is just the individual target organ predilection that appears to be unique** with each person. We need to keep this in mind, to avoid continued disservice to specific groups of patients. (Bjarnson I et al; Intestinal permeability in celiac sprue, dermatitis herpetiformis, schizophrenia and atopic eczema GASTROEN-TEROLOGY 86:1029, 1984. Hekkens WT, et al, Antibodies to wheat proteins in schizophrenia: Relationship or coincidence. In: THE BIOCHEMISTRY OF SCHIZOPHRENIA AND AD-DICTION, Hemmings G (ed), MTP Press, Lancaster PA, 125-133, 1980. Hekkens WT: Antibodies to gliadin in serum of normals, coeliac patients and schizophrenics. NATURE 199:259-261, 1963).

The doses of enzymes will be dealt with in Chapter 8. But the parameters tend to be 3-8 capsules two to five times a day. Be sure to lower the dose with any adverse reaction, such as stomach distress. And if money is a problem, it is more efficacious to use 6-8 capsules at 11 p.m. and 2-3 a.m. In other words, when there is no food competing for them. We do not want to waste them on digesting food if we only have the funds to have them dissolve tumor cells and antigen-antibody complexes. And it goes without saying that any time you are using enzymes for this purpose, you would be doing the coffee enemas to speed up the removable of the accelerated generation of waste materials.

JUICING

Juicing of vegetables and fruits was an important part of the

Gerson Treatment and it is as well an important part of the Kelley Treatment and you can understand why. You are getting live enzymes, oxygen rich fresh food, high in the correct kinds of electrons for energizing the body. It is not dead food and it is in an easily assimilable form. It is almost like getting an I.V. of precious nutrients.

The commonest juice to use is carrot, and don't worry about the carotenemia or the orange coloring of your skin. We all got it, but as your liver gets healthier it tends to fade. I have scoured the biochemistry literature and have not been able to find one article that points to any problem with this orange staining of the skin. In fact it should protect us against skin cancers and U.V.-induced skin pathologies.(Mathews-Roth MM, Gulbrandson CL, Transport of beta-carotene in serum of individuals with carotenemia, CLIN CHEM 20; 12: 1578-1579, 1974).

Other vegetables that are important to add to this drink periodically could include cabbage, beet, garlic (if you don't have leukemia). Dr. Robert Buist of Australia, and editor of INTERNATIONAL CLINICAL NUTRITION REVIEWS, reported 3 cases of prostatic cancer that cleared with beet juicing, among other things on the program.

Juicing is merely a way of (1) flooding the system with concentrated enzymes and nutrients and that is exactly what the person with severe illness needs to do in order to detoxify the body and allow it to heal sufficiently to get rid of stored toxins and materials that inhibit wellness; (2) furthermore, juicing is very alkalinizing, and most detox and healing enzymes function optimally when the body is slightly alkaline. Recall when it is injured or reacting or sick, it becomes more acid.

As stated in chapter 2, juices must be made from organic

vegetables, mixed thoroughly with the saliva for a minute, and drunk within 20 minutes of being made.

IMMACULATE INTESTINES: GUT GROOMING or CLEANSING

Every other month in the beginning of a healing program, it is also important to do a colon cleanse. This part of the program has been difficult for me to conceive, mainly because I have not gone to a pathology lab to look yet at the colons of people, but I plan to do this at some point. I never received information in medical school and cannot find it in the literature about caked-on concretions in the lining of the colon. If you read Jenson's book, TISSUE CLEANSING THROUGH BOWEL MANAGEMENT, you will see photographs of all sorts of material that comes out of the colon. I myself and many patients have done many of these cleanses and had similar results.

Basically you are using a psyllium or other fibrous material to rough up the lining of the intestine in order to try to remove the years of caked on material. As well, the psyllium is very hydroscopic, attracting moisture into the stool, thereby improving bowel function. It is usually taken in conjunction with bentonite or some other clay product which serves to absorb the toxins and help carry them out of the colon. But I would caution that nutrient levels should be assessed if 2 or more colon cleanse weeks are done in a 6 month period, as I have seen very low levels. We can't prove it is because of this, but have moderate suspicion.

These concoctions are best taken between meals, because if you take them with food, vitamins or juices, they will merely clump all these materials together and impair their absorption. So the colon cleansing materials are best taken on a fast when they can really clean out the intestine. But many people do it in between

123

meals when they are eating normally, because they cannot function at work and fast simultaneously. The directions for this cleanse follow.

COLON CLEANSE PROTOCOL

There are several ways to accomplish this protocol for scrubbing out the inside of the gut. For the beginner, purchase 2 items. One is a solution of bentonite or clay which is a great detoxifier, as it absorbs many times its weight in toxins. A good source is Sonne's #7, available at N.E.E.D.S. You will also need Sonne's powdered psyllium husks, which is the fibrous vegetable seed husk that serves as the scrubber or broom with which to loosen and sweep out the old material.

Next get any pint canning jar or food jar. Mix one tbs. (tablespoon) of the liquid bentonite solution #7 in the jar with 4 oz. of water. Then quickly add 1 tbs. of the powdered psyllium husks, cover, and shake vigorously. Quickly drink the mixture and follow it with 8 oz. of water. You must shake and drink it quickly, as it tends to clump and become even more unappetizing. It is not easy to drink, either, as it tastes like drinking thick mud, which is actually what you are doing. However, the results are so beneficial for so many, that it is well worth the aggravation.

Try to drink this three times a day, between meals, for 3 or 4 days. In other words, no food 2 hours before or after. If there is food present, it will merely be dragged out with the clay and not absorbed. When the clay absorbs onto food, it is not available to scrub the wall of the colon, which is the purpose. Likewise, do not bother to take freshly squeezed fruit or vegetable juices with it, as they too will be wasted. You may need to do a plain pint water enema or your coffee enema during these days, and for 2 days after, as it can be constipating.

Alternative directions:

Materials:

Psyllium seed husks, Pre-mixed bentonite liquid, sold under the Sonne's or V.E. Irons label. Or, you can mix your own starting with bentonite powder. Mix the powder in a solution of approximately 2 ounces of powder to 1 quart of water. Prepare the bentonite mixture the night before use, as it must sit for 12 hours before the powder completely dissolves. Bentonite is a clay mixture that efficiently absorbs toxins from the gut.

Procedure:

Add 1 tablespoon of psyllium seed husks to 8 ounces of water. Shake to mix thoroughly in a jar or shaker, then drink immediately (mixture will solidify if allowed to sit).

Follow with an 8 ounce glass of water. Then drink 4 ounces of the bentonite solution.

Repeat this three times a day for five days, for a total of fifteen doses. During the procedure, follow your regular diet; take the doses of psyllium and bentonite between meals, and continue your coffee enemas daily.

When you have finished your fifteen doses of psyllium, eat yogurt two to three times a day for the next five days to replenish your bacterial flora. We recommend only brands with active cultures, usually only available in health food stores.

Psyllium can absorb many times its weight in water, and in the gut enlarges much as a sponge does when exposed to water. The swollen mass of psyllium gradually works its way through the small and large intestine, filling every nook and cranny and forcing out all manner of stored wastes that would not otherwise be excreted.

During the procedure, you may feel discomfort the first day or two due to the expansion of the psyllium in the intestinal tract. This is a good sign, and means the psyllium is stretching the intestines to maximum diameter.

Most patients on this protocol pass a variety of exotic particles and substances. Many describe passing long casings, similar to a snake skin or sausage casing, that may represent dried mucous and dead cells from the surface of the intestines. These wastes can accumulate over a period of many years and seriously interfere with the absorption of nutrients. The colon cleanse is also often the most effective way of removing abnormal bacteria and other organisms from the gut that often take hold after antibiotic use. You could do this every other month for a total of three times a year.

I first became interested in bowel cleansing years ago when a very chemically sensitive young mother excitedly wrote to tell me how it had helped her chemical sensitivities. It makes sense that if the bowel wall contains caked-on concretions, and periodically just needs a good scrub, that the results should be better absorption of nutrients, and faster transit time in which to get rid of conjugated chemicals. Plus, if the intestinal wall is healthier, the cytochrome P-450 detox pathways that reside in the gut wall should function more optimally. This latter reason is why it helps chemical sensitivity symptoms.

FLUSHING

The **liver and gallbladder flush** is another entity which has been used to clean out the liver and the bile ducts and gallbladder. This one I find the most difficult to do and you will see why. But it is probably a good idea to do it once or twice a year at least, and if you are sicker, every other month for a while.

The rationale for this procedure is the blood stream is made very acidic for a few days with a phosphorous compound and apple juice so you can loosen a lot of the calcifications. Because phosphorous is anti-calcium, you must be sure to rinse your teeth carefully after having drunk the **phosphorous acid/ apple juice mixture for it can dissolve the calcium enamel from your teeth.**

You must also be sure to have enough calcium afterwards as described, so you do not risk depleting some of your own bone calcium stores. For as good as this regimen is for flushing out the detox organs, remember everything has its flip side of undesirable effects. **Calcium is one of the main buffers in the system to fight the acid that is generated from chemical exposures,** disease, allergic reactions, bad thoughts, infection, eating the wrong foods, and much more. **When our cells become too acid,** they then become weak, lose important minerals, and start to malfunction. **This is the beginning of chronic degenerative disease.** So we need excellent calcium stores.

Our problem is usually that we have taken too much of it in over the years without balancing it with the minerals that are necessary in order to put it in the proper storage organ, the bone. So instead we have made gallstones, kidney stones, and calcified our brain and coronary arteries. And calcifications and gallstones too small to be seen on x-ray can impair the function of this major detox organ.

The massive amounts of colon cleansing that accompanies this program serves to stimulate reflexes that facilitate the release of stored detox material and sludge from the liver bile ducts and gall bladder; some people are able to see this or identify this in the stool. And the reasons for the high amount of fat and oil is to make the ducts and gallbladder contract to release this material. There are many anecdotal stories of all sorts of things that people have released and how they have felt improved. I have not heard of one person who had a problem with this causing obstruction by gall stones, but I believe this could be a possibility.

In **summary**, the purpose of this protocol is to flush out the liver bile ducts and the gall bladder. It, like the colon cleanse should only be done every other month, **maximum three times a year.** It has improved the efficiency of the liver's detoxication ability for many and also relieved the gall bladder of accumulated sludge which could have gone on to form gall stones. It is involved, but again is worth the effort.

Above all, remember you are making the system very acidic for a few days in order to loosen calcified deposits from the liver ducts. The phosphorus drink is very acid, so it is important to rinse your mouth with a little baking soda solution after to avoid dissolving the enamel from your teeth.

The high intake of fat is to encourage the discharge of bile. The concentrated bowel flush is designed to cause the liver to dump out its bile accumulations which hold the conjugated chemicals and other products of metabolic waste. Also the forceful emptying of the gall bladder allows the discharge of sludge from here that otherwise could go on to form stones and gall bladder disease, and at minimum, compromise the efficiency of the gall bladder detoxification function.

Materials:

1 gallon of apple juice, organic
2 ounces of ortho-phosphoric acid (Phosfood from Standard Process or Orthophos from Nutri-Dyn)
Cal Amo (Standard Process) or calcium citrate 500 mg
Bentonite liquid

Procedure:

1. Add one-half bottle (one ounce) of ortho-phosphoric acid to the gallon of apple juice, and shake. Over the next three to five days, drink the full bottle of juice (this usually breaks down to about 3-4 full glasses a day, best taken between meals). Be sure to rinse your mouth out with baking soda or brush your teeth after drinking the juice to prevent the acid from damaging the teeth. While drinking the apple juice, eat normally. Take your coffee enemas as you normally would.

2. On the last day of the procedure (the day you finish the apple juice) take two capsules of Cal Amo immediately before breakfast and two capsules of Cal Amo immediately before lunch.

3. Two hours after lunch, take 1-2 tablespoons of Epsom salts dissolved in a small amount of warm water. Add juice to cover the taste, if desired. Warning: it is brutal.

4. Five hours after lunch, take 1 tablespoon of Epsom salts dissolved in warm water. Add juice if desired.

5. Six or seven hours after lunch, eat a dinner of heavy whipping cream and fruit, as much as desired. Any fruit is acceptable; most patients generally prefer a mixture of berries, either frozen or fresh. The mixture of fruit can be blenderized

to make a shake. With dinner, take one Cal Amo.

6. One half hour before bedtime, drink 1/4 cup of bentonite liquid.

7. At bedtime, drink 1/2 cup olive oil. A small amount of orange, grapefruit or lemon juice may be added if desired. Immediately after finishing the oil, go to bed and lie on the right side with knees drawn up for 30 minutes. You may feel nauseated during the night, due to the release of stored toxins from the gallbladder and liver. This is normal, and will pass. To us it is a good sign because it means the procedure is working.

8. On the next day, eat normally. Take two (2) Cal Amo with breakfast, two (2) Cal Amo with lunch and on Cal Amo with dinner.

The liver flush, in a simpler version, was first used during the 1920's as a means of improving liver function. The procedure is a refinement of the original technique, and serves several important functions. First, the ortho- phosphoric acid helps remove calcium and lipids (fats) from arteries, and normalizes cholesterol metabolism. The phosphoric acid, working with malic acid found in apple juice, also dissolves and softens gallstones in the gallbladder. The magnesium in the Epsom salts relaxes the sphincter of the gallbladder and bile ducts, allowing for easy passage of the softened, shrunken stones.

Finally, the cream and the oil cause a strong contraction of the gallbladder and liver, forcing out stored wastes, bile, and stones which easily pass into the small intestine. These wastes and stones are then excreted. The liver flush is a simple way of removing smaller gallstones without surgery, while at the same time lowering cholesterol levels and improving liver function.

An alternative procedure: Gallbladder flush, half ounce each of freshly squeezed lime juice and extra virgin olive oil, daily times one week and then one ounce daily times one week then one and a half ounces, daily until a tarry stool is passed, which represents gallbladder sludge, at which time the cleanse is over with. At whatever point it occurs, then it is done.

THE PURGE

The purge is one of the most important detoxification routines for cancer patients. Several versions of the technique exist, but the best is still that described in the original edition of Dr. Kelley's book ONE ANSWER TO CANCER. The purge puts the body at rest and aids the rapid removal of metabolic wastes from the body. In addition, the purge pushes the body into an alkaline state, in which repair and rebuilding of damaged tissues occurs rapidly. However, it is far too alkaline for many, and not recommended for those allergic to citrus or with eczema.

First, make a punch consisting of the following:

> Juice of 6 grapefruits
> Juice of 6 lemons
> Juice of 12 oranges

Put the juice from the above fruit into a gallon jug and add purified water until the jug is full.

Upon arising, drink one tablespoon of Epsom Salts dissolved in half a glass of purified water. One half hour later, take another tablespoon in half a glass of water. In another half hour, take a third dose of one tablespoon of Epsom Salts in half

131

a glass of water. You will now have taken three doses, over a one hour period.

Approximately two hours after the last dose of Epsom Salts, take a glass of the citrus punch. Thereafter, take a glass every hour. You are to eat no food that day except, if you wish, an orange for dinner.

You should take one capsule of Cal Amo three times during the day, spread out through the day.

During the purge, you may feel a variety of symptoms such as nausea, headaches, muscle aches and pains. Such symptoms indicate the body is mobilizing stored wastes, and should not cause alarm.

On day two of the purge, repeat the above.

BRUSHING

Another important parameter in helping the body clean up, detox and discharge it's unwanted accumulated waste is skin brushing. There is more about that in our 3 macrobiotic books. Use a warm wash cloth with water or a loufa sponge, preferably twice a day to wash the skin all over. Remember the skin is a discharge organ as well.

The stretching that is necessary so that you can reach all of your skin is also helpful in opening up lymphatics; much like yoga. Furthermore, exercises and even posturing, such as yoga and loving massages, network chiropractic and other bodywork modalities are good to help stimulate the lymphatics to facilitate removal of stored toxins in fat deposits. The body uses five main systems to excrete waste materials; the liver, the intestinal tract, the kidneys, the lungs and the skin. Too often, we forget that the skin can be used to help detoxify the body, and speed the removal of metabolic waste. On intensive healing programs, often cancer breakdown products and other metabolic debris tend to accumulate rapidly, and often patients develop all manner of skin eruptions in the form of oily excretions, discolored excretions, foul smells, and blemishes which can imitate acne, blisters, hives, eczema, boils, and much more. Such conditions may be worrisome, but should be viewed as a good sign. Read the 2 macro books for more explanation (YOU ARE WHAT YOU ATE, and THE CURE IS IN THE KITCHEN).

Dr. Kelley developed the following procedure 25 years ago, to stimulate waste release through the skin. It is a very valuable technique, and any toxic patient would be well advised to follow through with it regularly:

Once a week, rub your skin from head to foot with a mixture of equal parts of olive and castor oils (the castor oil is available at any pharmacy). Then, with the oil still intact on the skin, take a hot bath for fifteen minutes. The bath allows the oil to penetrate to the deepest levels of the skin. After the bath, go to bed under heavy cotton covers for one hour to sweat out the poisons. Be careful getting in and out of the bathtub as the oil will make you slippery. Finally, take a hot shower.

The oil soaks should be done weekly for the first three months of the program; at that time, they can be discontinued.

ADDITIONAL DETOXIFICATION ROUTINES

1. **Salt and Soda Baths**. During periods of intense toxicity, a warm bath with added baking soda and salt can greatly help to mobilize toxins out of the body through the skin. In a fairly warm bath, add one cup of baking soda (sodium bicarbonate)

and one cup of sea salt. Lie in the bath for 20-30 minutes. The bath should be repeated daily until symptoms diminish.

2. Mustard Foot Soaks. This particular remedy is very helpful for toxic headaches, generalized "goopy" toxic symptoms, muscle aches and pains, and water retention in the ankles or other parts of the body. In a basin of very warm water, add one tablespoon of mustard and a teaspoon of cayenne pepper. Sit in a comfortable chair and soak your feet in the basin for 20-30 minutes. The mustard soaks can be repeated 2-3 times each day, and should be continued during periods of intense toxicity. They may sound silly, until you realize that acupuncture meridians concentrate in extremities like the earlobe, hands, and feet. By stimulating the circulation to the feet, you therefore may open up blockages in this area that have a bearing on, for example, the same meridian that goes to the brain. That is how headaches can be relieved by foot soaks, massages, etc., that seem unrelated to the head.

3. Castor Oil Compresses. This is an old Edgar Cayce remedy, that does help draw out toxins from the body. The compresses are particularly useful when applied to the areas of pain, where tumors might be breaking down. Buy castor oil from your pharmacy and warm the oil in a pan. Soak a washcloth, towel, or other cloth in the oil and apply to tumors, areas of pain, and areas of inflamation. Keep the compress in place for 20-30 minutes. The castor oil poultices can be applied as often as you need relief, as they are not harmful. Do be careful not to overheat the oil or you might burn yourself when applying the compress.

CANDIDA AND THE LEAKY GUT SYNDROME

So why all this fuss to scrub out the gut? For many reasons, foremost of all being that the health of the gut determines the health of the rest of the body and its ability to heal expediently. First the gut is responsible for the **absorption of nutrients**. Plus it is responsible for the speed of the **detoxification system.** And it is necessary for clearing away wastes.

But let us not overlook other important roles, as it is a place where a large amount of **IgA** is secreted. This is an immuno-globulin or antibody that plays a strong **defense role.** Further-more, the gut has bacteria that **manufacture important vita-mins** like vitamin K and some B vitamins.

But when we eat a diet that produces too much of specific metabolic toxins, these can get absorbed into the system and create fatigue and other symptoms. Or if there is Candida overgrowth, as from years of sweets or antibiotics, prednisone, etc. (see THE E.I. SYNDROME), there can be a secretion of toxins from this mold or fungus that cause a variety of "undiagnosable" symptoms. Or Candida can elaborate an enzyme called thiaminase, which breaks down and destroys thiamine (vitamin B1) before it even gets absorbed. Thiamine is crucial in the body's ability to make energy.

Some people mistakenly think they have Candida-related complex of symptoms because their symptoms are brought on by or made worse by ingestion of sugars. But some of these have no Candida problems; in fact when we culture the stool on special media to foster the growth of Candida, there is none. Instead these individuals have sucrase deficiency or **abnormal gut fermentation of sugars** and we must deal with that prob-lem in a different way (Eaton KK. Sugars in food intolerance and gut fermentation, J NUTRIT MED, 3:295-301, 1992).

There are a host of other abnormal bugs (other yeasts, fungi, bacteria, protozoa, and more) that can also grow in the intes-tines. When there is an overgrowth of undesirable disease-producing organisms, we call this **dysbiosis**. Many reports in the scientific literature, for example, show that many people with a variety of types of arthritis and colon problems have abnormal bugs in the intestine. And they have an abnormal amount of antibodies to these bugs in their systems.

Sometimes when a person makes antibodies to some of these intestinal organisms, there are antigen receptor sites on the bug that resemble certain antigen receptor sites on our tissues. Hence once the demand for more antibodies arises because of overload in the gut of these bugs, sometimes the antibodies floating in out bloodstream make a mistake and start attacking our own tissues that resemble these bugs instead.

Hence you suddenly have antibodies that attack your thyroid for example. So one day the thyroid is normal and all the blood tests are fine. But the next day you are exhausted for no reason, or another day you are a mad woman who is so wired she can't stand herself, much less be able to understand how anyone else can tolerate her. **Thyroid antibodies** can do this.

If you saw a microscopic peek at a piece of the intestinal lining, you would see millions of microscopic finger-like projections along its surface. There are so many of these, that if you flattened them out, the square surface area of the gut would turn out to be something like the area of a tennis court. These microscopic finger-like projections, called **villi**, are where absorption of our precious nutrients occurs.

But imagine in your mind's eye years of waste material trucking down the gut, choking out these villi. After a while, there is such a **caked on build-up of debris,** that there is merely a channel down through the center of the intestinal tract or lumen through which the food rides. It rarely ever gets to have intimate contact with the villi of the gut wall anymore. And so

absorption is impaired.

This is one of the major reasons people feel so well or exhilarated after a colon cleanse, because not only do they no longer have the absorption of toxins from these caked on accumulations, but there is improved extraction of nutrients from food. Plus there is improved efficiency of detoxification, since a vast majority of the detox enzymes reside in the gut wall. Also the cleanse often gets rid of unwanted organisms and provides a fresh start. So now you see why cleansing the intestines can make a world's difference, and why it is just one more important part of the total package or total load of concerns in order to maximize health.

Nowhere is the concept of total load more important than in the cancer patient. But in truth, every single disease must embrace this concept. It seems to be thus far ignored by medicine, but once you step back and look at the broad scope of things, it makes you suddenly feel as though you are clairvoyant, because you get a different perspective of disease.

For example, many of you are already aware that **Candida** is a yeast that grows in intestines when people have had too many antibiotics, a high sugar diet, birth control pills, steroids, diabetes, etc. And you have learned that the overgrowth of Candida, or any other types of organisms that can grow in the bowel just as well, is called **dysbiosis** (living things growing where they do not belong). You learned that they can produce toxins that mimic diseases that are impossible to diagnose if the physician is not specifically looking for this problem.

But more importantly, these unwanted bugs can inflame the intestinal lining and cause what we call the **"Leaky Gut Syndrome"**. In other words, in response to the gut lining being inflamed or hyper-reactive to these bugs, the spaces between cells open up abnormally and allow the passage of materials that normally are not permitted into the blood stream from the gut. Hence the term , leaky gut syndrome.

When the gut is leaky or **hyperpermeable,** it allows things to pass through it into the bloodstream that normally would be restricted from entering. Cells that are assigned to protect the bloodstream see these "foreign" substances that normally were too big to get into the bloodstream when the cells were tighter. If they see a large particle of food, they attack. They make antibodies to it because it looks foreign to them, since their job is to attack foreign things (fight bacteria) to keep the body healthy.

However, when they attack food antigens and make antibodies to the food, this **creates food allergies.** These defense antibodies, once they have glommed onto an over-sized foreign food particle, can then attach to any target organ and cause literally any disease. Arthritis is a common result when these antigen-antibody complexes form and attach to the synovium of the joint. Once attached to the joint tissue, the antigen-antibody complexes cause the release of mediators that trigger inflamation, swelling, and pain.

But it does not occur right when you eat the food. Sometimes it **will not occur until days after you have eaten the food,** because it takes several days to make enough of the antigen-antibody complex to produce appreciable pain or swelling. And once it is attached, it may not leave the joints for months.

This is the source of much erroneous thinking about the food allergy and arthritis connection. For this type of antibody persists much longer than the regular hayfever antibody, which can disappear within hours or days, depending on dose. These antigen-antibody complexes that are firmly attached to

138

body tissues may last for **months**, rather than days.

Let's look at some of the other sneaky, yet common things that food antigens can do. Food antigens directed toward the urinary bladder will give **chronic cystitis** that no amount of antibiotics will clear up, but everytime the person eats the wrong food the bladder goes into painful spasms. Or the target organ can be the **vagina** and everytime the wrong foods are eaten the vagina discharges just like a runny nose would and it itches and burns just like the skin can in response to allergy. The problem is that medicine is not geared towards looking at other target organs. The **prostate** is a common target organ as well, for many food allergies as are rheumatoid joints and just about any part of the anatomy you can think of.

Of course, **the brain is one of the most common targets of food allergies** and symptoms can manifest in any way you can think of. They can manifest as depression, fatigue, schizophrenia, alcoholism, Alzheimer's, violent mood swings, learning disabilities, **ADD** (attention deficient disorder), **Tourette's**, brain fog and much more.

As we have referenced in other books, it is ironic that all the **non-steroidal anti-inflamatory drugs** (called **NSAIDs** in medicine) that are the premiere prescriptions for arthritis, actually **cause the leaky gut syndrome.** This has been well- referenced for years (LANCET, etc.) So the actual drugs that are the most commonly prescribed for arthritis are the ones that promote the pathology that causes the disease for many in the first place. So they are **guaranteed to never recover** and to **need progressively more medication** as their disease worsens, The old scenario repeats itself. For when drugs are used to mask symptoms, THE SICK GET SICKER, QUICKER.

As you can see, the hyperpermeable gut has far-reaching

ramifications in the pathophysiology of much disease. It deserves attention in resistant cases of arthritis, food allergy with its vast array of symptoms from fatigue to irritable bowel and even one of the worst forms of bowel disease, Crohn's disease (Hyatt F, Vogelsang H, Waldoer T, Lochs H, Intestinal permeability and the prediction of relapse in Crohn's disease. LANCET 341:1437-1439, 1993). Every symptom should make the physician consider ruling it out (Goldberg PA, Musculoskeletal complaints and intestinal permeability, NUTRITIONAL PERSPECTIVES 16:17-19, 1993).

And where disease of the gut is being considered, we should always consider if sufficient pancreatic and other digestive gland secretions are not also part of the bigger picture (Makc DR, Flick JA, Durie PR, Rosenstein BJ, Ellis LE, Perman JA, Correlation of intestinal lactulose permeability with exocrine pancreatic dysfunction, J PEDIATRICS, 120:696-700, 1992).

And as many of you Candida sufferers know, the "good bugs" in the intestine are just as important as the bad ones. There are hundreds of papers supporting the value of Lactobacillus acidophilus and other related **probiotic** organsims in good bowel ecology. These organisms promote better digestion, healthier bowel tissues, better intestinal manufacture of nutrients, less tendency toward cancer, longer life, and more. And we can assay for them now to determine if the numbers are adequate. (Mitsuoka T, Intestinal flora and aging, NUTR REV, 50:12, 438-4446, 1992).

And getting good levels can be difficult. Many people get excellent levels with Klaire Labs Vital Plex, for example, while others need to have the beneficial bacteria protected from gastric acid destruction by a capsule. In these cases we have had excellent results with Natren's Pro-BioNate-C.

The Leaky Gut has many more ramifications. For example, most minerals do not just "leak" or diffuse across the gut into the bloodstream. They must be carried across on specific carrier proteins. But these are damaged by an inflamed leaky gut. So it is a double-edged sword. You get leaking of toxins, bacteria, and large food antigens that make you sick, and you have impaired transport of the minerals you need in order to heal.

To make things more difficult, I only know of a couple of labs in the whole world that can diagnose the leaky gut syndrome. The brushing of skin and special baths merely help unload the work of the gut by shifting some of the overload clean-up to the skin. But the real clean-out of liver, gall bladder and intestines is, as you can now see, another simple, inexpensive way to improve the ability of the body to heal.

Resources

Gurchot C, The trophoblast theory of cancer (John Beard, 1857-1924) revisited, ONCOLOGY 31:310-333, 1975

Krebs ET, et al, The unitarian of trophoblastic thesis of cancer, MEDICAL RECORD, 149-174, July 1950

Rooney PJ, Jenkins RT, Buchanan WW, A short review of the relationship between intestinal permeability and inflammatory joint disease. CLIN EXP RHEUMATOL, 8:75-83, 1990

Smith MD, Gibson RA, Brooks PM, Abnormal bowel permeability in ankylosing spondylitis and rheumatoid arthritis, J RHEUMATOL 12:299-305, 1985

Navarro MD. The Unitarian or trophoblastic thesis of cancer,

PHIL J CANCER, 3:3-11, 1959

Taussig SJ, Yokoyama MM, et al, Bromelain, a proteolytic enzyme and its chemical application. A review, HIROSHIMA J MED SCI, 24: 185-193, 1975

Jackson PG, Lessof MH, Baker RWR, Ferrett J, MacDonald DM, Intestinal permeability in patients with eczema and food allergy, LANCET, 1285-1286, June 13, 1981

FitzGerald DE, Frisch EP, Milliken JC, Relief of chronic arterial obstruction using intravenous brinase, SCAND J THOR CARDIOVASC SURG 13:327-332, 1979

Weinberger S, HEALING WITHIN,Colon Health Center, P.O.Box 1013, Larkspur CA 94939, 1989 Meyerowitz, Steve,

JUICING, FASTING, AND DETOXIFICATION, The Sprout House, PO Box 1100, Great Barrington MA 01230.

Howell, Edward, ENZYME NUTRITION. Avery Publ, Wayne NJ 1985.

Howell, Edward, FOOD ENZYMES FOR HEALTH AND LONGEVITY,Omangod Press, P.O. Box 64, Woodstock Valley CN 06282, 1980.

Jensen, Bernard, TISSUE CLEANSING THROUGH BOWEL MANAGEMENT, Bernard Jensen Publ, Rt1 Box 52, Escondido CA 92025, 1981.

Santillo, Humbart, FOOD ENZYMES, THE MISSING LINK

TO RADIANT HEALTH, Hohm press Box 2501, Prescott AZ 86302.

For the cal amo: or call N.E.E.D.S. 1-800-634-1380
Standard Process   for substitute of calcium citrate,
1-800-225-4220   250 mg

For plant enzymes if you are intolerant of animal based ones:
(also available at NEEDS, 1-800 634-1380
Tyler Encapsulations
2204-8 NW Birdsdale
Gresham OR 97030
1-800-869-9705

Sources for organic glandular pancreatin

(1) N.E.E.D.S.
    527 Charles Ave.
    Syracuse NY 13209
    1-800 634-1380 or (315) 488-6300

(2) Klaire Laboratories
    1573 Seminole St.
    San Marcos CA 92069
    1-800-533-7255

[3] Nutricology, dba Allergy Research Group
    400 Preda St.
    San Leandro, CA 94577
    1-800-643-334

Also, for an excellent enzyme, Bromase, used for arthritis, thrombophlebitis, have your physician, health store or pharmacist call

Bio Tech
Box 1992
Fayetteville, AR 72703
1-800-345-1199

For tests on stool for intestinal dysbiosis and leaky gut syndrome:
Great Smokies Laboratory
18A Regent Park Blvd
Ashville NC 28806
1-800 522-4762

For encapsulated excellent quality intestinal flora,

Natrens Inc,
3105 Willow Lane
Westlake Village CA 91361
1 800 992-3323

Chapter 5

ATONING FOR THE BIOCHEMICAL SINS
OF THE 21st CENTURY

Fixing What's Broken

We the first generation to eat are these **processed foods,** which have **25%-75% of the nutrients removed.** We are also the first generation to have to detoxify hundreds of chemicals in our air, food, and water each day. This uses up nutrients at a faster rate than ever. So we have 2 major unprecedented conditions that make us the most nutrient-depleted generation ever. And nutrient deficiencies set the stage for all diseases, especially cancers.

There are numerous, well-documented studies of people who have cleared cancers without vitamin, mineral, amino acid and essential fatty acid supplements. However, there are those who have accomplished the same with nutrients. For my money, I would rather go in, assess the problem, see what's broken (see what vitamins, minerals, amino acids and essential fatty acids are missing in the system), fix what's broken and get out and get on with getting well as quickly as possible.

It makes a great deal more sense to me to try to make the person as healthy as possible, as fast as possible. For we must bear in mind, the longer the body is left deficient in specific nutrients, the more damage that can occur in other areas, from backup of undetoxified metabolites. And, sorry to say, in some individuals there seems to be a point of no return. These people have been damaged by a specific chemical, and have gone downhill ever since. And no one knows what to do for them. In others who are luckier, we can correct the deficiency, but it often takes many months to do so because they are so severely deficient.

145

For remember, the body can only take in so many minerals, for example, in a day.

Furthermore, **the statistics show that the vast majority of even"healthy, normal" people have one or more nutrient deficiencies, so it is nigh impossible to have cancer or serious disease and not have any deficiencies.** I can't imagine it happening and have certainly never seen it. As the first generation to eat all these processed foods, compounded by being the first generation to use up or waste nutrients detoxifying all these 21st century chemicals, **deficiencies are the rule,** not the exception.

The macrobiotic programs that have performed "miracles" with people disagrees with this and I am comfortable with people doing whatever they feel is best for their systems. However, I am a strong advocate of checking nutrient levels to find out what is missing and correcting them as quickly as possible. Perhaps having a medical license and the biochemical training to check nutrients has a bearing on this decision.

For example, without sufficient copper and zinc in the enzyme family of super oxide dismutases, gene mutations can occur that lead to **"Lou Gehrig's Disease"** or **amyotrophic lateral sclerosis.** It is a nasty disease that begins anytime in adult life and progresses to a profound degeneration in the spinal column and brain, and is usually fatal in five years.

But when we order rbc copper and zinc in our patients around the world, patients know from the reactions of the laboratory personnel that it is the first time they have ever drawn these tests. Yet this chemistry is so commonly abnormal in this era and responsible for the initiation of a vast number of end-stage disease states (Anonymous, Mutations in the copper- and zinc-containing superoxide dismutase gene are associated with

146

"Lou 'Gehrig's Disease, MUTR REV, 51:8, 243- 245, Aug 1993).

As you will learn, there is tremendous evidence in the regular mainstream scientific literature showing that nutrient deficiencies are more common than nutrient repleteness and an understanding of the biochemistry of disease, reveals that many nutrient deficiencies are responsible for most of the disease states that are instead commonly masked with medications.

DISPELLING ANOTHER MYTH: NUTRIENT DEFICIENCIES ARE RARE IN THE U.S.

As we saw in TIRED OR TOXIC? learning environmental medicine breaks many of the rules and models or paradigms upon which drug-oriented medicine is based. In fact it ushers in an exciting era of molecular medicine, where we can now usually find the causes of symptoms and get rid of them rather than merely druging them with endless years of expensive medications.

For one of the major problems for chemically sensitive individuals is that the xenobiotic (foreign chemical) detoxication system is not operating normally. And one of the reasons is that some of the nutrients (vitamins, minerals, amino acids and essential fatty acids) in the major detoxication pathways are deficient (too low). At first we had a tough time appreciating how this could happen in the land of plenty where foods are even fortified.

But when you look more closely, it's a testament to the integrity of the human biochemistry that we have done as well as we have in face of the prevalence of undetected deficiencies. For as you will see, unsuspected vitamin and mineral deficiencies

147

are rampant in the U.S. And these deficiencies not only explain why some have chemical sensitivity, but are also the cause of many other diseases.

HOW DO WE GET NUTRIENT DEFICIENT?

There are a number of ways, all of which are so subtle that nutrient deficiency is rarely sought as a cause of symptoms. For starters, the processing of foods to improve taste and extend shelf life is a major cause. When you process **brown rice to form white rice** by grinding, bleaching, and other processes, **you lose roughly 80% of many trace minerals**, like magnesium, manganese, copper, zinc, and more.

And an equivalent loss occurs when you go from whole wheat berries down to bleached white wheat flour, one of the mainstays of the **standard American diet (SAD)** in the form of white bread. So this last 50 years of processed foods is a vast experiment in what the human chemistry can adapt to. It is a huge experiment to see if by throwing out 80% of the nutrition of one of the major components of the diet, the health of mankind will suffer or not.

Nutrients can be lost a number of other ways, as various cooking techniques reduce nutrient content, like microwaving. Likewise, nutrients are lost with storage (time) and heat, but also with other techniques of preservation, such as irradiation of foods.

Nutrients are also lost from the soil with repeated growing of crops as well as harvesting before natural ripening has occurred, plus the forced ripening with chemicals like ethylene of produce picked green, before it has matured (one of the reasons a tomato in the winter can taste like cardboard, and difficult to believe that it is in any way related to that succulent vegetable

148

you grow in your garden). There are other factors that also reduce the nutrient value of foods, such as EDTA used to preserve the green color of frozen broccoli lowers the vitamin B6 in the vegetable.

But one more cause of nutrient loss is rarely mentioned or looked for in medicine: the loss from **overwork of the detoxica-tion pathways.** For every time you walk into a grocery store and detoxify even one molecule of pesticide, you use up or throw away forever, one molecule of glutathione or whatever other nutrient was silently used by your body to detoxify this chemical. This loss occurs even if you can't smell the chemical. Since we are the first generation of man ever exposed to such an unprecedented number of chemicals, detoxification is going on in most of us rather constantly. So most people are using up nutrients faster by being in a constant state of accelerated detoxification. Since the average person is exposed to and must detoxify in excess of 500 xenobiotics (foreign chemicals) in a day, it comes as no surprise that a vast majority of people are nutrient deficient, and the scientific literature bears this out with astounding repetitiveness.

In essence, most people are losing or using up specific nutrients in the daily work of detoxifying our 21st century chemical environment. The problem is that the loss of these nutrients then makes them sitting ducks for other medical problems, but medicine is still not training doctors to look for these curable causes of symptoms.

This becomes extremely important if you study the scientific research to learn that some incurable cancers, for example, have been literally cured by just giving vitamins. Take vitamin A, which is known not only to retard the development of malignancies (cancers) but to reverse some. But it is used up or depleted in the work of chemical detoxication.

Yes, you read that right. Scientists have discovered that **vitamin A and its related compounds can actually reverse or make go away some types of cancers,** like some forms of otherwise incurable leukemia. And being exposed to daily chemicals can use up this precious vitamin A. But rather than do good environmental controls to reduce chemical exposure and use inexpensive vitamins, many of the people with these types of leukemias are treated with expensive chemotherapy and bone marrow transplants, because they are in an experimental program or protocol that does not happen to be testing vitamin A.

Nutrient deficiencies are also common side effects of various drugs, yet medicine rarely looks at the nutrient levels that have been driven down by the drug. For example, magnesium deficiency is a common side effect of diuretic (fluid pills, blood pressure pills) therapy, yet an intracellular assay is rarely done, much less the more accurate magnesium loading test. And ironically, an initial undetected magnesium deficiency can be the very reason for the symptom for which the diuretic was prescribed in the first place (i.e., as in cases of magnesium deficiency-induced hypertension).

COPPER DEFICIENCY AS AN EXAMPLE

A literature search on just about any nutrient reveals a wealth of information substantiating widespread and unrecognized deficiencies. For example, let's look at **copper,** a mineral whose adequacy is not routinely checked for. When we think of copper, we often think of toxic or high levels from copper tubing and water pipes. But actually the **majority of Americans are deficient in copper.** A National Institutes of Health study showed that 81% of people have less than two-thirds of the RDA (recommended daily allowance) of copper.

Another study revealed that hospital meals provide only 0.76 mg of copper per day, whereas people need 2-4 mg for health, and even more for healing and chemical exposures. Another study by the F.D.A. showed that when they analyzed 234 foods which are the core of the American diet, they provided less than 80% of the RDA of copper. And yet another study of 270 United States Navy SEAL trainees (highly selected "healthy" young men) 37% had low plasma copper levels. And plasma copper is a very insensitive indicator of copper status.

Since they used an inferior test to assess copper adequacy, that means they missed some that were low. And when you realize that young "cream of the crop" healthy men are deficient, and that low copper can cause arteriosclerosis and high cholesterol, it comes as no surprise that they were baffled upon finding arteriosclerosis in young soldiers on autopsy.

What this means is that **nutrient deficiencies contribute to chronic degenerative diseases of old age, but they begin in teen-agers!** In other words, copper deficiency is an example of one of many very common mineral deficiencies that are rarely checked for, yet they begin in teen-agers; and when allowed to go undetected, can cause the very diseases we are treated for as adults, like high blood pressure and cholesterol. But instead of correcting the causes, medications are used to cover up the symptoms. Is it any wonder that **arteriosclerosis** continues to be the **number one cause of illness and death** in the U.S.?

Another study showed that 80% of Americans get 1 mg or less of copper per day, which is 1/4th of what they need. And yet another study which analyzed twenty different types of U.S. diets, showed only 25% of the people got 2 mg of copper a day (1/2 of what they need) and the majority of the diets provided only 0.78 mg of copper per day. So all copper studies seem to point to the fact that the majority of people are deficient. When we randomly studied 228 of our patients, 165 or 72% were deficient in copper.

So, no matter whose studies you look at over the last 20, years there is a wealth of data showing that copper deficiency is rampant in the United States. And among the symptoms that can stem from copper deficiency in its over 21 enzymes is hypercholesterolemia (**high cholesterol**) and arteriosclerosis (hardening of the arteries, which causes early heart attacks, high blood pressure, strokes, and Alzhiemer's), the number one causes of death and disease in the western world. Many copper enzymes are responsible for keeping us from chronic fatigue, depression, premature aging and much more. And furthermore, many of the enzymes of copper are needed to detoxify chemicals. And bear in mind copper is an example of but one of 40 essential nutrients.

And as you know, a number of minerals are commonly deficient that are crucial to the brain for on-going function, as well as protection against aging. For example we find copper low in 72% of our patients and a deficiency can impair myelin metabolism which is one of the defects of multiple sclerosis (Sandstead HH, A brief history or the influence of trace elements on brain function, AM J CLIN NUTR, 43:293-298,1986). And copper as well as manganese are two minerals that have been reported as better in vegans than those on the standard American fare, which may just be one more reason out of scores of reasons why many people with MS have improved on a macrobiotic diet.

One more common cause of copper deficiency is **iatrogenic,** meaning "caused by the treatment". Often the story goes like this:
A young woman will complain of fatigue. A cbc (complete blood count) will show a low hematocrit (percentage of red blood cells). So the doctor assumes that the blood is low

because she has an iron deficiency. So he gives iron, never checking iron or the other frequent cause of microcytic anemia (small cells and low red blood cell count) which is copper deficiency. If her anemia is in part due to a deficit of copper, not only will it fail to correct, but the more iron you give, the worse you make the copper deficiency, and the anemia. Unfortunately, the more resistant to correction she gets, the more iron he gives. So he drives the copper even lower!

And if the patient has an uncorrected anemia and continues to complain of fatigue, often more iron is pushed. Yet copper is necessary in the enzyme **cytochrome oxidase** for energy production. And it is necessary in converting thyroid hormone T4 to T3. I'll spare you the details of what the other copper enzymes do, but recall as one more example its use in super oxide dismutase for the chemically sensitive individual and those with inflammatory conditions like arthritis.

And giving too much iron can do a lot more besides worsen the hypocupremia. It can contribute to heart disease, Alzheimer's and deficiencies of other minerals, like manganese (Richardson JS, Subbarao KV, Ang LC, On the possible role of iron-induced free radical peroxidation in neural degeneration in Alzheimer's disease, ANN NY ACAD SCI, 648:326-327, 1992; Do diets high in iron impair manganese status?, NUTR REV 51:3, 86-88, 1993; Are we at risk for heart disease because of normal iron status?, NUTR REV, 51:4, 112-115, 1993).

But copper is not always easy to correct when it is deficient. Fortunately there are several forms to chose from since one is not perfect for eveyone. And often it is best absorbed when taken alone, that is at a meal but with no other minerals. In this way, there is minimal competition for the **mineral transporters,** which are specialized proteins that carry copper across the gut wall and into the blood stream.

So in essence, copper is a good example of a trace mineral that is slowly disappearing from the American diet. And because it is in 21 enzymes, many of which have to do with cholesterol metabolism, it has a role in why the number one cause of death and illness is on the rise and why so many people are foolishly on expensive drugs that do nothing to correct the underlying causal deficiencies.

THE NUTRIENT CONNECTION

When we look at **zinc**, literature reports indicate that unsuspected zinc deficiency is also relatively common. In one study only 13% of randomly selected patients had normal zinc levels, and 68% of the population ingested less than 2/3 the RDA for zinc. Zinc deficiency has been shown to be prevalent throughout the world, in all age ranges, in pregnancy, chronic disease, after surgery, and in chemical sensitivity.

Magnesium deficiency is even more prevalent when you consider that government surveys show the average American diet provides only 40% or less than half of the recommended daily allowance (RDA) for magnesium. Others confirm its widespread deficiency in over 54% of 1033 patients. And again, its deficiency in the chemically sensitive contributes to the total load of chemical sensitivity in the patient. And of course, this deficiency is also important in a variety of other diseases from arteriosclerosis, arrhythmia, and sudden death to osteoporosis, chronic low back pain and chronic fatigue.

Unfortunately, in U.S. medicine, there is currently a myth circulating, where it is not at all uncommon to hear a physician tell a patient that if he just eats a balanced diet, he need not concern himself about nutrient deficiencies. When in fact, nothing could be further from the truth.

And it is dangerously far from the truth as the **JOURNAL OF THE AMERICAN MEDICAL ASSOCIATION** article, June 13, 1990, shows us. Among 1033 patients who were hospitalized for a variety of ailments, some of which they died from, over 54 % of them were magnesium deficient. The most alarming part was that 90% of the physicians never ordered a magnesium assay. And of those who did, the worst and least sensitive assay was done. In other words, they used a test so old fashioned (serum magnesium, the same test that every doctor gets when he orders the chemical profile) that it looks normal even when a person is so low in magnesium that it can be the cause of life-threatening angina, arrythmia and even death.

Therefore, according to this study, it is **"reasonable and customary"** (a term insurance companies like to use to justify refusing to cover some items) for 90% of the physician population to fail to make the correct diagnosis for lack of assessing nutrient levels; and the result is that patients die of cardiac arrhythmias or sudden cardiac death because of these undetected deficiencies.

Obviously cases of solo deficiencies are rare, and multiple deficiencies are the rule. In other words, if a peson is deficient in one item, they are more likely to be deficient in some others as well. And the literature is full of reports of, for example, **hypercholesterolemia** from copper deficiency, or chromium deficiency, or magnesium deficiency, vitamin C deficiency, etc. The exciting part is that once the individual's own unique biochemical defects have been identified and corrected, you may have a patient who needs no medication. It is so logical: if you suddenly cannot properly metabolize cholesterol, in spite of dietary modifications, you had better find our what is missing in the biochemistry of your cholesterol metabolism

155

pathways.

It is known now that some **blood pressure pills actually increase blood lipids (cholesterol and triglycerides)**, and as well there is an **increase in suicide and accidental deaths with the cholesterol-lowering drugs.** We explained why in previous works. And, of course, all medications accelerate the loss of nutrients, because each medication is merely another chemical that uses up or lowers nutrients in the process of the body trying to detoxify it.

This in no way detracts from the fact that our armamentarium of drugs is fantastic in the benefits it creates. But they do deny us the opportunity of identifying the cause of many symptoms. As progressively more identifiable causes emerge for symptoms that we currently label as incurable, knowledge of the nutrient connection in medicine will grow. But not, regrettably, without many errors being made.

As one example, as of 1993, many clinical blood test laboratories are unfortunately adding a serum magnesium to their routine general chemistry panels. But studies reveal that many docs do not know that the serum magnesium makes up only 1% of the total body magnesium. So a person can be dangerously low and the test will be perfectly normal.

There is a physiology in the body called **homeostasis**. It is the body's attempt to make serum levels look good no matter how low the nutrient may be. For example, a person can be so low in calcium as to have severe osteoporosis, but the serum calcium will look normal. The reason the serum is protected (by homeostasis) is because it bathes all cells. If they are not bathed in enough calcium, you are probably in the emergency room with a seizure or heart attack. Better to "rob Peter to pay Paul" and keep the majority of the body's cells bathed in the proper mineral, and let just one organ system suffer.

So **do not have a serum magnesium test**. And if one is included in the chemical profile battery of tests, just ignore it. For this test will serve to give a false sense of security to those who do not yet know that the most accurate way to assess magnesium status is with a challenge test (described in **TIRED OR TOXIC?**).

Meanwhile, assessing and correcting nutrient deficiencies has been a major tool in overcoming chemical sensitivity. So when you hear someone saying, "There is no such thing as a nutrient deficiency in the United States if you just eat a balanced diet", I trust you can set them straight now. For without this knowledge, they have narry a hope of helping those heal who have severe chemical sensitivity and the seemingly endless array of symptoms that it can masquerade as. As for you, make sure that you at least have your daily anti-oxidants and multiple minerals (more on that later).

Clearly, **immune deficiency or dysfunction** can result from any single nutrient deficiency or excess, which is why it is so important to have levels assessed and balanced (Beisel WR, Edelman R, Nauss K, Suskind RM, Single nutrient effects on immunologic functions; Report of a workshop sponsored by the Department of Food and Nutrition and its Nutrition Advisory Group of the American Medical Association. JOURNAL OF THE AMERICAN MEDICAL ASSOCIATION 245:1, 53-58, January 2, 1981).

It will soon come as no surprise to any of you to know that for example, in the scientific literature there are studies demonstrating that if you look at some awful disease such as Alzheimer's, you find that if you compare these people with normal people, they have half the levels of protective vitamins A and E, for example; and yet this is not assessed (Zaman Z,

Roche S, Fielden P, Frost PG, Niriella DC, Cayley ACD, Plasma concentrations of vitamins A and E and carotenoides in Alzheimer's disease, AGE AND AGING 21:91-94, 1992).

Amino acid and essential fatty acid analyses can be done, but often are unnecessary once the minerals are corrected. Usually the most important nutrients are the minerals since these take the longest (along with essential fatty acids) to incorporate into body tissues. When vitamins are prescribed they can work immediately, but for minerals, the old enzymes must first be broken down, new enzymes must be synthesized and the minerals incorporated into them.

As you know from our previous writings, magnesium is the most important all around mineral. It is in over 300 enzymes and even government publications show the average American diet provides less than half of what everyone needs in an average day. As you now know, the serum magnesium test which is part of a chemical profile (which is a test that most doctors do when you have a physical or any complaint) is worthless.

Since less than 1% of the body's total magnesium is in the serum, if that test is abnormal, you are in deep trouble because you can even be severely deficient and the test will look normal. Likewise, the rbc magnesium, which is a step better, is still an inferior test. The best test is the magnesium loading test. The directions are described in the back of **TIRED OR TOXIC?**, and the complete paper we published with results and references for doctors is in the back of **THE CURE IS IN THE KITCHEN.** An I.V.(intravenous) test is even better, for some.

The next most important, and commonly deficient minerals are copper, zinc and manganese which among other things, are in enzymes called **superoxide dismutase** which have to do with neutralizing or gobbling up free radicals so that they do not go

158

on to destroy body tissues. In other words, the family of **S.O.D.** enzymes is one of the most important enzymes in the body, because it is endlessly working to negate the constant chemistry that is silently working non-stop to bring on aging, chemical sensitivity, and in fact all diseases, including cancer, etc.

The best assay for minerals that run these crucial enzymes are blood tests for these specific minerals done on **red blood cells** only, not serum or whole blood. In other words, when you see your report and it does not **specifically say rbc** zinc, rbc manganese, or rbc copper, if it merely says zinc, manganese and copper then you know that the wrong test was done. You should **make sure to see your test results** for this reason alone because, oftentimes even when the correct test was ordered, an incorrect test is done, but no one notices.

It is a fine point that has huge consequences. This is because the rbc test for minerals is rarely done, even though it is the most sensitive and the only one worth the money. Even when it is ordered, much of the time the less sensitive or inferior one is done. **So insist on seeing the result yourself.**

A third of the time when we mail prescriptions to our out of state patients to have their minerals checked, the labs do the inferior serum assay instead, even though it is clearly typed to do the rbc assay. These, done in serum or plasma are often normal even in the face of a serious deficiency. So have no hesitancy about seeing your laboratory results. It's your only safety mechanism. After all, who can you trust more than yourself to do a meticulous job in being sure the best was done?

We won't even begin to detail all of the **over 40 nutrients** in this treatis, except to say that having levels accessed and an appropriate prescription for you is the best route. There are glandulars, digestives and other **accessory nutrients** besides the 4 main categories of vitamins, amino acids, minerals, and essential fatty acids. Much of this is in **TIRED OR TOXIC?** and will tell you what tests to have your doctor draw.

Another important factor however, is that the body can only assimilate for so long. Whenever you are on a program to take supplements don't be afraid to listen to your innate body wisdom. When you get to one of those days when you feel like "Ugh, I can't take another vitamin!" you know it is time to give the body a rest. It can only take in so much before it has to then assimilate it and put it to work.

So, whether your body needs 2 weeks on and one week off the supplements, or to take them every other day, or to spread out what has been written for one day over 2 days, so be it. We must listen to our own individual biochemistry. At some point when you are off the supplements, at least once a month for the 3 to 7 days, you may want to take advantage of that interval to do either your bowel cleanse or gallbladder/liver flush. Because we don't want to make this book so big you'll need a wheel barrel to carry it to the beach, we are not putting in a great deal of information about supplements. This is mainly because they are so individualized. But allow me to just give you a sampling of the magnitude of this problem.

IF YOU FAIL TO IDENTIFY
AND CORRECT NUTRIENT DEFICIENCIES
THE SICK GET SICKER, QUICKER

When you think about it, the person with cancer or serious disease has to be even more compromised in his nutrient status in order to have gotten sick in the first place. Plus, when one is sick, nutrients are used up and depleted even faster, so it is a downward spiral where the sick get sicker quicker.

You have already learned that **vitamin A** has been found to reverse, turn off, turn around one of the most serious forms of leukemia for which there is no current medical treatment, including radiation, chemotherapy, bone marrow transplant or surgery and they think they know how it happens: it makes the genetic material correct itself and go back to normal. But could it be that the person is just making healthy cells now that merely out-number the bad ones?

Nevertheless, you will see later the voluminous references on how vitamin A does this; therefore it is important to begin with adequate levels. The trouble is that with prolonged, high doses, vitamin A can cause toxicity. As with everything, there is a **bell-shaped curve,** which changes with the person's condition. There is an optimal dose, on either side of which both an increase as well as a decrease in dose can lead to adverse effects that can culminate in death. So you must be very careful with it.

This toxicity is not a matter of just not feeling well. You see, in the brain there are some fluid filled cavities called **ventricles.** There are tiny canals through which this fluid flows into the spinal column and equilibrates, or equalizes pressure in the brain versus in the spinal column. If these tiny canals are plugged for any reason, the fluid builds up in the ventricles, they enlarge and they squash the brain against the immovable skull. This condition is called **hydrocephalus** and can lead not only to severe brain damage, but death.

One of the things that vitamin A does is cause endothelial proliferation, or excessive skin cell growth. Obviously, these delicate, tiny canals from the ventricles to the spinal column are lined with endothelial or skin type cells. If these hypertrophy, or grow too fast because of excessive vitamin A, they can plug off and hydrocephalus can result. Therefore, I would make sure that you are very carefully supervised when doing vitamin A levels in excess of 25,000 I.U. for longer than a month. And of course, remember there is so much biochemical individuality among people that there may be someone who has hypertrophy with lesser doses.

Beta-carotene is a precursor to vitamin A. In other words, it turns into vitamin A in the body and so, is a safer form because there is a limiting mechanism so that the body will not over convert more than it needs. However, this mechanism in some forms of cancer must be over-ridden with actual vitamin A. Besides knowing your actual vitamin A level, I would want to know as many nutrient levels as possible in order to fully balance your deficiencies with what is known to be needed because of a combination of your previous diet, life style, chemical exposures, genetic tendencies and the types of conditions from which you are now suffering.

We frequently find **vitamin B1 or thiamine** low, and of course it is crucial in the pathway for energy manufacture. **B2 or riboflavin** is crucial in the detoxification pathway as is **B3 or niacin.** It is also very important in lowering cholesterol. The flush that the niacin produces should also be useful in opening up or vasodilating areas and allowing more nutrient accessibility. **B5 (pantothenic acid)** is not easily measured but is easily supplemented. **B6, or pyridoxine,** is important in the metabolism of amino acids and in preventing and treating arteriosclerosis, carpel tunnel syndrome, post partum depression, nausea of pregnancy, and much more.

B12(cobalamin) of course, is important in pernicious anemia where the body fails to make intrinsic factor in the stomach. Therefore it cannot be absorbed and has to be given by injection, intravenlly, or sublingually. But more important and less known is that B12 has been found low in many psychiatric diseases, multiple sclerosis and other conditions where nerve function is not optimal. This by no means, represents a detailed analysis which can be found in scores of excellent nutritional books.

Vitamin C or ascorbic acid, as you will recall, is the first and the most important anti-oxidant that chemicals and noxious materials in the blood stream run into. Therefore, it is extremely important to always have exceptionally good levels of this since it is the **first guard** on the horizon. It runs many functions, one of which is also very crucial and that is in **putting the priceless minerals back in a useable form.** Everytime we use magnesium, copper, zinc, etc. in a reaction to help the body, they **loose an electron** and turn into a **oxidized form** which is no longer able to be used by the body. It is **vitamin C** that **restores it to the reduced form** so it is able to be utilized again. Dr. Linus Pauling, the only person to win two Nobel Prizes, is a biochemist (who is still working past age 90) who has done a tremendous amount of work to show that vitamin C is crucial in every avenue, from cancers to arteriosclerosis, high cholesterol and even the common cold. I have never heard his work criticized except by people who do not have a fraction of the biochemical expertise that he has. A tremendous amount has been written on how I.V.'s of vitamin C can improve recalcitrant conditions from hepatitis and AIDS to resistant infections.

Many people have too high a level of **vitamin D** from years of fortified milk products. It is a vitamin which will accentuate the calcifications of arteriosclerosis in the vessel walls. But we have encountered many people who also have had inferior levels and so like any other nutrient when in doubt, it is best to check it out. It is becoming increasingly clearer that it plays a role in preventing cancers, especially colon. It is great to get 20 minutes a day of **sun** on as much of your skin as possible to help

163

metabolize your own natural vitamin D.

Vitamin E of course, is the second most important vitamin in terms of it's anti-oxidant capabilities, because it **sits in the membrane of cells protecting** them from the penetration of chemicals that attempt to get in and destroy the function of the genetics enclosed in the nucleus. There are many forms of vitamin E, but the best for the body is **D-alpha tocopherol** accompanied by mixed tocopherols. I don't want to get into brand names in this book, but there are only certain brands that fulfill the requirements that we mention.

As with vitamin C, there were many pioneers in the field of vitamin E and its importance in the heart. The Shute brothers of Canada were way ahead of their time as well, since it is only in this decade that we have heard verification of the advantages of vitamin E in heart disease from major researchers. The two Dr.s Shute wrote books and papers decades ago about the protective effects of vitamin E on the heart. But researchers in the past denied these properties. And, as we have witnessed a multitude of times, when it is finally announced by these sources, it is as though they themselves discovered it. And they probably actually think they did, since it would be unheard of for them to stoop to read referenced health magazine articles of 2 and 3 decades ago.

(Stampfer MJ, et al, Vitamin E consumption and the risk of coronary disease in women, **NEW ENGLAND JOURNAL OF MEDICINE**, 328:1444, 1993. Rimm EB, et al, Vitamin E consumption and the risk of coronary heart disease in men, ibid: 1450. Steinberg D, Antioxidant vitamins and coronary heart disease, ibid: 1487.)

Vitamin F (there is no such thing) can be thought of as standing for **fatty acids** which you know from **TIRED OR TOXIC?** are essential and which make up the **membranes** of every cell and govern their functions. Most of us have years of the wrong fatty acids in our cell membranes including trans fatty acids from years of margarines, fast foods, processed foods, breads with hydrogenated vegetable oil, French fries, other fried foods and much much more.

These damage cell membranes and must be replaced with cold-pressed cis-form Omega 6 and Omega 3 oils. Flax oil, which is an Omega 3, seems to be one of the most healing (hence an important part of some programs, as Dr. J Budwig's).

Vitamin G (there is no such official entity) I like to use to remind me of the many beneficial effects of **glandulars,** (which include enzymes), that you just read about in the enzymes.

As you see, even though we have only mentioned a tad about the vitamins, and will go into depth with only particular minerals, all nutrients work in concert. And because no two people have the same deficiencies, and you do not even have the same deficiencies now as you had last year or will have next year, we cannot make blanket recommendations.

Add to that the fact that we could not physically take all the nutrients in a day that we would like. There are just too many. Besides we would probably get toxic overload effects from the capsular material and magnesium stearate(for ease of flow in the encapsulation machine). Thus, one more reason why your nutrient program must be individualized.

Once you get your individualized nutrient program, to save time, put your vitamins for the week in dixie cups taped together or ice cube trays. And you can buy tiny baggies that hold a day's worth for the office. For travel, I put one day's worth in a large baggie, use a twist tie, add the next day's, twist

165

tie, etc. It looks like a sausage of individual day's worth of vitamins.

As you know, with many of us there is only one door through our brain. It is not the logic door, it is not the common sense door; it's only the science door that is open. That is why we wrote **TIRED OR TOXIC?** for physicians and other people who must have the proof and references for all the statements in this book. In contrast, this book is for people who just must get well (although as you have seen, I just can't resist putting in some references, as there are so many).

This book attempts to fill in the blanks and help you continue growing from where we left off with the previous 5 books and the current ongoing newsletter, the **HEALTH LETTER**. In fact, as many of you have guessed, one of the reasons we started the newsletter was because this information about healing has been surfacing so fast that we find we cannot write books fast enough. And we must have a medium where we can get this information out to the people who so desperately need it.

As an example, the macrobiotic diet which has the best overall documented record for clearing the most impossible cancers is still scoffed by much of the medical profession. As of this writing it would be illegal for you or I to treat our own child with the macrobiotic diet, if he had a cancer. This applies even if you as the parent had had the same type of cancer and had cleared it with the macrobiotic diet. The laws would force us to use chemo, irradiation, surgery and/or bone marrow transplants, (and could cost over $200,000).

This is in spite of the fact that Carter's studies show that, for example, when people do everything medicine has to offer for cancer of the pancreas, the one year survival is 9%. If they do any amount of macro for 3 months or longer, the survival is over 52%. Likewise the median survival for prostate cancer goes from 72 months with all medicine has to offer to over 228 months from doing 3 months or more of macro (6 vs 19 yrs).

We would not have a legal right to chose for our child, but as you have seen the recommendations of the National Cancer Institute, the National Institutes of Health, the American Heart Association, the American Medical Association, and many other institutes are gradually moving toward the macrobiotic diet. Recall, Ornish's publication in the 1990 LANCET showed reversal of PET scans after one year on the diet. And this was in people who were at the end of their ropes, still clotting of ateries in spite of bypass surgery and cholesterol-lowering drugs. When medicine advances, it will embrace it with a passion and claim all credit for establishing it as it has with many other therapies in the past. The problem is you and I cannot wait for that to happen, for that may not happen in our lifetimes and we need all this information now.

Carter JP, Saxe GP, Newbold V, Peres CE, Campeau RJ, Bernal-Green L, Hypothesis: Dietary management may improve survival from nutritionally linked cancers based on analysis of representative cases. J AMER COLL NUTR 12:3, 209-226 (1993).

CHROMIUM DEFICIENCY CAUSES
THE CRAVING CYCLE AND HYPOYCEMIA

Chromium is not just for the chrome on bumpers; it also has to do with making very healthy surfaces on the inside of our blood vessels. Just as chromium plating protects bumpers from rust or oxidation and aging, it protects the lining of blood vessels against oxidation and premature aging or arteriosclerosis. It is one of over 40 nutrients that is essential for function of the body. We find a vast majority of our patients low in rbc (red blood cell or intracellular) chromium.

167

Chromium is essential for example, in **sugar metabolism** so people with diabetes, hypoglycemia (headache, mood swings, sweats, weakness, and fatigue, especially related to meals) should always be checked for a chromium deficiency. It is especially important in diabetes and insulin resistance. I have never seen a diabetic who has a normal chromium, nor have I ever met a diabetologist who checks the chromium, even though it has been in the scientific literature for over 2 decades (Mertz W, Chromium in human nutrition: A review, J NUTR, 123: 626-633, 1992).

Likewise, chromium is important in the metabolism of cholesterol and so people with **high cholesterol** or **triglycerides** should be checked for chromium repleteness. However, this is not routinely done in medicine as of this writing (Press RI, Geller J, Evans GW, The effect of chromium picolinate on serum cholesterol and apolipoprotein fractions in human subjects, **WESTERN JOURNAL OF MEDICINE** 152:41-45, January 1990).

Furthermore, **chromium deficiency** will make some people have horrible **cravings for sweets**, but the more sweets you eat the more you lower your chromium. The more you lower your chromium, the more you crave sweets. Chromium deficiency is one of the causes of sweet cravings. And the more you crave sweets, the more you eat sweets, and the more chromium you lose. Then other chromium problems develop like high cholesterol. It's a vicious cycle of getting fatter, more fatigued, and more disease and problems until someone steps in and breaks this vicious cycle.

THE VICIOUS CHROMIUM CYCLE:

eating sweets   ——> lowers chromium
low chromium   ——> triggers sweet cravings
sweet cravings   ——> cause one to eat more sugar
eating sugar   ——> triggers the loss of further chromium
low chromium   ——> triggers more sweet cravings,
      hypoglycemia, high cholesterol, mood swings,
        depression, poor digestion, obesity, etc.

But unfortunately, chromium deficiency is only one example of how a hidden or unsuspected common nutrient deficiency can have devastating snow-balling effects on the whole body and mind. Many other common mineral deficiencies, like manganese also can cause defective carbohydrate metabolism, complete with cravings and hypoglycemia.

Baly DL, et al, Effects of manganese deficiency on pyruvate carboxylase and phosphoenolpyruvate carboxykinase activity and carbohydrate homeostasis in adult rats, BIOLOG TR ELEMENT RES, 11:201-212, 1986

Mertz W, Chromium in human nutrition: A review, J NUTR 123:626-633, 1993

THE MAGNESIUM CYCLE OF DISEASE

When the United States Government knows that the average daily American diet provides less than half of the required magnesium we need for a day, and we know that magnesium deficiency is one of the causes of some folks' high blood pressure, and we know that hypertension is one of the major causes of sickness and death, it becomes important for you to know how to protect yourself.

It turns out that magnesium is crucial in the activity of the **sodium pump** so that when you are put on a **salt-free diet**, it's really because the pump in the cell membrane that is responsible for putting sodium on the right side of the cell is not working adequately because it lacks magnesium (It may well lack other things as well, like EFA's). But look at all the people suffering with a tasteless low sodium diet (salt is sodium chloride), only because no one checked their magnesium to see why the sodium pump was not working.

Also, magnesium is important for lipid metabolism. In other words, for the breakdown and proper metabolism of cholesterol and triglycerides. But look at the people who are denied the foods they like in attempt to bring their cholesterol and triglycerides down, when no one has done the magnesium loading test to find that it is the underlying magnesium deficiency that is causing their high cholesterol or triglycerides. Other mineral and nutrient deficiencies may be the cause, we're just using magnesium as an example, because it is one of the most common deficiencies(and causes of symptoms).

THE MAGNESIUM CYCLE OF DISEASE:

[1]

eating the American diet	——> causes mag deficiency
drinking alcohol	——> "
eating sweets, white sugar	——> "
eating bleached white flour	——> "
eating bleached white rice	——> "
medications like diuretics	——> "

170

[2]

magnesium deficiency——>causes cardiac arrhythmia, chronic back spasms, bladder spasms, asthma, migraine, irritable bowel, PMS, depression, fatigue, insomnia, sudden death, hypertension, etc.

[3]

hypertension is treated with a diuretic, which ——> causes mag deficiency which worsens, causing any of above symptoms

[4]

as more symptoms appear ——> more medications are used

[5]

the metabolism of medications uses up magnesium ——> worsens magnesium deficiency

[6]

meanwhile mag deficit is not diagnosed and ——> continues to worsen, creating more symptoms, until a person has a heart attack and dies; and no one ever knows why.

So bare minimum, regardless of what your disease or symptoms are, and in fact even if you are well, please do the magnesium loading test (in Tired or Toxic?) and an RBC chromium and an RBC manganese.

References:
Dyckner T, Wester PO, Effect of Magnesium on Blood pressure, **British Medical Journal** 286, 1847-1849 June 11, 1983.

Zawada ET, Ter Weeja, Mc Clung DE, Magnesium Prevents Acute Hypercalcemic Hypertension. **Nephron** 47:109-114, 1987.

Motoyama T, Sano H, Fukuzaki H, Oral Magnesium Supplementation in Patients With Essential Hypertension. **Hypertension** 13:227-232, 1989.

Motoyama T, Sano H, Suzuki H, Kowaguchi K, Saito K, Furuta Y, Fukuzaki H, Oral Magnesium Treatment And The Erythrocyte Sodium Pump In Patients With Essential Hypertension. **Hypertension** 4(Suppl 6): S682-S684, 1986.

Ahmad A, Bloom S, Sodium pump and calcium channel modulation of mg-deficiency cardiomyopathy, AMER J CARDIOVASC PATHOL 2:4, 277 (1989).

"WHY LEUKEMICS NEED
HIGH CALCIUM PRESCRIPTIONS

As much as I would like to lay out a specific nutrient program for people to follow, I must give caution and a few examples to demonstrate how much knowledge is really required about the individual's condition. But more important is an assessment of the **uniquely individual biochemistry of each person.** Their heredity, their disease, their previous diet, etc. are all important in making the **nutrient prescription** for each individual.

For example, as much as I have shown that magnesium is important, if someone has a bleeding disorder like leukemia, for example, magnesium should be restricted because **magnesium inhibits the clotting of blood.** But, for someone with arteriosclerosis you want a higher than normal level of magnesium. This is because with arteriosclerosis, (narrowing of the blood vessels from accumulations or deposits of cholesterol), the slowed blood flow through narrowed vessels can not only cause hypertension, but can clot.

For when blood trudges through narrowed vessels, there is slowing of the flow and sometimes stagnation. And stagnated blood clots. Therefore, you want the blood not to coagulate very easily, because a clot can then lodge in a vessel and choke off the blood supply to something further downstream, causing a stroke or a heart attack, for example.

But, in the person with leukemia, he doesn't clot well because he has a deficiency of platelets and often other blood factors. So, you want his nutrient schedule to downplay magnesium and in fact, magnesium can be quite lethal for him. As well, vitamin B6 is very important for the coagulation of blood so you want the B vitamins to be down played in a condition such as leukemia, but up regulated for arteriosclerosis.

173

So, you can see from this one small example how important it is for the clinician to be aware of all this voluminous research and this one tiny example that I'm giving is among thousands. I just gave this one because the references happen to be handy on my desk at the time of this writing. But suffice it to say, that a book that purports to give a general prescription of nutrients, must take many different conditions into account. In addition, the prescription for each individual must take many other factors about the individual into account above and beyond the condition or diagnosis.

(Nadler J, Hwang D, Yen C, Rude R, Magnesium plays a key role in inhibiting platelet aggregation and release reaction. ARTERIOSCLEROSIS AND THROMBOSIS 11:5,1546a September/October 1991).

Parvez Z, Speck U, Effect of vitamin B6 derivatives on blood coagulation and platelet function. J DRUG DEV, 4(2):65-69, 1991.

Remember how in the coffee break chapter we discussed how vitamin A and it's derivatives can modify oncogene expression? The translation of this means **vitamin A can actually turn off leukemia** by putting the genes or the DNA material back into normal position or configuration; this is extremely important. Remember how I said also that there was a bizarre syndrome that they couldn't figure out because they didn't know the toxic metabolic products from the breakdown of the cancer had to be gotten rid of and to speed this up they could have used coffee enemas? Instead, some people died from the accumulation of toxic metabolites.

You have just learned how important it is to have low magnesium levels in leukemia, because high magnesium inhibits the coagulation and leukemics have a problem with that. Well, let me take you even further along to remind you that **calcium is magnesium's antagonist.** So, if you want to make sure the magnesium is low, you give a great deal of extra calcium. Well, there is an even more important reason for high calcium to be given to leukemics and that is because high **vitamin A causes the calcium to be drawn out of the bone and wasted.**

It turns out that **vitamin A,** even though it is necessary to **promote cell differentiation to reverse leukemia,** in high doses stimulates the secretion of parathyroid hormone which secondarily sucks out more calcium from the bone. In order to replace this calcium, leukemics need a high level of prescribed calcium, as well as a physician, (as do all cancer patients), with a very good knowledge of all this biochemistry.

I would suggest that whomever you choose for your therapy, you make sure they are well-versed with the information in this book and you might even give them a verbal test that will satisfy you that indeed, they are familiar with it in a very specific manner. For it may make the difference between your life and death.

Another problem of high **vitamin A is that it causes the release of** a great deal of **histamine** and of course histamine is very **immunosuppressive.** In other words, it stifles the immune system and in fact, it has been shown that it can weaken the immune system and set the stage for other allergies, other diseases and cancers. Those of you who are knowledgeable in the total load will recognize this also as one more reason why disregarding one's allergies when they have a serious illness will serve only to put one more nail in their coffin.

Luckily, **a high dose of vitamin C is a good antihistamine.** And you know now that the enzyme **histaminase, necessary to break down histamine, must have a molecule of copper in it** to function. So, you can begin to understand how extremely knowledgeable the person must be who is prescribing your nutrient corrections as you are healing.

In future books and in regularly appearing articles in our on going newsletter, the **HEALTH LETTER,** we hope to keep people abreast of all these newer findings so that hopefully we can put more and more of this knowledge and control in the lap of whomever needs it.

Another important aspect for the person with high blood calcium such as a leukemic or a person with metastatic cancer is to have enough of Omega-3 oil (flax being the best), since it turns out that it inhibits the synthesis of cyclooxygenase and has an anti-inflammatory effect. It tends to decrease the bone resorption mediated by prostaglandin E2. (Hence another reason why many leukemics are carnivores).

And **do not be fooled by a high serum calcium, as seen in many cancers.** It can mean many things, for example, (1) the cell membrane is damaged, so the calcium pump is defective, (2) calcium is being pulled from the bone to buffer the extreme acidity of rapidly growing cancer cells, (3) the cancer may be ectopically producing parathyroid hormone, or (4) the boney metastases may elevate levels. So suffice it to say that the high calcium often seen in cancer patients, may be fictitious, and may just mean the calcium is in the wrong place, and it can still actually be deficient.

Some leukemics heal on the alkaline macrobiotic, while others need carnivore. The high calcium, needed for the carnivores, probably serves to buffer and alkalinize the cell environment, since cancer cells are notoriously acid and anaerobic (pushed to low oxygen fermentative chemistry, which is acidic). And, whenever you need to increase one element, you know there are many balancing acts that must be performed elsewhere. For example, vitamin D is increased when calcium needs are increased. And do not forget nature's best source is natural sunshine.

There is a plethora of evidence now that calcium, as much as 2.5 gms a day, has been preventive in colon cancer. But it must be balanced, or the calcium will merely go on to cause arteriosclerosis, renal and gall bladder stones, and other unwanted calcifications which hasten degeneration and aging.

But there is much more to be learned, and appreciation of the calcium factor in disease will be a long time in coming, when you consider that it is already known that **vitamin A and its analogs actually hault and reverse (as well as prevent) many cancers.** Yet many sufferers are not on it and researchers are stumped as to what the retinoic acid syndrome means yet, as you read. As of this writing, clinicians have decided to treat the potentially lethal retinoic acid syndrome with corticosteroids, because they have no other idea, or even hint of what is causing it or how to treat it.

And I shudder to think of the reaction that the suggestion of coffee enemas would bring. But, if the people who have the thousands of lives in their hands would only read through this book, its references, and the previous 5, we could probably make a tremendous difference in the cancer mortality in this country within the next year. What an exciting thought.

However, people with large financial interests vested in the current program where 1/3 of the populus will die of cancer and the average amount of money spent trying to control the cancer is $200,000.00 per person, may not be enthusiastic about a program of vitamins, coffee enemas, organic foods, juices and enzymes. I am afraid we will not see the day when these natural

God-given and life-saving therapies will enthusiastically be embraced by the medical/pharmaceutical conglomerate.

As proof of that, much of this has already been around since the turn of the century, while much has been written about it for over 75 years. I'm not so naive to think that just because I'm the first one to collate it all, that they will run out and enthusiastically embrace these principles, or even incorporate them into on-going programs.

For all you have to do is recall that it was well over 50 years between the time that Dr. James Lind discovered that limes prevented scurvy and they were routinely included in the ships' larders. In the interim, thousands of men needlessly died.

References:

Akiyama H, Nakamura N, Nagasaka S, Sakamaki H, Onozawa Y,Hypercalcemia due to all-trans retinoic acid, **LANCET** 339:308-309, February 1, 1992.

Anghileri, **THE ROLE OF CALCIUM IN BIOLOGICAL SYSTEMS, VOL I,**CRC Press, Boca Raton, 1985

Barefoot RR, Reich CJ, **THE CALCIUM FACTOR,** Bokar Consultants Inc., P.O.Box 21270, Wickenburg, AZ 85358

Koike T, Tatewaki W, Aoki A, Yoshimoto H, Yagisawa K, Hashimoto S, Et al, Brief report: Severe symptoms of hyperhistaminemia after the treatment of acute promyelocytic leukemia with tretinoin (all-trans retinoic acid), **NEW ENGLAND JOURNAL OF MEDICINE** 327:6 385-387 August 6, 1992.

Johnston CS, Martin LJ, Caix, Antihistamine effect of supplemental ascorbic acid and neutrophil chemotaxis, J AMER COLL NUTR, 11:2, 172-176 1992.

Liotta LA, Cancer cell invasion and metastasis, SCI AMER, Feb 1992

Lipkin M, Calcium and colon cancer, NUTR REV, 51:7,213-214, July 1993

Robinson DR, Eleviation of autoimmune disease by dietary lipids containing omega-3 fatty acids, NUTR & RHEUM DIS, 17:2 213-220, May 1991.

Frankel S, Eardley A, Lauwers G, Weiss M, Warrell RP, The "Retinoic Acid Syndrome" in acute promyelocytic leukemia, ANN INT MED, 117:292-296 1992.

POTASSIUM AND IT'S RELATION TO HEALING

You'll recall from the Gerson Therapy that raw vegetable, fruit and liver juices were used every hour while the person was awake, and also potassium was prescribed. Not only is **potassium** very high in vegetarian diets (as opposed to high sodium in carnivore type diets), but it is crucial to healing.

Even conventional medicine is now picking up on the importance, as can be seen in published articles. Unfortunately, however, it is not part of standard diagnosis yet. Since potassium is so crucial in healing, it is not unexpected that it should have a bearing on the number one cause of disease and death. For example, potassium deficiency has been found to be important in determining whether or not some people have high blood pressure. But still rbc potassium is not routinely checked in patients suspected of hypokalemia, much less as part of the diagnostic workup for hypertensive patients.

(Khaw KT, Barrett-Connor E, Dietary potassium and stroke-associated mortality. NEW ENGLAND JOURNAL OF MEDICINE 316:5 235-240, January 20, 1987, and Singh RB, Sircar AR, Rastogi SS, Singh R, Dietary modulators of blood pressure in hypertension. EUROPEAN JOURNAL OF CLINICAL NUTRITION 44:319- 327 1990).

As many of you have seen, we have found an extremely high incidence of people with abnormally low erythrocyte or red blood cell, or rbc potassium. Unfortunately, the majority of medicine only measures the serum or plasma potassium which, like the serum or plasma levels of any nutrient, are not very sensitive tests and make people look normal when they are abnormal.

Low potassium (called hypokalemia) is a manifestation not of actual potassium need so much as an indicator of abnormal cellular function. What I mean by this is, if a person is on a diuretic or a fluid pill say for blood pressure control, that type of medication usually does waste and lower the potassium. But if they are not on a medication that loses potassium, but nevertheless have a low potassium, you want to question why the potassium is low.

For the majority of people, not having a high vegetable diet is one of the reasons for low potassium. But another reason is that the potassium pump, which is in the cell membrane, is damaged. The reason the cell membrane is damaged, is because it does not have the correct fatty acids in its walls that contribute to its electrical and other physiological processes.

Instead, it has abnormal fatty acids, called trans fatty acids that damage the function. They come from years of eating foods

180

high in trans fatty acids (the label will say hydrogenated oil) like margarines, processed foods, commercial cookies, breads, french fries, etc., foods that are considered the standard in the American diet. Remember these are all high in trans fatty acids, which are more damaging to the cell membrane than eating saturated fats from bacon, steak, etc.

After this knowledge had been in the scientific literature for over 2 decades, the NEW ENGLAND JOURNAL OF MEDICINE (Aug. 16, 1988) finally published it and I naively thought this would make the news and cardiologists world wide would stop the ridiculous recommendation of margarines and other plastic foods that they and hospital dietitians routinely recommend to cardiac patients. It is unconscionable because the use of these causes damage to the cell membranes that actually shortens lives by accelerating arteriosclerosis, degeneration, aging and cancer development. But it did not make news until 1993. I can't figure out who has control over this stuff. Anyway, I have not noticed any hospital dieticians or cardiologists change anything yet as a consequence.

References

American Academy of Environmental Medicine, Box 16106, Denver CO 80216 (for physician courses on nutritional biochemistry)

Anonymous, New misgivings about magnesium, SCIENCE NEWS 133:23, 356, 1988

Elsborg L, The intake of vitamins and minerals by the elderly at home. INTERN J VIT NUTR RES 53:321-329, 1983

Freeland-Graves J, Mineral adequacy of vegetarian diets, AM J CLIN NUTR 48:859-862, Sept 1988 (3 suppl)

Gregor JL, Prevalence and significance of zinc deficiency in the elderly. GERIATR MED TODAY. 3:1, 24-10, 1984

Halstead CH, Rucker RB, NUTRITION AND THE ORIGINS OF DISEASE, Academic Press, San Diego, 1987

Hambridge KM, Zinc nutritional status during pregnancy: a longitudinal study. AM J CLIN NUTR 37:429-442, 1983

Holdener EE, Retinoids in cancer prevention and therapy, ANN ONCOL 3:7, 513-526, 1992

Hum S, et al. Varied protein intake alters glutathione metabolism in rats. J NUTR 122:2010-2018, 1992

Jacques PF, Effects of vitamin C on high-density lipoprotein cholesterol and blood pressure, J AMER COLL NUTR, 11:2, 139- 144, 1992

Lardinois CK, Neuman SL, The effects of antihypertensive agents on serum lipids and lipoproteins, ARCH INTERN MED 148:1280-1288, 1988

Leo MA, Lowe N, Lieber CS, Potentiation of ethanol-induced hepatic vitamin A depletion by phenobarbital and butylated hydroxytoluene. J NUTR 117:70-76, 1987

Lindenbaum J, Healton EB, Savage DG, Brust JCM, Garrett TJ, Podell ER, Marcell PD, Stabler SP, Allen RH, Neuropsychiatric disorders caused by cobalamin deficiency in the absence of anemia and macrocytosis, NEW ENGL J MED 318:1720-1728,1988

Klevay LM, Reck SJ, Barcome DF, et al, Evidence of dietary copper and zinc deficiencies. JAMA 241:18, 1916-1918, 1979

Mensink RP, Katan MB, Effect of dietary trans fatty acids on high-density and low-density lipoprotein cholesterol levels in healthy subjects, NEW ENGL J MED 323:439-445, 1990

Prasad AS, ZINC IN HUMAN NUTRITION, CRC Press, Boca Raton FL 33431, 16-30, 1979

Rea WJ, Johnson AR, Smiley RE, Maynard B, Dawkins-Brown O, Magnesium deficiency in patients with chemical sensitivity. CLIN ECOL 4:1, 17-20, 1986

Rea WJ, Nutritional status and pollutant overload. Chap 6 in CHEMICAL SENSITIVITY, 221-479, CRC Press, Boca Raton FL 1992

Rogers SA, Unrecognized magnesium deficiency masquerades as diverse symptoms: Evaluation of an oral magnesium challenge test. INTERN CLIN NUTR REV, 11:3, 117-125, 1991

Rogers SA, Chemical sensitivity, Part I, INTERNAL MEDICINE WORLD REPORT, 7:3, pp 1, 15-17, Feb 1-15, 1992; Part II, , 7:6, pp 2, 21-31, Mar 1-15, 1992; Part III, INTERNAL MEDICINE WORLD REPORT, 7:8, pp 13-16, 32-33, 40-41, Apr 15-30, 1992

Rogers SA, Zinc deficiency as a model for developing chemical sensitivity. INTERN CLIN NUTR REV 10:1253-259, 1990

Rogers SA, TIRED OR TOXIC?, Prestige Publishing, Box 3161, Syracuse NY, 13220

Sanstead HH, Henriksen LK, Gregor JG, Prasad A, Good RA, Zinc nutriture in the elderly in relation to taste acuity, immune response and wound healing. AM J CLIN NUTR 36:1046-1059,

1982
Schroeder JA, Nason AP, Tipton IH, Essential metals in man. Magnesium. J CHRON DIS 21:815-841, 1969   Seelig MS, MAGNESIUM DEFICIENCY IN THE PATHOGENESIS OF DISEASE, Plenum Publ, 227 W 17TH St, NY, 1980

Simon JA, Vitamin C and cardiovascular disease: A review, J AMER COLL NUTR, 11:2, 107-125, 1992

Van Rij AM, Zinc supplements in surgery. "Current Topics in Nutrition and Disease. Chemical, Biochemical and Nutritional Aspects of Trace Elements", Prasad AS, ed., Alan R. Liss Inc., 150 Fifth Ave, NY 10011, 6:14, 259-256, 1982

Wang R, Prevalence of magnesium deficiency, in Giles TD, Seelig MS. MONOGRAPH: THE ROLE OF MAGNESIUM CHLORIDE IN CLINICAL PRACTICES, 5-6, Oxford Health Care Inc.(through Searle Pharmaceuticals), Clifton NJ 1988

Wang R, Ryder KW, Frequency of hypomagnesemia and hypermagnesemia, requested versus routine. JAMA 363:3063-3064, 1990

VITAMIN A CURES SOME CANCERS

In reviewing the scientific literature on **vitamin A**, I was shocked to find that researchers across the world have actually caused "complete remission" in acute promyelocytic leukemia with vitamin A or a vitamin A like compound, retinoic acid. It turns out they think that the vitamin A causes a rearrangement of the genes.

The thing is that even though there were numerous papers substantiating "dramatic therapeutic effects" with "very high rate of complete remission" as well as "excellent results in the treatment of squamous cell carcinomas of the skin and the cervix", the researchers were puzzled by relapses. Indeed, anyone comprehending all of the preceding would be very excited by the possibility that these relapses were unnecessary and that coffee enemas and complementary nutrients, enzymes and attention to the diet and total load would have been very effective in cleaning out the metabolic waste products of the cancer and promoting healing.

One recurring mistake is that drug oriented researchers keep trying to treat nutrients as though they are drugs. So they study the effects of them one at a time. As you recall from our other books and the HEALTH LETTER articles, there are numerous papers showing that when you give, for example, vitamin A but neglect to balance it with other nutrients, that you lower other crucial nutrients. Thus the net effect is that the nutrient in question that is being studied appears to be only marginally effective at best. High doses of A are known to compromise the level of E, and since they operate synergisticly, the erroneous conclusion drawn from some studies was that A was just not that effective.

There were indeed, multiple other types of cancers that were either reversed or were inhibited from occurring with vitamin A or vitamin A analogs (a vitamin A analog is a molecule that looks a lot and acts a lot like vitamin A, but it has been changed chemically; sometimes done so that it can be manufactured as a drug at a much higher profit than inexpensive natural vitamin A would be).

The types of cancers that have been either inhibited or cleared with vitamin A or it's analog include acute promyelocytic leukemia, juvenile chronic myelogenous leukemia, T cell malignancies, squamous cell (skin cancers) carcinomas of the head, neck and cervix, basal cell carcinomas, bladder tumors and pre-cancerous and cancerous conditions of the skin, mouth, larynx, lung, bladder and vulva.

Chemicals deplete vitamin A. Therefore a **knowledge of environmental medicine and environmental controls are just as important for the cancer patient as the E.I. patient.** (Leo MA, Lowe N, Lieber CS, Potentiation Of Effomol-Induced Hepatic Vitamin A Depletion By Phenobarbital And Butylated Hydroxytoluene, JOURNAL OF NUTRITION 117:70-76, 1987.

BHT, is a common food additive, depletes vitamin A. Thus an example of the importance of organic and unprocessed foods in attempting to treat a cancer as well as any other disease. (Halsted CH, Rucker RB, Eds, NUTRITION AND THE ORIGINA OF DISEASE, Volume 7. Academic Press, NY 1987). I strongly reccommend this book for any doctor treating cancers. It includes such chapters as: Evidence of Vitamin A and gene expression, Omega 3 Fatty Acids And Regulation Of Lipoproteins, Vitamin A Deficiency In Cancer, Environmental Chemicals Lowering Vitamin A, Depleting It, Role Of Gastrointestinal Hormones In Adaptation, etc.

CANCER PATIENTS ARE CHEATED

There is a plethora of evidence, as you can see for using vitamin A not only to prevent cancers, but more importantly to treat them. But it is not done because expensive drug protocols pay for research that in turn supports the increased use of expensive chemotherapy. Once more, the medical literature is replete with articles showing severe, often fatal side effects of chemotherapy. For **chemotherapy works by poisoning every cell. It is taken up faster by cancer cells, because they are growing faster,** thus they get a higher dose of it. But many types of chemotherapy damage the heart so much that it is the failure of the heart to survive that kills the patient, not his cancer.

And it is known that doses of the anti-oxidants like vitamins A, C, and E can prevent this, but they are not incorporated into all protocols! (Stahelin HB, Brubacher GG, Preventive potential of antioxidative vitamins and carotenoids on cancer, INTERN J VITAMIN & NUTR RES SUPPL, 30:232-241,1989). So when it comes to the lesser known nutrients, it is no surprise that they, too are neglected. It is criminal not to prescribe nutrients for patients on chemotherapy in this age with all that is known about anti-oxidant chemistry and the universal cell damage created by chemotherapy, as well as its ability to knock the bottom out of remaining nutrient levels.

Take **carnitine** as an example of a lesser known nutrient. Carnitine is an **aminated butyrate**, essential to the body, and found in highest amounts in meats. Its purpose is to carry acyl groups across the mitochondrial membrane. What this amounts to in terms of symptoms is that it can correct "uncorrectable hypoglycemia" (low blood sugar), hyperlipidemia (high cholesterol and /or triglycerides), and is necessary for energy synthesis.

But in terms of the chemotherapy patient, **carnitine is crucial in protecting him from death from chemotherapy** (Albert DS, et al, Carnitine prevention of adriamycin toxicity in mice, BIOMEDICINE, 29:265-268, 1978).

The bottom line is that the cancer patient, more than anyone, needs meticulous nutrient assessments and corrections.

References

Smith MA, Parkinson DR, Cheson BD, Friedman MA, Retinoids in cancer therapy. JOURNAL OF ONCOLOGY 1992 May;10 (5):839-864.

Degos L, Retinoic acid in acute promyelocytic leukemia: a model for differentiation therapy. CURRENT OPINION IN ONCOLOGY 1992 Feb;4(1):45-52.

Muindi J, Frankel SR, Miller WH Jr, Jakubowski A, Scheinberg DA, Young CW, Dmitrovsky E, Warrell RP Jr, Continuous treatment with all-trans retinoic acid causes a progressive reduction in plasma drug concentrations: implications for relapse and retinoid "resistance" in patients with acute promyelocytic leukemia. BLOOD 1992 Jan 15;79(2):299-303.

Degos L, All-trans-retinoic acid treatment and retinoic acid receptor alpha gene rearrangement in acute promyelocytic leukemia: a model for differentiation therapy. INTERNA-TIONAL JOURNAL OF CELL CLONING 1992 Mar;10(2): 63-9.

Bollag W, Holdener EE, Retinoids in cancer prevention and therapy. ANNALS OF ONCOLOGY 1992 Jul;3 (7):513-526.

Byers T, Perry G, Dietary carotenes, vitamin C, and vitamin E as protective antioxidants in human cancers. ANNUAL RE-VIEW OF NUTRITION 1992;12:139-159.

Frankel SR, Miller WH Jr, Dmitrovsky E, Retinoic acid and its rearranged receptor in the etiology and treatment of acute promyelocytic leukemia. ONCOLOGY 1992 Aug;6(8): 74-78.

Hill DL, Grubbs CJ, Retinoids and cancer prevention. AN-NUAL REVIEW OF NUTRITION 1992;12:161-181.

Frankel SR, Eardley A, Lauwers G, Weiss M, Warrell RP Jr, The "retinoic acid syndrome" in acute promyelocytic leukemia. ANNALS OF INTERNAL MEDICINE 1992 August

15;117(4):292-296.

Chow JM, Cheng AL, Su IJ, Wang CH, 13-cis-retinoic acid induces cellular differentiation and durable remission in refractory cutaneous Ki-1 lymphoma. CANCER 1991 May 15;67 (10):2490-2494.

Warrell RP Jr, Frankel SR, Miller WH Jr, Scheinberg DA, Itri LM, Hittelman WN, Vyas R, Andreeff M, Tafuri A, Jakubowski A, Differentiation therapy of acute promyelocytic leukemia with tretinoin (all-trans-retinoic). NEJM 1991 May 16;324(20): 1385-1393.

Kramer ZB, Boros L, Wiernik PH, Andersen J, Bennett JM, Cassileth P, Oken M. 13-cis-retinoic acid in the treatment of elderly patients wit acute myeloid leukemia. A phase II pilot study of the Eastern Cooperative Oncology Group. CANCER 1991 Mar 15;67(6):1484-1486.

Dorgan JF, Schatzkin A, Antioxidant micronutrients in cancer prevention. HEMATOLOGY-ONCOLOGY CLINICS OF NORTH AMERICA1991 Feb;5(1):43-68.

Singh VN, Gaby SK, Premalignant lesions: role of antioxidant vitamins and beta-carotene in risk reduction and prevention of malignant transformation. AM J CLIN NUTR 1991 Jan;53(1 Suppl): 386S-390S (yes SR it's "S" not 5).

Stich HF, Mathew B, Sankaranarayanan R, Nair MK, Remission of precancerous lesions in the oral cavity of tobacco chewers and maintenance of the protective effect of beta-carotene or vitamin A. AM J CLIN NUTR 1991 Jan;53(1 Suppl):298S-304S.

Fontana JA, Burrows-Mezu A, Clemmons DR, LeRoith D, Retinoid modulation of insulin-like growth factor-binding proteins and inhibition of breast cancinoma proliferation. ENDOCRINOLOGY 1991 Feb;128(2):1115-1122.

Oikarinen A, Peltonen J, Kallioinen M, Ultraviolet radiation in skin ageing and carcinogenesis: the role of retinoids for treatment and prevention. ANN MED1991; 12(5):497-505.

Mayne ST, Graham S, Zheng TZ, Dietary retinol: prevention or promotion of carcinogenesis in humans? CANCER CAUSES & CONTROLS 1991 Nov;2(6):443-450.

Clarkson B, Retinoic acid in acute promyelocytic leukemia: the promise and the paradox. CANCER CELLS 1991 Jun;3(6):211-220.

Black HS, Mathews-Roth MM, Protective role of butylated hydroxytoluene and certain carotenoids in photocarcinogenesis. PHOTOCHEMICSTRY&PHOTOBIOLOGY1991 May;53(5):707-716.

De Luca LM, Retinoids and their receptors in differentiation, embryogenesis, and neoplasia. FASEB JOURNAL 1991 Nov;5(14): 2924-2933

Krinsky NI, Effects of carotenoids in cellular and animal systems. AM J CLIN NUTR 1991 Jan;53(1 Suppl):238S-246S.

Mathews-Roth MM, Carotenoid functions in photoprotection and cancer prevention. JOURNAL OF ENVIRONMENTAL PATHOLOGY, TOXICOLOGY & ONCOLOGY 1990 Jul-Oct;10(4-5):181-192 (this one shows that carotenemia, the yellow skin color from carrot juice, has no serious toxicity).

Mayne ST, Beta-carotene and cancer prevention: what is the evidence? CONNECTICUT MEDICINE 1990 Oct;54(10):547-

551.
Whelan P, Retinoic acid and prostatic cancer cell growth. PROGRESS IN CLINICAL & BIOLOGICAL RESEARCH 1990;357:117-120.

Mettlin C, Selenskas S, Natarajan N, Huben R, Beta-carotene and animal fats and their relationship to prostate cancer risk. A case-control study. CANCER 1989 Aug 1;64(3):605-12. (Animal fat related to increased risk of prostatic cancer.)

Stahelin HB, Gey F, Brubacher G, Preventive potential of antioxidative vitamins and carotenoids on cancer. INTERNA-TIONAL J VIT & NUTR RES, Supplement 1989;30:232-241.

Santamaria L, Bianchi A, Cancer chemoprevention by supplemental carotenoids in animals and humans. PREVENTIVE MEDICINE 1989 Sep;18(5):603-623.

Krinsky NI, Carotenoids as chemopreventive agents. PREVENTIVE MEDICINE Sep;18(5):592-602.

De Vet HC, The puzzling role of vitamin A in cancer prevention (review). ANTICANCER RESEARCH 1989 Jan-Feb;9(1): 145-151.

Ziegler RG, A review of epidemiologic evidence that carotenoids reduce the risk of cancer. JOURNAL OF NUTRITION 1989 Jan;119(1):116-122.

Mettlin C, Levels of epidemiologic proof in studies of diet and cancer with special reference to dietary fat and vitamin A. PROGRESS IN CLINICAL & BIOLOGICAL RESEARCH 1988;259:149- 159.

Hayes RB, Bogdanovicz JF, Schroeder FH, De Bruijn A,

Raatgever JW, Van Der Maas PJ, Oishi K, Yoshida O, Serum retinol and prostate cancer. CANCER 1988 Nov 1;62(9):2021-2026.

Prince MR, LaMuraglia GM, MacNichol EF Jr, Increased preferential absorption in human atherosclerotic plague with oral beta carotene. Implications for laser endarterectomy. CIRCULATION 1988 Aug;78(2):338-344.

Lippman SM, Shimm DS, Meyskens FL Jr, Nonsurgical treatments for skin cancer: retinoids and alpha-interferon. JOURNAL OF DERMATOLOGIC SURGERY & ONCOLOGY 1988 Aug;14(8):862-869.

Behan PO, Behan WMH, Horrobin D, Effect of high doses of essential fatty acids on the postviral fatigue syndrome, ACTA NEUROL SCAN 82:209-216, 1990

Tate G, Mandell BF, et al, Suppression of acute and chronic inflammation by dietary gamma linolenic acid, J RHEUMATOL, 16:729-733, 1989

Chandra RK, Effect of vitamin and trace-element supplementation on immune responses and infection in elderly subjects, LANCET 340:1124-1127, 1992

HOW THE SICK GET SICKER, QUICKER, BY FOLLOWING CURRENT MEDICAL PROTOCOL

(a referenced summary for physicians and advanced readers)

Medicine is a strange field. Even though one of the roles of research biochemists is to make important discoveries about human health, doctors in general do not read the biochemistry research journals. Instead, they read medical journals which are often between 10 and 45 years behind the actual scientific discoveries. And should anyone take a preview peak into the literature and report it before some mysterious self-appointed authority in medicine does, they have down through history (and into this very moment in history) been proclaimed as quacks or the information is branded as unsubstantiated.

Oddly enough, this mysterious self-appointed keeper of the facts can rely on being believed, because rarely does anyone go to the scientific literature to see if indeed what was said is true. This innominate group actually decides what shall be publicized and what shall not, despite the obvious benefits to mankind. It is almost as though there is an unwritten rule, "It shall not be discovered and announced and taken for common knowledge until we are ready."

For example, most grocery store cooking oils and margarines are purified and hydrogenated. This means the oils and margarines have been processed with strong chemicals that remove most of the vitamins and minerals. This is so that the product can last for months on a shelf and not spoil. Unfortunately, these nutrients, like vitamins E, B6, and minerals like magnesium, chromium, and copper are the very ones that are necessary to prevent arteriosclerosis (to include early heart attacks, high blood pressure, impotence, Alzheimer's presenile dementia, strokes and premature aging), the number one health problem in the United States.

But more importantly, hydrogenation means that the product has been exposed to a temperature often in excess of 400 degrees Fahrenheit. This causes a twisting of the molecule. In chemistry terms, this changes the configuration or shape of the molecule from a **cis** form to a **trans** form. Normally, lipid (fat or oil) molecules fit into the membranes of cells as part of the structure, upon which all function depends. When these heat twisted molecules (trans fatty acids) are ingested, they fit into the membranes like a broken key. They get locked into the structure, but they stop it from functioning properly, and they compete with natural cis form fatty acids that are necessary for membrane function.

Meanwhile, the trans form fatty acids are capable of doing the very same damage that saturated fats (bacon, cheese, steaks, and other saturated fats, etc.) do. After decades of scientific journal articles warning of this, it was reported in the medical literature in the NEW ENGLAND JOURNAL OF MEDICINE in 1990, but never made the lay news.

Margarines, recommended by cardiologists to prevent cardiovasculare disease, are as much as 35% trans (the bad twisted molecules) fatty acids. Corn oil, artificial ("plastic") egg substitutes and most "natural whole grain health breads" contain significant amounts as well. So the cardiologists of the U.S. have been actually accelerating disease by recommending corn oil margarines, egg substitutes, corn and safflower oils, etc. all of these years. I designate U.S. cardiologists, because medicine in Europe is neither so ignorant of biochemistry, nor so egocentric that they cannot listen to docs who do read the latest science, or perhaps not as controlled financially by other interests, like food and chemical manufacturers. I suggest this because Europe won't even allow the sales of our margarines there because they are so high in trans fatty acids, and notoriously bad for the health of the populus.

Now that this has been known for over 20 years, the NEW ENGLAND JOURNAL OF MEDICINE finally published it in 1990. They showed physicians across the world that margarines and grocery store polyunsaturated oils are at least as harmful to the body as saturated oils. That was 3 years ago. But I do not yet know of one cardiologist who has caught on and stopped recommending margarines, plastic eggs, processed foods and corn oil. And the farce persists on T.V., too.

What did make national news, however, from that issue was a study designed to refute a technique to test for food and chemical sensitivities. In spite of this technique having been published in over half a dozen reputable journals, including the United States government's National Institutes of Health medical journal, ENVIRONMNENTAL HEALTH PERSPECTIVES, no one acutally studied the article to find its 13 flaws. An overwhelming publicity was manufactured for this study (over 2 dozen major newspapers across the U.S. were alerted by the journal 2 days before doctors received their copies in the mail——I know because I was personally telephoned by these 2 dozen papers for a comment). Interestingly, the publicity that this article had was way out of proportion to its importance, even if the conclusions had been correct. But in the very same August 16, 1990 issue was the article showing the dangers of trans fatty acids, and not a peep was heard about this.

The most outrageous flaw of all was the fact that because the researchers were so unknowledgeable about the technique that they had set out to disprove, **they had the technique backwards.** They actually used the dose that is supposed to cause symptoms or provoke them in place of the dose that is supposed to turn off the symptoms. So no wonder they were successful in showing the technique does not work.

If you have it absolutely backwards, it is not the technique. But that is neither here nor there. The point is that there is some power in medicine so influential and at the same time dangerously unfamiliar with the scientific literature, while concomitantly being under the influence of those with their own agendas that the best is not done for the American people.

Let's get back to the cardiologist (since he specializes in the treatment of the number one cause of death and illness in the U.S.) and see another example of how he has been hoodwinked by this mysterious governing body.

MAGNESIUM LEADS THE WAY AS AN EXAMPLE

With the processing of foods such as going from whole wheat or brown rice down to bleached white rice and bleached white flour, over 75% of the magnesium is lost [Schroeder,1969]. U.S. government surveys confirm that the average American diet provides only 40% of the recommended daily amount of magnesium [Anonymous, 1988]. In another study 39% of the populus had less than 70% of the RDA for magnesium (Marier, 1986). Add to this the fact that sugar, phosphates (high in processed foods, soft drinks), alcohol, stress, and a high fat diet further potentiate magnesium deficiency [Seelig, 1989], and it is not surprising that leading authorities in magnesium estimate that 80% of the populus is magnesium deficient.

There is no blood test to adequately rule out magnesium repleteness. The **serum level** is the most commonly performed, but is far **too insensitive** to be of any value except in cases of severe deficiency, since only 1% of body magnesium is extracellular [Rhinehart,1988]. A major disservice has been done since this has become a member of the chemical profile so commonly done on patients, because it allows the doctor who does not know how insensitive the test is to assume magnesium repleteness when he sees it reported as normal. This is a serious assumption, especially in light of the JAMA study (Whang, 1990) showing that 90% of physicians never even think of looking at even the least sensitive test (a serum magnesium) in over 1000 patients who were so ill as to be hospitalized (and many of whom died as a consequence of a magnesium deficiency not being diagnosed and corrected).

The intracellular erythrocyte (red blood cell) level is the best currently available blood test [Elin, 1987], but that also is too insensitive to be of reliable value. **The best test is a loading test** [Rasmussen, 1988, Seelig, 1989, Rea, 1986, Nicar, 1982, Ryzen, 1985, Rogers, 1991]. **Magnesium causes muscle relaxation, while calcium causes muscle contraction or spasm**, which is especially pronounced if unbalanced in the face of an undiagnosed magnesium deficiency. If the spasm is in the smooth muscle of the vascular tree, it can lead to hypertension [Altura,1984, Seelig,1989], peripheral vascular disease [Howard, 1990], angina, arrhythmia, and **sudden death** [Singh, 1982, Leary, 1983]. Magnesium deficiency also damages the sodium pump [Cachs, 1988], providing a dual mechanism for hypertension.

But if a magnesium deficiency is causing hypertension and the cause is not sought, or just as bad, a mere serum magnesium is done and found to be normal, often the first drug to be prescribed is a diuretic; known for its ability to not only induce hypokalemia, but a magnesium deficiency as well, thereby accentuating the underlying cause of the symptom for which the drug was prescribed. Hence the hypertension can worsen, requiring other drugs, or go on to cause other symptoms such as refractory hypokalemia [Whang, 1992] or recalcitrant cardiac arrhythmia [Seelig,1980, Marino, 1991]. The latter spurs the use of calcium channel blockers, but magnesium is nature's calcium channel blocker [Iseri, 1984] and controls the calcium pump [Abraham, 1982].

So even though the calcium channel blocker ameliorates the symptoms, the undiagnosed magnesiunm deficiency continues, plus the calcium channel blocker can cause further magnesium deficiency by itself [Ebel,1983]. We get into the familiar downward spiral of disease where the SICK GET SICKER. And this is only the beginning.

For not only does the diuretic accentuate hypomagnesemia, but it causes the loss of other nutrients used in the daily work of detoxifying it. If that were not enough, diuretics raise lipids [Lardinois, 1988]; but magnesium deficiency itself also disturbs proper lipid metabolism [Rayssiguier, 1981]. So now disordered lipid metabolism is added to the initial problem of hypertension. Therefore, **by using drugs to mask symptoms, the path of illness is accelerated.** Multiple mechanisms intertwine and snowball and we get, just as in chemical sensitivity, the spreading phenomenon where the SICK GET SICKER.

With the exercise craze, our unsuspecting patient may decide to jog, but sweating accelerates the loss of magnesium through the skin [Stendig-Lindberg, 1987]. Sudden death from magnesium deficiency-induced cardiac arrhythmia may result [Anonymous, 1990], and may indeed have been the cause of sudden death among famous athletes.

There are many examples in the literature that demonstrate medicine's serious neglect of the facts regarding nutrient biochemistry. For example, in one study of 22 cardiac arrest victims, 59% had abnormal serum magnesium levels. 100% of those with abnormal serum magnesium died. In the "normomagnesemic" group (many were not actually magnesium replete because the least sensitive indicator of magnesium status, a serum level, was used), 66% died [Cannon, 1987]. So magnesium status (determined by the inadequate serum value) still made a significant difference between 0% versus 44% survival.

In another study of 103 patients with documented acute myocardial infarction, patients were randomized into two groups: one received intravenous magnesium, the other group received placebo. The in-hospital mortality of the placebo group was 17% compared to 2% for the magnesium group, leaving the magnesium-treated group with a reduction in mortality of 88.2% [Schecter, 1990]. Yet with all this data, magesium status is not routinely and optimally evaluated to this date. At least many (but not all!) hospitals and emergency rooms are now giving a bolus of magnesium stat to MI victims.

But it is not yet universally routine for physicians to check the magnesium status of patients currently under indefinite treatment for chronic diseases of the vascular system, despite reports where hypokalemia, hypocalcemia, and/or hypophosphatemia could not be corrected until the hypomagnesemia was diagnosed and corrected [Whang,1984, 1992]. And, of course magnesium deficiency has a major bearing on the development of arteriosclerosis, the number one cause of morbidity and mortality (Orimo, 1990)

Despite the fact that there are over 30 million hypertensive Americans [Kaplan, 1986], and despite the fact that magnesium deficiency is a part of the cause for many [Altura, 1981, 1984, 1985, Resnick, 1984], 90% of physicians do not check for a magnesium deficiency in the United States in patients so sick as to be hospitalized [Whang, 1990]. And in an era where such phrases as **"reasonable and customary"** dictate what the patient can have as his standard of care, it becomes clear that the standard is not in the best medical interest of the patient or the

199

society that picks up the medical tab.

As another example of how we tend to undervalue nutrient biochemistry in medicine, in an issue of a popular internal medicine journal there was an article on muscle cramps, one on Raynaud's phenomenon, and one on the correction of hypokalemia. All three problems can be classic symptoms of magnesium deficiency, yet magnesium deficiency was not mentioned in the entire issue [ARCH INT MED,1990].

Since diseases of the cardiovascular system are the number one cause of death and dying in the United States, and consequently a major part of the **12% of GNP** expenditures that go for medical care, this is no small matter. And bear in mind that magnesium is an example of but one of over 40 nutrients that we are limiting this whole discussion to for simplicity.

In one study that did not use sophisticated nutrient analyses, 59 patients with a mean age of 82 and a recent hip fracture were studied. One half of the group received a few nutrient tests and supplements, while the other half of the group did not. The rate of medical complications for the group that had attention to its nutrients was 44% compared with 87% for the other, nearly double. And the mean duration of hospital stay for the nutrient group was 24 days versus 40, nearly half. The death rate in this highly fragile, aged and injured group was 24% for the nutrient group versus 37%. Yet still in spite of the enormous health and financial benefits, this is not standard care [Delmi, 1990], in an era where patients and their physicians are penalized for deviating from the "standard" of care.

Furthermore, chronic magnesium deficiency has been implicated in some cases of TIA or mini-strokes [Fehlinger, 1984], organic brain syndrome [Hall,1973], and contributing to the pathology of Alzheimer's disease. And we haven't begun to touch upon the over 40 other symptoms that this one deficiency, magnesium, can produce. Intestinal spasms mimicking colitis [Main 1985], cerebral vascular spasms called migraine, bronchial spasms of asthma [Rollo, 1987], chronic fatigue [Cox, 1991], unwarranted depression, or the fallopian spasms of infertility are possible. And, of course, the symptoms of chemical sensitivity can be wholly or in part produced by magnesium deficiency [Rogers, 1991].

It is interesting that emergency injections of magnesium have been the time-honored treatment for often tragically fatal toxemia of pregnancy for over 60 years [Lazard, 1925], for example, but the correct prophylactic determination of magnesium status, so easy to do with a urine loading test [Rogers, 1991], is not routine with pregnancy, before this sometimes fatal event.

Other common magnesium deficiency symptoms include a host of psychiatric symptoms like irritability, anxiety, aggitation, panic attacks, and more [Hall, 1973]. You can begin to appreciate how one almost feels clairvoyant when he/she sees an article on panic disorder in cardiology patients [Beitman, 1991]. And again, with no mention of the one common deficiency that could be the cause of both symptoms, an undiscovered magnesium deficiency. But remember, magnesium deficiency isn't the only thing that can cause panic disorder, as chemical sensitivity can cause this.

Yet the recent National Institutes of Health Consensus Statement on panic disorder mentions neither environmental triggers nor nutrient deficiencies in the differential diagnosis [Anonymous, 1992]. Nor do they mention that stress and magnesium deficiency are mutually enhancing [Seelig, 1981, Boullin, 1967], in that stress through catecholamine induction enhances magnesium deficiency, while magnesium deficiency causes irritability, aggitation, and panic, which in turn push

201

more on the catecholamines, etc.; another spiral mechanism of how the SICK GET SICKER when environmental and bio-chemical causes are not sought.

IS THERE A CONSPIRACY
OF IGNORANCE AND ARROGANCE?

By now you see that medicine is forging ahead in the wrong direction, in spite of voluminous evidence. For example overt **malnutrition is seen in 40% of patients hospitalized for cancer**(Landel AM, Hammond WG, Meguid MM, Aspects of amino acid and protein metabolism in cancer-bearing states, CANCER, 1:55 (1 Suppl):230-237, 1985). And it is known that surgery, radiation and chemotherapy can result in further deterioration in nutritional status in patients (McAnena OJ, Daly JM, Impact of antitumor therapy on nutrition, SURG CLIN NORTH AMER, 66(6):1213- 1228, Dec 1986).

They also know that many foods contain nutrients that help induce detoxification enzymes and inhibit cancer (Steinmetz KA, Potter JD, Vegetables, fruit, and cancer . II.Mechanisms, CANCER CAUSES AND CONTROL 2(6):427-442, Nov 1991. Wattenberg LW, Inhibition of carcinogenesis by minor nutri-ents constituents of the diet, PROC NUTR SOC, 49:2, 173-183, Jul 1990).

And they know that **many vitamins and minerals can prevent or treat cancers** (Wargovich MJ, Lointier PH, Calcium and vitamin D modulate mouse colon epithelial proliferation and growth characteristics of a human colon tumor cell line, CANAD J PHYSIOL & PHARMACOL, 65:3, 472-477, Mar 1987. Lippman SM, Meyskens FL, Vitamin A derivatives in the prevention and treatment of human cancer, J AMER COLL NUTR 7:4, 269-284, Aug 1988. Prasad KN, Mechanisms of action of vitamin E on mammalian tumor cells in culture, PROGR CLIN BIOLOG

RES, 259:363-375, 1988. Kallistratos GI, Fasske EE, Karkabounas S, Charalambopoulos K. Prolongation of the survival time of tumor bearing Wistar rats through a simultaneous oral adminstration of vitamins C and E and selenium with gluta-thione, PROGR CLIN BIOL RES, 259:377-389, 1988.)

And we know that the National Cancer Institute has grown from a budget of $2.5 million in 1974 to $55 million in 1988. Where are the oncologists who are recommending diets and correcting nutrient deficiencies (not to mention the other techniques in this book)? We know **there is a controlling factor in what you the consumer and I the medical professional are to be taught and told.** Could this controlling body be so misguided that you have to learn about these techniques from a non-oncologist? (Greenwald P, Light L, McDonald SS, Stern HR, Strategies for cancer prevention through diet modification, MED ONCOL &TUMOR PHARMACOTHERAPY, 7 (2-3):199- 208, 1990).

When you try to discuss these exciting facts with someone in the field, there is a mixed reaction of (1) arrogance at the idea that someone should try to invade their field and (2) feigned ignorance of the facts. I say feigned, for I find it difficult to believe they are truly ignorant of scores of years of exciting work in their own field. Judging from this unbalanced reaction when you try to make this material known (I would be gleefully excited if someone told me how chemically sensitive people could be well faster and cheaper), I can but conclude that there is a controlling body (as in every field) that does not want the tide turned. It even **controls how physicians think**, it is so powerful. We saw it with Candida, chemical sensitivity, Love Canal, Dr. Linus Pauling's vitamin C, etc. Logic and evidence become strangers as denigrating remarks are assumed to be correct only because of the name of the institution commenting. And if unsuccessful, character assassination, and trumped up

FDA and IRS investigations suddenly appear, making Karen Silkwood a fairy tale in comparison.

But remember from Chapter 3, for example, the evidence for coffee enemas was published in the JOURNAL OF THE NATIONAL CANCER INSTITITE in 1981! Do you have any idea how many people died since then, not of their cancer, not from the metastases, not from the chemo or irradiation or surgery, but from the **toxicity of tumor breakdown products?** But there is no glamour, nor **money** in research that does not result in the sale of very expensive drugs.

Once you know a little nutritional biochemistry and the principles of environmental medicine, current articles in the literature and the continued practice of medicine as though a headache is a darvon deficiency becomes ludicrous. I would be embarrassed to publish an article such as the following. They found that a 58 year old man with extensive total body dermatitis and Crohn's disease (a serious condition of the bowel) cleared his dermatitis with zinc supplementation. My gosh, if I wrote about all the conditions that cleared with nutrient corrections I would not have time to practice.

And I bet you are even laughing and saying to the researcher, "Gee whiz doc, did it surprise you that a man with chronic bloody diarrhea might be deficient in a mineral that then has a bearing on his developing a terrible skin condition?"

The sad part is that dermatitis is still regarded in general as a mysterious problem that often accompanies severe bowel disease. This paper is regarded as a cute anomaly and is passed by by the majority of gastroenterologists and dermatologists. Find it hard to believe? Call 10 of each specialists and ask what tests they would do on you if you came into the office for severe dermatitis, and by the way you have Crohn's disease.

A more conscientous doc would recall the case when someone comes in with the same problem, but the scenario might go like this. "I recall an article of a man who cleared with zinc. Why don't you try some?" No levels to see if you are low, no recommendation of dose, no balancing with other nutrients, no appreciation that just because zinc was the answer for that gentleman, it does mean that all the rest of the people in the universe with dermatitiis have that specific deficiency. I hear these stories everyday. **It is as though the drug industry owns our brains in medicine. We find it difficult to conceive of any other form of medicine.** And the most discouraging aspect of this is that when we get someone well with these logical techniques, it is regarded as close to quackery because we didn't use drugs. Or, as in this case, it is regarded as an isolated peculiarity. (Heimburger DC, Tamura T, Marks RD, Rapid improvement in dermatitis after zinc supplementation in a patient with Crohn's disease, AMERICAN JOURNAL OF MEDICINE 88:1, 71-74, 1990)

BEWARE OF CROOKED SCIENCE!

There is no limit to how low medicine will stoop to discredit nutrients. You know that most work showing the benefits of vitamin E gives a therapeutic dose from 400 I.U. to 800 I.U. This includes studies to show low vitamin E protects against chemotherapy (adriamycin) damage to the heart, reperfusion injury (heart-lung machines), etc, etc.

Even the well-publicized NEW ENGLAND JOURNAL OF MEDICINE studies in the fall of 1993 showed that 85,000 nurses had half the cardiac risk when on a measley 100 I.U. of vitamin E.

So you can imagine our surprise to hear of a paper that "proved" that vitamin E is of no use to diabetics. Anyone who

205

understands the most primitive chemistry of vitamin E would find that utterly impossible to believe. But when we read the "scientific" paper, we found out how they reached that conclusion. The dose they used was less than 10 I.U.. Yes, it was even less than the scant RDA for vitamin E.

The bottom line is, if you hear anything on CNN, or read it in USA TODAY, that goes against your gut level intelligence, check it out. You can't trust any "data" today. It seems the powers that decide what gets in the press have their own agendas. And your health is not factored in. (Schoff SM, et al, Glycosylated hemoglobin concentrations and vitamin E, vitaminC, and beta-carotene in diabetic and non-diabetic older adults. AM J CLIN NUTR, 1993; 58:412-6).

"IF YOU EAT A BALANCED DIET, YOU CAN'T GET DEFICIENT"

This commonly offered medical advise overlooks the fact that the majority of the **SAD (standard American diet)** is processed, leaving only **25-75% of the original nutrients** in food. We are the first generation to ever be continually detoxifying such an unprecedented number of daily chemicals (over 500, average). Add to that the fact that the work of detoxication loses or uses up nutrients, and it is really a tribute to the design of our bodies that we do as well as we do. In a Food and Drug Administration study to analyze 234 foods over 2 year, they found the average American diet to have less than 80% of the RDA (recommended daily allowance) of one or more: calcium, magnesium iron, zinc, copper, and manganese [Pennington, 1986].

In one study of patients admitted to an acute medical service, 23- 50% had undiscovered deficiencies, and this was not a sophisticated analysis Roubenoff, 1987] . When other studies have demonstrated magnesium deficiency in well over 50% of the population [Rogers, 1991, Whang, 1990], it behooves any of of us to condemn any symptom to a lifetime of medications without ruling out deficiencies. For as you can appreciate, even the most seemingly minor of symptoms, like anxiety or insomnia can herald a magnesium or other nutrient deficit that can begin to insidiously disrupt arterial and cardiac integrity and consequently increase the vulnerablity to life-threatening events [Seelig, 1989]. But if they are unknowingly masked with a seemingly harmless tranquilizer or hypnotic, the opportunity to prevent more serious sequelae is lost or at best delayed.

For in fact it is fortunate that a magnesium deficiency can manifest as a plethora of symptoms, since many other nutrient deficiencies that contribute to arteriosclerosis often do so silently, like chromium [Boyle,1977, Schroeder, 1970, Fuller,1983, Press,1990, Elwood,1982]. And when a chromium deficiency does cause one of its classic symptoms, like hypoglycemia [Anderson,1984,1986, Uusitupa,1983, Offenbacher,1980], that symptom is still not a routine trigger to asses the adequacy of the rbc chromium.

If this were not enough, look at how we compound some of these **biochemical blunders** in medicine. Magnesium deficiency plays a major role in the development of arteriosclerosis [Orimo, 1990, Seelig,1980]. Vitamin E is deficient in the average processed diet. And vitamin E deficiency is also important in the development of cardiovascular disease [Gey,1990], in fact it can even protect against a magnesium deficiency-induced cardiac myopathy [Freedman, 1990] as well as reduce the size of experimentally-induced myocardial infarct [Axford-Gatley,1991] and the extent of reperfusion injury [Ferreira, 1991, Reilly,1991]. And as you might guess, magnesium deficiency can be induced by vitamin E deficiency [Goldsmith, 1967, Haddy 1960]. Another way for the downward spiral where once symptoms are masked with drugs and the environmental trigger and nutritional defect are not found and corrected, the SICK GET SICKER.

And it should come as no surprise that **both deficiencies, magnesium and vitamin E, also promote chemical sensitivities as well as cancer** [Seelig, 1979], in addition to arteriosclerosis, since the pathologies of many diseases are similar: **it just depends upon the hereditary target organ predisposition and environmental vulnerability, the individual biochemistry, and the xenobiotic dose and time frame. In other words, the causes are different for each individual, each having his own unique total load.** Somehow in medicine, because one drug type will ameliorate the symptoms in most people with similar symptoms, the thinking has erroneously led physicians to assume that when a cause is found, it too, must be the same for all sufferers. But nothing could be further from the truth, and this one fact has enormously slowed progress in conquering many diseases, especially cancer.

A similar error has occured when **researchers have attempted to study nutrients like they would study a drug: alone.** They ignore the fact that the total load is crucial. For example, some studies on vitamin A were inconclusive for its cancer-sparing effect, in spite of its well-known anti-oxidant properties. This was is part because they tried to study it alone as though it were a drug. But high **doses of vitamin A alone, or unbalanced, tend to suppress the level of vitamin E** by as much as 40% (Meyskins, 1990), making the person vitamin E deficient.

Since vitamin E is a necessary complementary anti-oxidant that keeps the carcinogen out of the cell, omitting it from the study (ignoring its synergistic acitivity with vitamin A) negates the benefit of A. Likewise, when you do a study on vitamin E, for example, and do not include sufficient **vitamin C**, you cannot

regenerate tocopherol from the tocopheroxyl radical to **recycle and restore** its usefulness [Bendich,1986]. The result is that vitamin E, in a study with this poor design, does not manifest its full potential. It then, likewise, comes out looking less beneficial than it is, because of iatrogenic deficiencies.

To ignore the chemistry of the body, is like trying to study an engine without a carbeurator.

It is no small wonder that so many drugs stifle symptom manifestations when you see how similar the biochemical pathologies are. And yet how individually unique the cause and treatments are if a search is made for the nutritional or biochemical defects and environmental triggers (Mago 1981, Rea 1977, 1978, 1981, Rogers 1992), or deficits and toxicities. And you can readily appreciate that **by resorting to drugs, we set the patient up for the inevitable worsening,** like the ultimate premature failure in the form of a fatal cardiac event [Marino, 1991].

You can begin to appreciate how clairvoyant you become as you read such article titles as "Excess mortality associated with diuretic therapy in diabetes mellitus" [Warram, 1991]. There was no mention of magnesium in this article either. But yes, diabetes does foster the loss of magnesium [Lau, 1985, Martin,1947] and vice versa, magnesium deficiency potentiates diabetes [Zonszein, 1991]; and you know the diuretic causes magnesium loss, and so it comes as no surprise, in fact it is inevitable that a person with not one, but two mechanisms to potentiate magnesium loss would succumb faster, probably of sudden death. **They are so behind, they think they are first!** Now you are beginning to think like a specialist in environmental medicine when you see the connectedness. For enviromental medicine forces the practitioner to relate all events in the body to the total load, or he simply cannot help people heal, and the SICK GET SICKER, QUICKER.

As one appreciates the complexity of this, it becomes easier as you learn how interrelated everything is. And this knowledge helps the physician to avoid further blunders that only serve to potentiate illness. The recommendation of calcium for the prevention of osteoporosis is one of a multitude of examples.

Many people are deficient in calcium because the standard acidic **processed diet is high in hidden phosphates** (most processed foods, but soft drinks especially). Also by eating large quantities of meats and sweets, this requires a huge amount of buffering. **When the plasma buffer reserves are exhausted, the body calls upon the calcium from the bone to buffer**. When building bone, calcium is laid down in bone only when enough of the complementary minerals are present, such as zinc, copper, boron, and magnesium [Abraham, 1991]. But when these are not present, taking extra calcium merely deposits the calcium in the toxic waste heap of the body, the blood vessel wall [Tanimura, 1986].

In other words, by haphazardly recommending calcium to a nation of people who are already consuming vaste quantities of cheese, milk, ice cream and meats, and without measuring the erythrocyte (rbc) zinc, rbc copper, magnesium loading test, etc., **we are potentiating the development of vascular calcifications instead of bone calcification.** We are enhancing the deposition of extra calcium in the vessels of the heart and brain to hasten coronary artery disease and senile brain disease, two items already taking their toll on the economy.

And all because we fail, in an era of unprecedented high tech medicine with powerful prescription medicines, to analyze an individual's nutrient biochemistry and then prescribe a balanced correction. So it matters not whether we address a symptom, a disease, a metabolic process, or even an endocrine problem [Fatemi, 1990]; **a complete workup has not been done if a nutritional defect is not sought.**

In **summary,** we see (1) that by not reading the current biochemical and environmental literature, the physician is helping the SICK GET SICKER, QUICKER, and one nutrient has served as an example of how (2) when drugs are used in the current medical system to mask symptoms, that by ignoring the underlying cause, it is left to worsen and inevitably leave new symptoms in its wake, and (3) that medications also have effects of their own that induce further nutrient deficiencies, thus potentiating the decline in health of the patient. Of course, it is not the physician's fault as much as that of the system with this mysterious unnamed governing board.

So in the meantime, a good rule of thumb would be for the physician to recommend minimum processed foods, nothing that contains hydrogenated oils, and no margarines. Instead, have non- farmed ocean fish twice a week, cut down on saturated fats from red meat, eat butter on breads (and select breads that contain no hydrogenated oils), dress salads with flax oil, and cook with olive oil. And it goes without saying that he should be recommending meal plans with a preponderance of fresh vegetables, whole grains, and beans, as well as nuts and seeds, fresh vegetable juices, and sea vegetables. Then start to assess the nutrient levels of all sick patients in attempt to identify some of the biochemical defects that are the basis for many symptoms (Rogers, 1990, 1991, Gallinger 1992).

REFERENCES

Abedin Z, et al, Cardiac toxicity of perchloroethylene, S MED

J 73:1081-1083,1980

Abraham GE, The calcium controversy. J APPL NUTR 34:2,69-73, 1982

Abraham GE, The importance of magnesium in the management of primary postmenopausal osteoporosis. J NUTR MED 2,165-178, 1991

Altura BM, Altura BT, Gerrewold A, Ising H, Gunther T, Magnesium deficiency in hypertension: Correlation between magnesium deficient diets and microcirculatory changes in situ. SCIENCE 223,1315-1317, 1984

Altura BM, Altura BT, New perspectives on the role of magnesium in the pathophysiology of the cardiovascular system: I. Clinical aspects. MAGNESIUM 4:226-244, 1985

Anderson RA, Poansky MM, Bryden NA, Canary JJ, Chromium supplementation of humans with hypoglycemia. FED PROC 43:471,1984

Anderson RA, Chromium metabolism and its role in disease processes in man. CLIN PHYSIOL BIOCHEM 4:31041, 1986

Anonymous, New misgivings about magnesium. SCIENCE NEWS 133:32,356, 1988

Anonymous, Magnesium deficiency: A new risk factor for sudden cardiac death. INTERN MED WORLD REPORT 5:9,18,1990

ARCHIVES OF INTERNAL MEDICINE v.150: p519-522, p613-617, p496-500, 1990

Axford-Gatley RA, Wilson GJ, Reduction of experimental myocardial infarct size by oral administration of alpha-tocopherol. CARDIOVASCULAR RES 25:89-92,1991

Boyle E, et al, Chromium depletion in the pathogenesis of diabetes and arteriosclerosis. SOUTH MED J, 70:12,1449-1453,1977

Cachs JR, Interaction of magnesium with the sodium pump of the human red cell. J PHYSIOL 400,575-591, 1988

Cannon LA, Heiselman DE, Dougherty JM, Jones J, Magnesium levels in cardiac arrest victims: Relationship between magnesium levels and successful resuscitation ANN EMERG MED 16,1195-1198, 1987

Cox IM, Campbell MJ, Dowson D, Red blood cell magnesium and chronic fatigue syndrome. LANCET 337,757-760,1991

Delmi M, Rapin CH, Bengoa JM, Delmas PD, Vasey H, et al., Dietary supplementation in elderly patients with fractured neck of the femur. LANCET 335:1013-1016, 1990

Ebel H, Guenther T, Role of magnesium in cardiac disease. J CLIN CHEM CLIN BIOCHEM 21:249-265,1983

Elin RJ. The status of mononuclear blood cell magnesium assay, J AM COLL NUTR 6:2,105- 107, 1987

Elwood JC, Nash DT, Streeten DHP, Effect of high-chromium brewer's yeast on serum lipids.J AM COLL NUTR 1:263, 1982

Fatemi S, Ryzen E, Flores J, Endres DB, Rude RK, Effect of experimental human magnesium depletion on parathyroid hormone secretion and 1,25-dihydroxyvitamin D metabolism.

213

J CLIN ENDOCRIN METAB 73,1067-1072, 1991

Fehlinger R, Fauk D, Seidel K, Hypomagnesemia and transient ischemia cerebral attacks. MAGNESIUM BULL 6:100-104, 1984

Ferreira RF, Milei J, Llesuy S Flecha BG, et al, Antioxidant action of vitamins A and E in patients submitted to coronary artery bypass surgery, VASCULAR SURG 25:191-195,1991

Freedman AM, Atreakchi AH, Cassidy MM, Weglicki WB, Magnesium deficiency-induced cardiomyopathy: Protection by vitamin E. BIOCHEM BIOPHYS RES COMM 170:3,1102-1106,1990

Fuller JH, Shipley MJ, Rose Gm Harrwett RJ, Keen H, Mortality from coronary heart disease and stroke in relation to degree of glycaemia: the Whitehall Study. BR MED J 287:867-870,1983

Gallinger S, Rogers SA, MACRO MELLOW, Prestige Publ., Box 3191, Syracuse, NY, 13220, 1992.

Gey KF, Lipids, lipoproteins and antioxidants in cardiovascular dysfunction. BIOCHEM SOC TRANS 18:1041-1045,1990

Goldsmith LA, Relative magnesium deficiency in the rat. J NUTR 93,87-102,1967

Haddy FJ, Local effects of sodium, calcium and magnesium upon small and large blood vessels of the dog forelimb. CIRCULATION RESEARCH 7,57-70, 1960

Hall RCW, Joffee JR, Hypomagnesaemia, physical and psychiatric symptoms. JAMA 224:13,1749-1751, 1973

Howard JMH, Magnesium deficiency in peripheral vascular

disease. J NUTR MED 1:39-49, 1990

Iseri LT, French JH, Magnesium: Nature's physiologic calcium blocker. AM HEART J 108:1,188-192, 1984

Kaplan NM, Dietary aspects of the treatment of hypertension. ANN REV PUBLIC HEALTH 7:501-519,1986

Kline K, Cochran GS, Sanders EG, Growth-inhibitory effects of vitamin E succinate on retro virus-transformed tumor cells in vitro, NUTR CANCER 14:27-41, 1990

Kremer JM, Michaler AV, et al Effects of manipulation of dietary fatty acids on clinical manifestation of rheumatoid arthritis. LANCET 189-197, Jan 26,1988

Lardinois CK, Neuman SL, The effects of antihypertensive agents on serum lipids and lipoproteins. ARCH INTERN MED 148. 1280-1288, 1988

Lazard EM, A preliminary report on the intravenous use of magnesium sulphate in puerperal eclampsia. AM J OBSTET GYNECOL 26,647-665, 1925

Leary WP, Reyes AJ, Magnesium and sudden death. SA MED J 64,697- 698,1983

Mago L, The effects of industrial chemicals on the heart, 206-207 in Balazo T, ed., CARDIAC TOXICOLOGY, CRC Press, Boca Raton, FL, 1981

Main AN, Morgan RJ, Russell RI, et al, Magnesium deficiency in chronic imflammatory bowel disease and requirements during intravenous nutrition. J PARENTERAL NUTR 5:151985

Marier JR, Magnesium content of the food supply in the modern-day world. MAGNESIUM 5:1-8,1986

Marino PL, The hidden threat of magnesium deficiency. INTERN MED 12:6,32-46,1991

Martin HE, Wertman M, Serum potassium, magnesium and calcium levels in diabetic acidosis. J CLIN INVEST 26,217-228, 1947

Nicar MJ, Pak CYC, Oral magnesium deficiency, causes and effects. HOSPITAL PRACTICE 116A-116P, 1987

Offenbacher EG, Pi-sunyer FX, Beneficial effects of chromium-rich yeast on glucose tolerance and blood lipids in elderly subjects. DIABETES 29:919-925,1980

Orimo H, Ouchi Y, The role of calcium and magnesium in the development of atherosclerosis. ANN NY ACAD SCI 598:444-457, 1990

Ornish D, et a;, Can life-style changes reverse coronary heart disease? LANCET 336:129-133

Pennington JA, Young BE, The selected minerals in foods surveyed from 1982 TO 1984, J AMER DIETETIC ASSOC 86:7,876, JULY 1986

Press RI, Geller J, Evans G, Effect of chromium picolinate on serum cholesterol and apolipoprotein fractions in human subjects. WEST J MED 152: 41-45,1990

Rasmussen HS, McNair P, Goransson L, Balslov S, Larson OG, Aurup P, Magnesium deficiency in patients with ischemic heart disease with and without acute, myocardial infarction uncovered by an intravenous loading test. ARCH INERN MED 148: 329-332, 1988

Rayssiguier Y, Gueux E, Weiser D, The effect of magnesium deficiency on lipid metabolism in rats fed a high carbohydrate diet. J NUTR 111:1876-1883,1981

Rea WJ, Environmentally-triggered small vessel disease. ANN ALLERGY 38:245-251, 1977

Rea WJ, Environmentally-triggered cardiac disease. ANN ALLERGY 40:4, 243-251, 1978

Rea WJ, Recurrent environmentally triggered thrombophlebitis: A five-year follow-up. ANN ALLERGY 47:333-344, Nov 1981, Part I

Rea WJ, Johnson AR, Smiley RE, Maynard B, Dawkins-Brown O, Magnesium deficiency in patients with chemical sensitivity. CLIN ECOL 4:1,17-20, 1986

Rea WJ, Brown OD, Cardiovascular disease in response to chemicals and foods. In: Brostoff J, Challacombe R, eds FOOD ALLERGY AND INTOLERANCE. Balliere Tindall/Saunders, London/NY, 737-753, 1987

Resnick LM, Gupta RK, Laragh JH, Intracellular free magnesium in erythrocytes of essential hypertension: relation to blood pressure and serum divalent cations. PROC NATL ACAD SCI USA 81:6511-6515, 1984

Rhinehart RA, Magnesium metabolism: A review with special reference to the relationship between intercellular content and serum levels. ARCH INT MED 148:2415-2420,1988

Rogers SA, TIRED OR TOXIC?, Prestige Printing, Box 3161, Syracuse NY 13220, 1990

Rogers SA, THE CURE IS IN THE KITCHEN, ibid, 1991

Rogers SA, Chemical Sensitivity, Parts I, II, III INTERNAL MED WORLD REP, Feb 1992, Mar 1992, Apr 1992

Roubenoff R, et al, Malnutrition among hospitalized patients: problem of physician awareness. ARCH INTERN MED 147:1462-1465.1987

Ryzen E, Elbaum N, Singer FR, Rude RK, Parenteral magnesium tolerance testing in the evaluation of magnesium deficiency. MAGNESIUM 4:137-147, 1985

Schroeder JA, Nason AP, Tipton IH, Essential metals in man, magnesium. J CHRON DIS 21:815-841, 1969

Schroeder HA, Mason AP, Tipton IH, Chromium deficiency as a factor in arteriosclerosis. J CHRON DIS, 23:123-142,1970

Seelig MS, Magnesium (and trace substance) deficiencies in the pathogenesis of cancer. BIOLOGICAL TRACE ELEMENT RESEARCH 1:273- 197, 1979

Seelig MS, MAGNESIUM DEFICIENCY IN THE PATHO-GENESIS OF DISEASE. EARLY ROOT OF CARDIOVASCU-LAR, SKELETAL, AND RENAL ABNORMALITIES. Plenum Med. Book Co., NY, 1980

Seelig MS, Magnesium requirements in human nutrition. MAGNESIUM BULL 3:suppl 1A:26-47, 1981

Seelig MS, Nutritional status and requirements of magnesium.

MAG BULL 8:170-185, 1986

Seelig M, Cariovascular consequences of magnesium deficiency and loss: Pathogenesis, prevalence, and manifestations — magnesium and chloride loss in refractory potassium repletion. AM J CARDIOL 53:4g-21g, 1989

Seelig CB, Magnesiuum deficiency in hypertension uncovered by magnesium load retention. J AM CLIN NUTR 8:5,455, abs.113, 1989

Shecter M, et al, Beneficial effect of magnesium sulfate in acute myocardial infarction. AM J CARDIOL 66:271-274, 1990

Singh RB, Cameron EA, Relation of myocardial magnesium deficiency to sudden death in ischaemic heart disease. AM HEART J 103:3,399- 450, 1982

Stendig-Lindberg G, Graff E, Wacker WE, Changes in serum magnesium concentration after strenuous exercise. J AM COLL NUTR 6:1,35-40, 1987

Tanimura A, McGregor DH, Anderson HC, Calcification in atherosclerosis. I. Human studies. J EXP PATHOL 2:4, 261-273,1986

UUsitupa MIJ, Kumpulainen JT, Voutilainen E, Hersio K, et al, Effect of inorganic chromium supplementation on glucose tolerance, insulin response and serum lipids in noninsulin-dependent diabetics. AM J CLIN NUTR 38:404-410,1983

Warram JH, Lori LMB, Valsania P, Christlieb AR, Krolewski AS, Excess mortality associated with diuretic therapy in diabetes mellitus. ARCH INTERN MED 151:1350-1356, 1991

Whang R. Qu TO, Aikowa JK, Watanabe A, Vannatta J, Fryer A, Markanich M, Predictors of clinical hypomagnesmia, hypokalemia, hypophosphatemia, hyponatremia and hypocalcemia. ARCH INTERN MED 144:1794-1796,1984

Whang R, Ryder KW, Frequency of hypomagnesemia and hypermagnesemia, requested versus routine. JAMA 263,3063-3064, 1990

Whang R, Whang DD, Ryan MP, Refractory potassium repletion. ARCH INTERN MED 152,40-45, 1992

Zonszein J, Magnesium and diabetes. PRACT DIABETOL, 10:1-4, Mar/Apr 1991

*****

BOOKS OF INTEREST

Budwig, Johanna, FLAX OIL AS A TRUE AID AGAINST ARTHRITIS, HEART INFARCTION, CANCER AND OTHER DISEASES, Apple Publishing Company, 220 E 59th Ave, Vancouver, British Columbia Canada V5X 1X9.

Halsted CH, Rucker RB, NUTRITION AND THE ORIGINS OF DISEASE. Acedemic Press, NY 1987.

Haas EM, STAYING HEALTHY WITH NUTRITION, Celestial Arts Publ. PO box 7327, Berkley CA 94707, 1992.

Moss RW, CANCER THERAPY, THE CONSUMER'S GUIDE TO NONTOXIC TREATMENT AND PREVENTION, Equinox Press, 331 W 57th St., Ste 268, New York, NY 10019, 1992

Werbach MR, Nutritional Influences on Mental Illness, Third

Line Press, INC., 4751 Viviana Dr., Tarzana CA 91356, 1991

Pauling L, HOW TO LIVE LONGER AND FEEL BETTER, W.H.Freeman & Co., NY, 1986 (born 1901 and still working !)

Feuer G, de la Iglesia FA, MOLECULAR BIOCHEMISTRY OF HUMAN DISEASE VOL III, CRC Press, Inc., Boca Raton FL, 1990

Hausman P, THE CALCIUM BIBLE, Warner Books, Box 690, NY,NY10019, 1985 Anderson RA, Wellness Medicine, American Health Press, P.O.B.5388m Lynnwood WA 98046-5388, 1987

HELP! I'M BEING MAGNESIUMED TO DEATH!

I don't blame you one bit for feeling that way. But you will understand in a moment, for there are several reasons why I am so "hung up" on magnesium:

(1) I know of over a dozen people under the age of 45 who died in the last year alone, probably of magnesium deficiency.

(2) Even a casual glimpse of T.V. tells you that Hank Gathers, Jim Fixx, Reggie Lewis, and others had cases that reaked of magnesium deficiency. And, of course, athletes lose it faster, because of their copious sweating.

(3) There is voluminous evidence that everyday in the U.S., people are dying of magnesium deficiency, yet a few places are just now deciding to do the worthless serum test. How long before the rbc value is routinely done and finally the loading test? And how many will needlessly suffer or die between then and now? It is no big deal to do these tests.

(4) Even as I go through this morning's mail, I see that the state

of the art in teaching doctors how to treat atrial fibrillation does not have even one word about magnesium! They only talked about drugs! (Hancock EW, Atrial fibrillation and regular rhythm in an elderly woman, HOSPITAL PRACTICE, 37-38, Aug 15, 1993). When I read these cases I want to call up the patients and tell them they do not have to die, but there is no way of finding them (and they are probably dead).

This is in spite of multiple articles showing vast reduction in arrhythmias and death if magnesium is checked or even given empirically (Horner SM, Efficacy of intravenous magnesium in acute myocardial infarction in reducing arrhythmias and mortality, CIRCULATION, 86:774-779, 1992. Ceremuzynski L, Hao NH, Ventricular arrhythmias late after myocardial infarction are related to hypomagnesemia and magnesium loss: Preliminary trial of corrective therapy, CLIN CARDIOL, 16:493-496,1993. Leone A, Biondo L, et al, Low dose lidocaine combined with magnesium sulfate in warning ventricular arrhythmias, JPN HEART, 34:23-28, 1993).

A recent study reported that of 143 patients admitted to a major regional coronary care unit, 40% were low in magnesium, and they are still using the worst assay, a serum magnesium. And of the few doctors who actually treated their patients to correct the magnesium deficiency, they used too small a dose (Seelig CB, Montano CE, Ranney JE, Physician recognition of magnesium status in patients with coronary artery disease admitted to a regional medical center, AMER J CARDIOL, 72:226-227, July 15, 1993.).

(5) I do not want anyone who takes the time and effort to read through these books to die from magnesium deficiency (which you will recall is a cause of **sudden cardiac death**).

Chapter 6

THE ECOLOGIC TRINITY:
CLEAN AIR, FOOD AND WATER

THE TOTAL LOAD

At first, when I started learning about these alternatives for people who could not do macro or who did not do well on it, I thought the **previous 5 books** were unimportant for those people who were trying to heal by the Gerson or Kelley or other methods. But I couldn't have been more wrong. They **provide a necessary background about the total load** and of environmental well-being, as well as instructions on how to prepare nutritious foods. In other words, it is all very necessary background. To be unaware of all that is in the previous 5 books, is like trying to go to medical school, but skipping the first the two years of anatomy, physiology, pharmacology, biochemistry, etc.

For example, you don't have much of a chance of healing a cancer if you are eating an excellent diet, but it doesn't have a good preponderance of organic foods. Studies show that organic foods have often 2 1/2 times the minerals of non-organic. But more important is what they do not have: the unwanted pesticides and antibiotic residues that only serve to add to the burden or total load of an already ailing system.

Nor do you have a chance of getting well if you have a bedroom that is chemically contaminated with high levels of trichlorethylene, formaldehyde, xylene, benzene, toluene, etc. out gasing from a new carpet. Nor do you if you are electro-magnetically sensitive and have your bed up against the wall, an electric blanket, and your head next to the night stand where there is a clock radio and a few other gadgets all plugged in.

223

Nor do you have a very good chance of succeeding on your program if you live in a very moldy environment and don't know about diagnosing and treating this. And because no doctor can go home with you at all times to see what other environmental stressors may be elevating your total load, you need to know all about it so you can police it for yourself.

And regardless of what kind of program you are on, you need to know a great deal about whole, organic foods, their selection, and preparation, storage, and eating. Therefore, I cannot recommend strongly enough that if you are putting yourself through THE UNIVERSITY OF HARD KNOCKS, you want to make darn well sure that your education has left no holes barred. For we live in a world that not only most likely contributed to your illness, but serves to perpetuate it for the uneducated.

Researchers estimate that 80-90 % of human cancers may be attributable to environmental factors, and that the etiology of about 35% (range 10-70%) of human cancers may be related to dietary factors. And estimates by the United States Department of Health and Human Services have been similar. **So we can never learn too much about the role of diet and environment in healing,** for it is the reverse process that got us into trouble in the first place.

Doll R, Peto R, 1981. The causes of cancer: quantitative estimates of avoidable risks of cancer in the United States today. J NATL. CANCER INST. 66:1191-1308

Ross AC, Evaluation of publicly available scientific evidence regarding certain nutrient-disease relationships: 8A VITAMIN A AND CANCER, Dec 1991, FDA contract #223-88-2124)

WHAT YOU CAN DO TODAY ?

Create a bedroom in which you can heal:

1. Get all cotton bedding, sheets, pillow cases, and mattress pad. If new, wash several times in baking soda to remove the formaldehyde (new smell).

2. Put several layers of old cotton blankets over the mattress, be sure they are washed in baking soda. If unable to do this, go to a restaurant supply and get a large roll of heavy duty aluminum foil, and put 6 layers over the mattress (under the sheets and cotton mattress pad), shiny side up.

3. Get a room air cleaner and put a molecular absorber (available from N.E.E.D.S.) in the room, but not near the bed, but across the room.

4. Remove as much from the bedroom as possible, especially dry cleaned clothes, polished or new shoes, cosmetics, dust catchers.

5. Open windows in the early dawn to allow fresh air in, free of traffic pollutants. If the air quality is not good, build a filter (a simple wood frame the size of the opened window with screening on both sides and fill the middle with purafil, (available from the E.L.Foust Co. or from N.E.E.D.S).

6. Reorganize the room to minimize your head being near electromagnetic fields of wall wiring and the particle board head board.

7. This is the hardest for most, but often the most therapeutic: get rid of smelly drapes and carpet (most had no idea how much they reeked of formaldehyde and other chemicals until

they got rid of them and got clear enough to be able to smell things properly again).

8. Read THE E.I. SYNDROME, then TIRED OR TOXIC ? for further environmental controls and a multitude of important details, then plough through YOU ARE WHAT YOU ATE, THE CURE IS IN THE KITCHEN, and MACRO MELLOW for more pearls. I would suggest the HEALTH LETTER (subscription from the same publisher) as well. As I have said, I am not into selling books, but it is the cheapest way I can think of for **sending the intelligent consumer to medical school for an education in the 21st century medicine,** so that he and she can claw their way out of the drugs and surgery-oriented medicine and start healing the impossible.

Start a diet with which you can heal:

1. DO NOT EAT ANY sugar, white flour products, alcohol, tea, coffee, soda, chocolate, processed foods, or smoke. If you can't stop these, you had better back up and ask yourself how you were so severely emotionally damaged that you do not want to live any longer. Then start addressing that. There are many terrific resources for this (Siegel, LeShan).

2. Eat as organic as possible. Most health food stores have organic whole grains, beans, sea vegetables, sunflower and other seeds, almonds and other nuts. The above and below ground vegetables, if not organic, should be purchased as fresh as possible, usually from the local Saturday morning farmers' market.

3. Do not drink city chlorinated, fluorinated water.

4. Drink only clean non-chlorinated water in glass bottles, or from reverse osmosis unit, distiller, or a nearby spring or well.

Check source of water, as there can be problems with all of the above.

5. Read YOU ARE WHAT YOU ATE, MACRO MELLOW, then THE CURE IS IN THE KITCHEN, even if your diet prescription is not macrobiotic or vegetarian.

Start with a body which can heal:

1. Do not use any fragrant soaps, cosmetics, shampoos, after shave, deodorants, fabric softeners.

2. Do body scrubs daily

3. Get some exercise in fresh air, even if it is raining or snowing; if you are too sick, do mild stretching and massage.

4. Get into the sun at least 1/2 hour a day, with no glasses, sun or otherwise.

Start with a mind that is ready to heal:

1. Get rid of old guilt, anger, jealousy, hate, and fear.

2. Practice seeing the bright side of everything.

3. Sing happy songs each day.

4. Get some laughter each day.

5. Get and give some physical hugging each day.

6. Do something unexpectedly nice for someone else each day that brings them joy. Random acts of kindness are a must.

7. Read about getting well each day so that you are continually growing.

8. Find out what your passion is .....what fills you with a zest for living, and DO IT.

9. Renew your spirituality as you have never done before. For example, if it is harmonious with your beliefs, read your BIBLE each day, and if it is meaningless, start with some fellowship study groups through your church or synagogue, and read some of the books suggested here, like Colson's.

10. Spend time with God each day. Let him hold you in his arms. Learn to pray, learn to **listen to Him** and hear His messages, and then do it daily.

******

WHAT IS WRONG WITH CHLORINATED WATER?

Chlorine is a halogen that damages body enzymes. It does not belong in our bodies as part of our water needs. Water is a God-given crucial nutrient for the body. But we have been hood-winked into accepting a product that is of progressively more inferior composition. It is well-known that the average city water today contains over 500 chemicals that do not belong in it. But chlorine is intentionally added, and there are alternatives to purify it, like ozone and ultra-violet light.

I have personally seen people experience a set-back in their healing of a cancer either by drinking chlorinated water, or swimming in chlorinated pools. All municipal water supplies in the U.S. have at least 1 ppm chlorine, and pools are even higher. And remember any thing on your skin is like drinking it, because of dermal absorption. In some cities of the U.S., the chlorine level is so high, that taking 3 showers a day puts you over the government standard for exposure.

Chlorine for starters **potentiates magnesium deficiency**, which you know can cause just about any symptom you can think of, from high blood pressure, to chemical sensitivity or sudden death. Furthermore it also decreases the absorption while increasing the excretion of calcium and phosphorus. (Kaup SM, Greger JL, Effect of various chloride salts on the utilization of phosphorus, calcium and magnesium, J NUTR BIOCHEM 1:542, Oct 1990).

All these years we've been putting people on low sodium diets for control of high blood pressure. But it turns out the sodium is not the problem as much as the chloride (Wyss JM, et al, Exacerbation of hypertension by high chloride, moderate sodium diet in the salt-sensitive spontaneously hypertensive rat, HYPERTENSION, 9[Suppl III]:III-171-III-175, 1987).

It is now known for example that the chlorinated water which is the "normal" drinking water of nearly all U.S. cities, not only **contributes to hypertension**, but also **cancers** of the pancreas, colon, bladder and much more. It also increases the loss of calcium into your urine, thus promoting osteoporosis.

A much better way of cleaning the water of bacteria would be ozonation which is indeed done widely throughout Europe. There are many other things they do, such as not allow our dyed oranges that contain carcinogenic dye just so naturally green oranges of Florida can compete with naturally orange California oranges. Nor do they allow our margarines, full of trans fatty acids, and known to promote arteriosclerosis.

Could it be this does not make the news because our water is chlorinated? As usual, the Europeans are ahead of us in preserving natural health, and they use ozone extensively to kill the bugs in water as opposed to chlorine. It does a beautiful job, you have none of the free radical damage to the body of chlorine, and there are multiple other benefits of ozone for those who wish to seek them out. But research now shows that there is indeed a correlation of chlorine with many diseases, including cancer. For starters, chlorine can interfere with and damage the activity of many enzymes.

Likewise, the dangers of **fluoride** are often ignored. It too can be very damaging to enzymes and can cause a host of symptoms, as it is an aging factor (Yiamouyiannis J, FLUORIDE THE AGING FACTOR, Health Action Press, 6439 Taggart Rd, Delaware OH 43015, 1986). And although a discussion of it is beyond the intended purpose of this book, please do not go on fluoride, for example, on the recommendation that it is good for osteoporosis, until you have all the facts, comprehensive nutrient levels, and a consultation with a physician who is knowledgeable in biochemistry. And have a good filter system on your water.

Raloff J, Chlorination products linked to cancer, SCI NEWS, 143:343, 1993.

Sselmuidencb IJ, Gaydos C, Feighner B, Novakowski WL, Serwadda D, Caris LH, Vlahov D, Comstock GW, Cancer of the pancreas and drinking water; A population-based case-control study in Washington county, Maryland. AMERICAN JOURNAL OF EPIDEMIOLOGY 136:7,836-842 1992.

Sato Y, Ogata O, Fujita T, Importance of chloride in the development of salt-induced angiotensin II hypertension in Rats, AMERICAN JOURNAL OF HYPERTENSION 1991:4:615-617.

Kurtz TW, Morris RC, Dietary chloride as a determinate of

disordered calcium metabolism in salt-dependent hypertension, LIFE SCIENCES 36:921-929 1985.

Kurtz TW, Al-Bander HA, Morris RC, "Salt-sensitive" essential hypertension in man, NEW ENGLAND JOURNAL OF MEDICINE 317:1043-1048,1987.

Miki T, Sano H, Suzuki H, Cawahara J, Hattori K, Saito K, Yutake F, Fukuzaki H, Defective chloride on blood pressure and sympathetic nervous system activity in deoxycorticosterone acetate-treated rats, AMERICAN JOURNAL OF HYPERTENSION 2:253-255, 1989.

AN ENVIRONMENTAL MEDICINE APPROACH
TO CHRONIC BACK PAIN

A 46 year old physician presented with a history of chronic back pain. In his 20's he had lifted a boat sustaining a rupture of the L5 disc. Bed rest and analgesics were successful. A few years later he began having recurrent pain while doing home landscaping and eventually had so much pain that he was steadily on analgesics, muscle relaxants, and non-steroidal anti-inflammatory drugs.

After ten years of drugs to mask the pain whenever he engaged in gardening, tennis, motor cycle riding and other activities, he got to a point where he could no longer function in spite of medication. At that point he had his first set of x-rays since the original injury 15 years prior. They showed that there was no longer any disc at L5, and diseased discs at L4 and L3, with arthritic spurs about all three vertebral bodies.

At that point in time he began a series of prescribed devices designed for immobilization of the lumbar area, beginning with corsets with steel stays and ending with a fiberglass cast

231

that he could strap himself into daily. He also began back-strengthening and stretching exercises, chiropractic adjustments, and still required medications as well. And he had stopped all activities because of pain.

For six years he managed like this, having frequent radiologic examinations, and living on three classes of medications. He was in daily pain and had no activities outside of his medical practice. He was offered a lumbar fusion but feared surgery.

At this point he decided to see what environmental medicine could do for him. Workup revealed he had predictably 3 types of triggers: [1] foods (red meat, wine, and nightshades), [2] chemicals (formaldehyde and natural gas), and [3] nutrient deficiencies (magnesium and manganese deficiencies). He learned how to compensate for the food and chemical sensitivities and corrected the nutrient deficiencies. He now has been pain-free for 5 years, and has been able to resume all prior activities and uses no medications, and has had no surgery.

Let's look at some of the most prominent lessons to be learned from this approach. First, acute pain in the back serves a useful purpose to tell us to allow it to rest and heal. But **chronic pain** for years later after healing should have been complete, **serves no useful purpose.** There is no teleologic reason I can think of to have to endure pain 20 years after an injury. The body should be able to heal this sort of thing.

There must be something perpetuating it. And usually the **target organ** for environmentally-induced symptoms is an **area of weakness or previous damage.** Indeed scar tissue can disturb the flow of not only lymphatics but energy meridians. So in essence, flair of old injury sites usually indicates current (nutrient) imbalances and allergic intolerances, not something you "have to learn to live with".

232

Numerous studies show that many individuals with arthritis and body pain have hidden food sensitivities. For back pain and arthritis, red meats and the nightshade family are particularly common. The nightshades include potatos(including soups and breads made with potato water or modified food starch), tomatos, all peppers,(red, yellow, green, jalapeno, pimento, etc.), cayenne, chili, eggplant, paprika, curry, MSG, and tobacco. As you see, the generic term "spices" can hide many nightshades. And the hooker is that for many, no relief comes until the diet has been totally free of all of these for at least 6-12 weeks. So you can appreciate why if someone gives them up for a couple of weeks and sees no improvement, that he could easily be convinced to abandon the diet and indulge in his favorites again, never to discover the culprit.

You will also recognize that for many, steak and potatoes, pizza or hamburg and fries with catsup are the backbone of the diet. But some people are fortunate in that hidden food sensitivity is their only trigger, so they can do a specifically structured elimination diet to identify the food and that is all they need to accomplish to be pain-free.

Others have nutrient deficiencies that serve several mechanisms. For example, government studies show the average American diet provides only 40% (less than half) of the RDA for magnesium. One of the symptoms of magnesium deficiency is unopposed muscle spasm. If the back is an area of previous damage and becomes the target organ, that's often where the spasm is or pain shows up when someone is deficient.

If the spasm is due to magnesium deficiency yet is undiagnosed and the spasm is treated with muscle relaxants, then the magnesium deficiency goes undetected and can eventually exacerbate. Perhaps the next target organ will be the coronary artery smooth muscles and angina will begin, or arrhythmia, or

233

it can precipitate one of the newer "unexplainable" syndromes like chronic fatigue or sudden death.

There are several problems still to be overcome, once magnesium deficiency is entertained. For example, the choice of tests to assess magnesium status; for commonly the least sensitive test is used, the serum magnesium, leaving an erroneous impression. A loading test is optimum, but rarely performed. Another example of common pitfalls is that intracellular manganese deficiency is also quite common. Furthermore, if it is undiagnosed and uncorrected, it may inhibit magnesium from correcting, regardless of how much is given.

Some individuals are so magnesium depleted that they require an intravenous dose of magnesium to jump-start the system, so to speak. Others need a liquid magnesium solution because they do not assimilate magnesium efficiently from tablets and capsules due to digestive inadequacies.

And, of course in addition to the magnesium deficiency causing spasm, a deficiency of it in the xenobiotic detoxication pathway can lead to the inability to detoxify chemicals as well as the normal person; this in part is what creates chemical sensitivity. So as an example, one nutrient deficiency can cause spasm directly, it can lead to chemical sensitivity whereby a chemical exposure can cause the spasm, and if the proper test is not done or the companion nutrients are not tested, then the deficiency can be unidentified or uncorrected and go on to cause even additional and sometimes fatal symptoms.

As the individual starts to have less pain by eliminating some of the hidden foods that trigger pain, he no longer endures constant pain. And as he uncovers hidden nutrient deficiencies that also perpetuate his symptoms, the symptoms now begin to be intermittent rather than chronic. Once they are intermittent,

234

it makes it easier to identify the most difficult of all triggers, chemical sensitivity.

Provocation tests, both intradermally and in a booth, as well as measurement of body stores of undepurated(undetoxified and harbored) xenobiotics can give an indication of chemical sensitivity or inability to metabolize these foreign substances. But once the total body burden of stressors (i.e. unmasking of hidden food sensitivities, correction of nutrient deficiencies) has been reduced, often the chemical sensitivities can be diagnosed without needing any tests.

For example in this patient, he was then able to realize that for years, after he had been in shopping malls for an hour or more, he had marked exacerbation of his back pain. Also when helping out with the cooking in the kitchen with the gas burners and the oven going (as well, they had gas heat) that he would get a flare of his pain. These exposures brought on even more dramatic pain once he began to simmer down the other triggers (a phenomenon known as unmasking). This new knowledge caused him to reflect on how previous exposures had mysteriously worsened his symptoms, when he was unaware of the connectedness.

Eventually he began to appreciate how much the total accumulation of stressors (their dose, duration and intensity) determined the threshold at which his symptoms would worsen. And the major advantage was that it taught him how to keep his pain quiet by addressing the total load or total body burden of stressors contributing to his symptoms.

It is well-known now that non-steroidal anti-inflammatory drugs increase intestinal permeability and can cause the leaky-gut syndrome. This hyperpermeable gut in turn allows the passage of larger food molecules than usual into the blood stream. Since these are foreign to the immune system (never having been encountered before) an antibody response can be mounted in which case food allergies mysteriously appear seemingly overnight. As well, antibodies may be made to bowel flora. And the target organ for any of those antigens may be the musculo-skeletal system or be totally different, thereby introducing a new set of symptoms to the patient.

If the development of food-induced symptoms were not enough, often the hyperpermeable gut is defective in its ability to handle nutrients (damaged mineral carrier proteins), and deficiencies begin which of course eventually may cause a deficiency in the function of the xenobiotic detoxication pathways; hence, chemical intolerances begin as well. As with the example of undetected magnesium deficiency, you can begin to appreciate how the sick get sicker as the processes snowball. And we haven't even begun to explore how an inflamed gut can contribute to increased chemical sensitivity by the mere fact that the majority of the body's cytochrome P-450 detoxication enzymes reside in the intestinal lining, an area whose function is compromised if the gut is inflamed.

Once more the burgeoning era of molecular medicine has enabled man to begin to identify the deficiencies and triggers and get rid of symptoms rather than merely masking them. The cost effectiveness of this form of medicine, worthy enough as it stands alone, pales in comparison to the increase in productivity and improvement in quality of life, as any of us who have suffered chronic low back pain can attest. Once more environmental medicine demonstrates a recurring theme, that when everything else has been ruled out and your back is against the wall, it behooves you to look at what the specialty of last resort can offer.

Many patients who were signed, sealed and ready for surgery, instead opted to try to find a cause for their symptoms, and were successful. They never did have surgery and they are free of pain. They realized that **an old injury should not make us forever dependent on the pharmaceutical industry.** Chronic back pain should not be a motrin deficiency. Like myself, they could not see why God would create such a magnificent piece of biochemical equipment as the body, only to have it dependent upon drug companies for function.

And, of course, the proof of the pudding has been that with **principles of good clean air, food and water, the body can heal** an incredible array of problems. These are **God-given remedies** that anyone should be able to acquire. It is merely a sign of our warped times that we have made them such unusual and difficult commodities to acquire.

RESOURCES

Bjorenson K et al: Effect of nonsteroidal anti-inflammatory drugs and prostaglandins on the permeability of the human small intestine. GUT 27:1292-1297, 1986

Brostoff J, Challacombe SJ (eds.): FOOD ALLERGY AND INTOLERANCES. WB Saunders, New York, 1987

Ebringer A, et al: Antibodies to Proteus in rheumatoid arthritis. THE LANCET 305-307, Aug 10, 1985

Ebringer A, et al: Klebsiella antibodies in ankylosing spondylitis and Proteus antibodies in rheumatoid arthritis.
BR J RHEUM 27 (suppl II):72-85, 1988

Kjeldsen-Kragh J et al: Controlled trial of fasting and one-year vegetarian diet in rheumatoid arthritis. THE LANCET 338:8772, 899-902, Oct 12, 1991

Panush RS: Food-induced ("allergic") arthritis: clinical and serologic studies. J RHEUMATOL 17:291-294, 1990

Prescott L: Magnesium deficiency: A new risk factor for sudden cardiac death. INTERN MED WORLD REP 5:9, 18, 1990

Rea WJ, et al: Magnesium deficiency in patients with chemical sensitivity. CLIN ECOL 4:1, 17-20,1986

Rea WJ: CHEMICAL SENSITIVITY, VOLUME I, CRC Press, Boca Raton, 1992

Rogers SA: Diagnosing the tight building syndrome. ENVIRON HEALTH PERSP 76:195-198, 1987

Rogers SA: Unrecognized magnesium deficiency masquerades as diverse symptoms. Evaluation of an oral magnesium challenge test. INTERNAT CLIN NUTR REV 11:3, 117-125, 1991

Rogers SA: Chemical Sensitivity: Breaking the paralyzing paradigm, part 1. INTERN MED WORLD REP 7:3, pp 1,15-17, Feb 1-14, 1992

ibid, part II, 7:68,pp 8,21-31, Mar 15-31, 1992

ibid, part III, 7:8, pp 13-16,32-33, 40-41, Apr 15-30, 1992

Seelig CB: Magnesium deficiency in hypertension uncovered by magnesium load retention. J AM CLIN NUTR 8:5, 455, ABS.113,1989

Singh RB, Cameron EA: Relation of myocardial magnesium deficiency to sudden death in ischemic heart disease. AM HEART J 103:3, 399-450, 1982

Sullivan JG, Krieger GR: HAZARDOUS MATERIALS TOXI-
COLOGY. CHEMICAL PRINCIPLES OF ENVIRONMENTAL
HEALTH, Williams & Wilkins, Baltimore, 1992.

HEAVY METAL TOXICITY

One important cause of many people's total load and resultant
symptoms is heavy metal toxicity. What are **heavy metals?**
Metals are some of the oldest toxins known to man, and they
come from many sources. They come (as do most all toxins)
from the air, water, soil and food. They are chiefly the
combustion products of fossil fuels.

For example, **lead poisoning** or toxicity can result from exposures to lead based paint, hair dyes, and auto and industrial
exhaust. It can cause anemia, toxic encephalopathy (abnormal
brain function, poor concentration, thought process, and
memory, lowered I.Q., depression) abdominal colic, and many
other symptoms. In fact, these minerals or metals are great
masqueraders because they can mimic just about any symptom
imaginable, including cause or potentiate cancer.

Cadmium is another heavy metal, also coming from auto
exhaust and industrial exhaust primarily, and cigarettes. It is
well known for its ability to cause kidney damage and high
blood pressure. **Aluminum** is another well-known heavy
metal which can be obtained not only from exhausts but
cookware, deodorant, beer, soda and food cans, prescribed
antacids, and even hemodialysis or "kidney machines". It is
well known as a cause of Alzheimer's presenile dementia.

Arsenic comes mostly for pesticides, herbicides and cigarette
smoking or second hand cigarette smoke. **Mercury** can come
not only for industrial exhaust and incinerator exhaust, but

items such as dental amalgams, Preparation H, and the old calamine teething powder, (it's a common preservative in many prescribed injectable medications and immunizations) plus fungicides and seafood. It too, can cause any symptoms from headache to bloody diarrhea to multiple nervous system disorders and many other symptoms.

Why are heavy metals important? Mainly because they can **cause any symptom** and they are rarely thought of or looked for because there are really no good diagnostic tests for chronic heavy metal poisonings. **Fatigue** is probably the number one symptom because many of these heavy metals sit in the enzymes, on the membrane and inside the mitochondria where energy is synthesized inside cells. Also these **heavy metals** will **displace good minerals** such as zinc, magnesium, manganese, copper, iron, etc., **and sit in the enzymes in their place.** When they do so, **the enzymes are no longer normally functional.**

How does one know if they have heavy metal toxicity? Not so easily. Because these metals accumulate slowly over a period of many years, toxicity is rarely expected unless there is a large acute poisoning. Fatigue, numbness and tingling or paresthesias, abdominal pain and other body pains, headaches, bizarre palsies or nerve disorders and difficulty walking or ataxia, poor I.Q., poor ability to think straight, confusion, depression, panic, kidney damage, immune system damage, and cancer are just some of the many symptoms that can accrue from heavy metal toxicity.

How is it diagnosed? Right now heavy metal toxicity enjoys a diagnostic status similar to that of nutritional deficiency and chemical hypersensitivity. Even though it **can masquerade as nearly any symptom, it is rarely considered.** Blood and urine tests are much too gross and only reflect abnormality if the exposure has been exceedingly large and over a very short time but just recently. But for the average case, heavy metals accumulate in very small amounts over a period of many years and it's only when the amount becomes appreciable, that symptoms start occurring.

As heavy metals are accumulated over the years, they leave the blood, so that they are no longer measurable there, and they start compartmentalizing. Some have a predilection for kidney tissue, such as cadmium, others are predisposed toward going primarily to the bone, such as lead. But this does not mean that this is where it always goes. It depends much upon the individual susceptibility. Many people have healthy enough bodies that they are able to ward off heavy metal toxicity. As with any disease, there are multiple factors influencing the susceptibility.

Some factors are obviously exposure time, dose and duration. Others are genetics, lifestyle (whether someone smokes or not, hobbies), diet, the nutritional status of the patient, the total body overload of this metal, plus the home, occupational, and leisure environments.

For example, a person who has higher levels of vitamin C, will not absorb cadmium and lead as easily as someone who has low levels. Likewise, a person who is deficient in zinc will absorb cadmium much more readily.

Hence, we have another indolent cause of "undiagnosable" symptoms. We have metals that are in the air, food and water most all of the time, and can cause just about any symptom. But because they do so slowly, over a period of ten to twenty years, they are not afforded the attention that an acute exposure is, and yet, for example, arsenic can cause chronic dermatoses, cardiac disease, chronic upper respiratory infections, periph-

241

eral neuropathy, anemia, liver disease, and Raynaud's phenomenon. And it can cause chronic fatigue because it uncouples oxidative phoshorylation, otherwise known as the main chemical reaction in the body of energy metabolism.

Cadmium, for example, which someone in the electroplating or galvanizing industry, or someone who works with color pigment paints and batteries would have an exposure to, can cause various forms of kidney disease leading to the need for dialysis or anti-hypertensive medications. It can cause emphysema, it can cause amino aciduria or **loss of amino acids** in the urine which then can go on to cause numerous symptoms from **chronic fatigue** to **chemical sensitivity** or **toxic brain syndrome.**

Cadmium toxicity can also cause **cancer of the prostate**. It has a half life in the body of 30 years and one cigarette provides one to two micrograms of cadmium. Other sources of cadmium are industrial exhausts, but incinerators provide a majority of it. Fifty to 75% of the body burden is in the liver and kidneys, so it will rarely show in a blood test. **Lead is the most ubiquitous** toxic metal and the one that has probably been studied the most. It's toxic to most living things. Food is the major source for exposure, then air and water. Lead comes from auto exhaust, industrial exhaust, soldered linings of food cans, pains, and many foods, and 90% of it collects in the red blood cell. With time, more of it then is deposited into the bones, as well as kidneys and brain and other nervous tissue. It can be responsible for **hyperactivity, attention deficit disorder** and a **low IQ,** it can cause **peripheral neuropathies or foot drop or wrist drop.** Among the U.S. cities with the highest lead levels in the city drinking water is Utica, New York, right in our own backyard (USA TODAY, 1993).

And as for **mercury**, no other metal better illustrates the diversity of symptoms that it can present as, and it has a particular affinity for brain and kidney tissue. Inside a cell it binds to enzymes and causes cellular injury and death. It can result in bizarre tremors, gingivitis, abdominal pain, bloody diarrhea, ulcers, ataxia, visual disturbances, it inhibits the chemistry of the brain, even before there are any other signs of poisoning. Many people have had remarkable healing of resistant conditions after having replaced their silver-mercury amalgam tooth fillings with composites, for example (Kolata G, New suspect in bacterial resistance: Amalgam, NEW YORK TIMES., C1, Apr 27, 1993).

Aluminum is known to be associated with increased neurofibrillary degenerate tangles and brain degeneration and progressive encephalopathy, as only seen in **Alzheimer's** presenile dementia, as well as **convulsions** and other symptoms.

In essence, heavy metal toxicity has been known since before 200 B.C., but it is only now, as we are entering the era of molecular medicine, that we are becoming interested in finding the causes of diseases and so heavy metal toxicity is now being investigated. Before, medicine was mainly interested in finding drugs to cover up the symptoms of diseases. Now in this modern era, we are more focused on finding the causes, so that we can get rid of the diseases and not have to rely on medications. In other words, a headache is no longer a Darvon deficiency.

An inexpensive medication, and its dose, used for heavy metal toxicity will be explained in Chapter 8.

Much of the above information is from CASSARETT'S AND DOULL'S TOXICOLOGY, Klaassen CD, Amdur MO, Doull J, eds, 3rd edition, McMillan & Co., New York, 1986.

243

HOW TO DIAGNOSE HEAVY METAL TOXICITY

The original meaning of the word chelate (pronounced key' late) is a claw. Hence a **chelating drug is like a claw.** It is taken for the express purpose of **grabbing onto a substance that you want removed from the body and dragging it out through the detoxification system** of the liver and disposing of it through the bile and into the gut or into the urine. Small amounts can also be depurated through the sweat, tears, menstrual and breast and mucous secretions of the body as well as hair.

A major problem with most chelators, is that they remove more than just the drug, mineral, chemical or metal you want. They also cause the loss of many important minerals. So a physician who has training in chelation is mandatory for this. For he must know really the chemistry of detox and all the nutrients of the body. If you feel unsure, as always there are simple little tests you can give to assure yourself that the physician in question is in the same ballpark as you.

For example, you could ask what minerals are lost or jeopardized when you give or take too much zinc. The answer is many minerals, but the most commonly affected are iron, copper, molybdenum. The way in which you are answered is also important, for if it is as though you are a real pain for asking, it makes me wonder if this doctor really likes intelligent patients, which you are much better off being.

Anyway, there are many types of chelators, and they all have their own problems, and uses. Some chelators are better for some heavy metals, while others are preferred for different ones. So it depends on what you are trying to get rid of. Often, however, you don't even know what it is you are toxic with or what needs removing or chelating.

The best way to find out is a trial of a chelator. The basic theory is logical: You obtain a 24 hour urine collection and have it analyzed for heavy metals. Be sure it includes lead, mercury, arsenic, cadmium, and aluminum at least. Then you take 2 days of a chelator, chosen for what you suspect you are looking for and doses according to your weight and liver enzyme status.

On the 2nd day, you collect another 24 hour urine for the same heavy metals and see what the difference is. If you put out twice as much mercury, for example, it is a good sign that your body was harboring excessive amounts of stored mercury and that you might be considerably healthier once you got rid of this burden and enzyme paralyzer.

Halstead BW, THE SCIENTIFIC BASIS OF EDTA CHELA-TION THERAPY, Golden Quill Publ., Box 1278, Colton CA 92324, 1979.

PARKINSON'S DISEASE AS AN EXAMPLE OF A HEAVY METAL TOXICITY DISEASE

Parkinson's disease is an example of the nasty symptoms that can occur with heavy metal poisoning. Serious neurological diseases like multiple sclerosis and Parkinson's disease are noted for their steady progression to a point of no return. You can slow down the progression of the disease, but you usually cannot reverse them. Often times there is evidence that in some cases, heavy metal toxicity is one of the damaging causes.

Remember, when metals get into enzymes they severely damage their function in many ways. Some people have aluminum toxicity from years of aluminum cookware, especially if they had highly acidic food from this cookware such as coffee or spaghetti. Worse, many have exorbitant levels from years of aluminum antacids for stomach troubles, or buffered (with aluminum) aspirins for joint disease. Aluminum is another cause of Alzheimer's (McLachlan DR, Crapper DR, et al, Would decreased aluminum ingestion reduce the incidence of Alzheimer's disease?, CANAD MED ASSOC J, 145:7, 793-802, 1991).

Of course, many **pesticides** do their damage not only by the very nature of the pesticide itself, but also by the incorporation of heavy metals such as arsenic into the pesticide, and this adds further to the damage. Parkinson's disease is one such disease where they are finding increasingly more evidence of multiple environmental triggers. Pesticides seem to be one of the sneakiest yet most damaging of causes for many "incurable" neurological diseases like Parkinsons's. And, of course, many prescription drugs have as a known side effect, Parkinson-like symptoms, since chemicals that overload the detox system often show up as damage in the nervous system.

As well, it is well known by researchers that people with Parkinson's (and many other diseases) have abnormal activity of the detoxification system and its enzymes, which is certainly what one would expect. For low levels of nutrients in the detox pathways initially would serve to make one more vulnerable to damage of the system when exposure to a heavy metal or metal-containing pesticide occurs.

Then once the damaging substance is in the system, you would expect it to consume or waste more detox nutrients in the work of trying to get rid of the stuff. But even worse, some of it eludes the detox chemistry and **strongly attaches to enzymes and regulatory proteins, acting like a monkey wrench** in a delicate clock mechanism. And when the enzymes paralyzed by the metals are in the detox pathways, we are in real trouble. For in addition, the detox capabilities of the body are now further compromised for other chemicals that formerly caused no problem; so the **spreading phenomenon** occurs (Where the SICK GET SICKER).

And it will come as no surprise to those of you who have read about E.I., that Parkinson patients have a 60% deficiency in their detoxication pathways as compared with normals, since impaired detoxication and nutrient deficiency are common precipitating factors to most diseases.

 So, **the worse the disease, the more the total load must be taken into effect** and a checklist for the total load will never be complete because we keep adding new chemicals, heavy metals and problems to our environment (irradiated foods, leaky atomic reactors, etc.).

References:

Semchuk KM, Love EJ, Lee RG, Parkinson's disease and exposure to agricultural work and pesticide chemicals, NEUROLOGY 42:1328-1335, July 1992.

Steventon GB, et al, Xenobiotic metabolism in Parkinson's disease, NEUROL 39:883-887, 1989

Editorial, Parkinson's disease: One illness or many syndromes?, LANCET, 339:1263-1264, May 23, 1992.

Armstrong M, Daly AK, Cholerton S, Bateman N, Idle JR. Mutant debrisoquine hydroxylation genes in Parkinson's disease. LANCET 339:1017-1018, 1992.

NEVER UNDERESTIMATE THE IMPORTANCE
OF A TINCTURE OF TIME

Besides organization, a commitment to getting well, and support from a loving spouse, friends or relatives, another important part of healing is to appreciate the **time** it takes to heal. I remember so well when my attorney girlfriend was healing her leukemia the second time. She was religiously following her carnivore diet this time and suddenly about after 9 months, everything just clicked into place. She was well, she looked wonderful, she had a glow about her, boundless energy, and her counts were normal. We would gallop through the woods on horseback, carefree as children, a dangerous thing to do for a leukemic if we were not absolutely sure that she was well.

Yet that 8 or 9 months of steadfast religious plugging away at the program was one of the most important parts of getting well. Just imagine if you were nurturing a little plot in your garden and you went out and haphazardly watered it once a week without checking on it or weeding it. What do you think your chances of growing good vegetables would be? But if you begin by checking on it everyday, clean out any weeds, see if it needs water, check the soil pH (whether it is too acid or alkaline), make sure the soil is the most fertile possible and nurture it along, you will have the best crop possible. The same should be applied to the body.

A major part of the total load is **consistency.** And somehow we need to appreciate that there is a **period for healing** that requires much **dedication to persevere.** I have seen people die who had kicked death in the teeth against all odds. Some of them did it more than once. Then they suddenly lost the perserverence, the consistency, and let it all slide. In some circumstances being able to control cancer breeds a cockiness where you feel that it was almost too easy, or that the disease can be turned on and off any time you want.

For cancer victims, this is just not so. You only get so many chances. Try not to let yourself get so bored or cocky that you go off your program, thinking it will be a breeze to duplicate. When you have something that works for you when nothing else did, stick with it. Consistency and time are two more components of the total load.

FOOD ALLERGY AND GLUTEN-SENSITIVITY CAN MIMIC MANY "UNDIAGNOSABLE AND INCURABLE" DISEASES

In chapter 4 you learned about the leaky gut. One of the many things that can inflame the gut and cause the leaky gut syndrome, which then goes on to cause all types of diseases, is unsuspected food allergy. The strange thing that many do not understand is that THE LEAKY GUT CAN CAUSE FOOD ALLERGY, AND FOOD ALLERGY CAN CAUSE THE LEAKY GUT. Once leaky, then this can go on to cause any number of **auto-immune** diseases like arthritis, colitis, thyroiditis, etc. Now you can begin to appreciate that **the health of the gut is tantamount to a healthy body.** And anyone who is constipated, has spastic colon or other bowel disorders is just like an accident waiting to happen.

Food allergy that anyone can diagnose can manifest as hives after strawberries, for example. But the outside skin is not the only organ. In fact any part of the body can be the target for food allergy, including **our inside skin lining, the gut.** Commonly missed food allergy symptoms are chronic fatigue, arthritis, migraine, visual problems, chronic cystitis, chronic vaginitis, mood swings, hyperactivity, learning disorder, asthma, and much more. Food allergy can also manifest with the gut as the target organ, as in ulcerative colitis.

249

Some people are highly sensitive to **gluten.** Gluten is a protein part of some types of grains and non-grains. Gluten is particularly high in **wheat, rye, barley** and **oats.** People who are sensitive to gluten (actually the **gliadin**) in these grains have a bizarre reaction when they eat even 1/2 of a spoonful of anything that has even the slightest amount of it. But the most bizarre part of this sensitivity is that most people who have it are totally unaware of it. And they would never guess that it could be the cause of their chronic fatigue or depression or colitis or arthritis, or a myriad of other incurable symptoms.

For the gluten-sensitive, there can be serious reaction in the intestine where the absorbing surface is damaged. You recall from chapter 4 that crucial absorption takes place on this surface through its covering of finger-like projections, called **villi.** As much as 75-99% of the surface area can be so damaged that it severely compromises the absorption of precious vitamins, minerals, amino acids, essential fatty acids, in other words, all the nutrients necessary for a normal functioning body.

Furthermore, gluten-sensitivity makes the gut even more inflamed and leaky so that now the body makes antibodies to all sorts of intestinal bacteria and chemical additives in foods or anything that leaks through. This is in part how the body makes **auto- immune diseases.** For some of these antigens on intestinal bugs are similar to antigens on our own tissues in the body. Therefore once an antibody is made to a particular substance, and leaks across the gut wall into the blood, it then attaches to body tissues that have the same types of receptors, or similar appearing antigens.

But once our antibodies are attached to our cells, it causes a **chain reaction** of chemicals being released (like histamine) that then go on to causes any symptom, from swelling to pain and itching. And if the damage is in the cells of a particular organ, like the kidney, then it appears predominantly as a kidney disease. But if it is in a tissue that goes to every organ, like blood vessels, then you can have hypertension, vasculitis, or again a specific organ damage.

Likewise if the antibody is directed to nervous tissue, then you could have multiple sclerosis, Alzheimer's, neuritis, and paresthesias (pain, numbness and tingling). An example is, many people with certain types of arthritis (like **ankylosing spondylitis**) have antibodies to certain bacteria in the intestine,(Klebsiella is one). It is thought the antibodies to these intestinal bacteria then leak through the gut wall into the blood where they attach to the joint synovial membrane and inflame it and cause arthritis. As well, when the gut is hyperpermeable, the normal barriers do not exist and cancer is more prevalent; and of course when you are nutrient deleted because of poor absorption of intestinal nutrients, that also predisposes one to cancer. So, it's a **downward cycle where the sick get sicker.**

There is an excellent book that I would recommend that you read entitled CAN A GLUTEN FREE DIET HELP? by Lloyd Rosenvold, M.D. (published by Keats Publishing Inc, 27 Pine St, Box 876, New Canaan CT 08480-0876).

In here you will see that **Celiac Disease,** which is what **gluten sensitivity or gluten enteropathy** is called, can masquerade as anything from fatigue to depression to irritable bowel to MS (multiple sclerosis) and much more. One of the problems is that it is extremely difficult to avoid gluten because it is one of those hidden antigens.

Besides being in anything that contains **wheat, rice, barley or oats,** and sometimes **buckwheat** and **millet** (depending upon how sensitive the person is), it's in anything that says it has

modified food starch or MSG or just plain **spices**. It can be in prescription medications as a binder, filler or bulking agent. It can be in vitamin tablets, it can be in sausages and textured protein meat extenders and substitutes, as well as in canned meat. It can be in imitation cheeses and malt extract which is used in many beverages as well as foods. It can be a hidden ingredient in ice creams, catsup, mayonnaise, instant coffee, whiskeys, and much more.

As you see from this list, to avoid gluten you would practically be on a macrobiotic diet or at least a diet of whole foods such as the carnivore diet. You can begin to see how many of the healing diets of the world overlap.

As the author points out, many celiac victims also have a concomitant lack of the enzyme **lactase** which breaks down milk sugar, and do very well avoiding milk. As you recall, milk and wheat are among the commonest antigens in the American diet to produce symptoms, so merely avoiding those helps many people feel better.

So, you can see that we have come full cycle in avoiding many of the things that we began teaching people to avoid two decades ago. But at that time we were merely trying to help them figure out their possible food sensitivities. Now you can appreciate that these principles can carry you much further in your quest for wellness, against all odds.

That's why I reiterate again, that if you are serious about getting well, you need more than this solo book; you need to refresh your knowledge of environmental medicine principles. And if you are going to diagnose some of your own 21st century environmental sensitivities, you must know a great deal, as no doctor is going home with you to figure out what is wrong there. Fortunately, as many people can verify, once you know these facts and figure out how to get yourself well, it is yours forever.

For example, how could anyone hope to be clearing their cancer, for example that might have been triggered by heavy metal toxicity if they are still using aluminum pots and pans and cooking with aluminum containing baking powder. If they have not read, they will not know all the "nitty gritty' about healthful eating.

If they do not know how to make normal bowel flora and to have the bowel checked so that they can be sure they have the good types of bacteria in the bowel for optimal function, then they do not have as good a chance of healing. For example, if the bowel is inflamed, then there may be an impairment of the **sucrase** enzyme which breaks down sugar. So, everytime the person eats anything with sucrose (ordinary table sugar), he can have all sorts of undesirable symptoms, because the body is not able to properly break this down. He may even erroneously blame the problem on Candida.

The intestinal bacteria also have a role in making or synthesizing certain vitamins such as **vitamins K and B12**, and if you have too much yeast for example, then you can have elaboration of the enzyme **thiaminase** which actually breaks down and destroys thiamine in the gut, even before it gets absorbed. **Thiamine or vitamin B1** is necessary for the energy pathways. So, you can see how convoluted and how important it is to have a healthy gut as one of the multiple entities that must be addressed when looking at the total load.

There is an antibody test for gluten, but I would consider a trial off gluten as much more reliable. Also, there is an in office test of **malabsorption** that can be done called the D-Xylose test.

D-XYLOSE TEST

Purpose:

The purpose of the D-Xylose test is to check for intestinal malabsorption. Many people do not absorb their nutrients from food and supplements properly because of a variety of problems in the intestine. This can range from actual cancers to allergies, to immunoglobulin deficiencies, Candida overgrowth, parasitic diseases, amyloid, blind loop syndrome, radiation poisoning, gluten enteropathy or sensitivity, intestinal dysbiosis, and much more.

Contraindication to doing the test:

There are no known contraindications to this test, however we know that anyone can be sensitive to anything at anytime. It is also not known whether it can cause fetal harm, so therefore you should refuse the test if you are pregnant.

How to do the test:

1. Be fasting for 8 hours including no water.

2. Bring at least 250cc (ml) or one cup of your own tolerated water. If you are not sure, Mountain Valley or another non-carbonated, non-chlorinated glass-bottled mineral water will do.

3. When you arrive at the office for your designated test time, empty your bladder and then the nurse will dilute the xylose in your water. (Xylose is like a sugar that the body makes. It is not related in any way to xylene, a damaging everyday chemical.) You drink the entire amount quickly and then a blood test is drawn at 1 hour and 2 hours. You will not have

anything to eat or drink additionally during that time. We collect urine for 5 hours during the test as well. After the 5 hour urine has been received, you are free to go and eat and drink whatever you want. The lab will analyze the results and then we will be able to more definitively tell if you have any absorption problems effecting your health.

So, you can see that sensitivity to one tiny, little fraction of the wheat kernel can leave the gut inflamed and cripple the chemistry of the body. And as you will read in the gluten book, it is a diagnosis that is often missed. When we see how important the total load is, you can understand why we are loosing the war on cancer, because medicine not only fails to routinely look for correctable biochemical defects and environmental triggers, but it does not address the total load very often, especially in cancers or any other serious diseases.

Part of the problem is because of our infatuation with labelitis and also our decision to divide medical men up into specialists where one takes care of uteruses and breasts, the other one takes care of bones, another one takes care of lungs, another one takes care of the right kidney and one takes care of the left kidney.

There couldn't be a sillier approach to medicine, because the only person left who takes care of the whole body (the Generalist), does not have knowledge of environmental medicine and nutritional biochemistry either. So he can't deal with the total load (Epstein SS, Bingham B, Ral D, Bross ID, Loosing The "War Against Cancer": A Need For Public Policy Reforms. INT J HEALTH SERV:455-469, 1992, and Meyerskins FL Jr, Coming Of Age—The Chemo Prevention Of Cancer. NEW ENGLAND JOURNAL OF MEDICINE 323:825-826, 1990).

SILENT PESTICIDE POISONING
CAN RUIN YOUR LIFE IN A DAY

If I had to pick one chemical class that has **caused the most E.I.,** and some of the most severe cases, it would be **pesticides**. As a class of chemicals that possesses multiple diverse structures, they were initially manufactured for chemical warfare. So they are **anti-life, biological poisons** to begin with. As usual, there are multiple reasons why they can be so dangerous, yet permeate every aspect of our environment.

(1) Most were synthesized over 50 years ago, **with minimal or no tests of safety.** In spite of Rachel Carson's SILENT SPRING and a multitude of activist groups over the decades, the testing has been meager, and when carried out, done by the chemical companies' own laboratories. When the EPA set a time limit years ago by which these should be corrected, it was never followed up on. We are still waiting for the tests, but meanwhile the pesticides continue wide use (and high profits). And since the chemical companies now have even more financial resources and stables full of attorneys, ethical efforts move even more slowly these days.

(2) Most people think that the worst ones have been removed from the market. But, as an example, you can get DDT in the states, and in fact I have patients with abnormally high levels of it after their offices were sprayed!

(3) The most carcinogenic pesticides that are not allowed in the U.S. are still made here, and sold to third world countries. We in turn buy their winter produce for consumption. Ironically by their use of our illegal pesticides, they can undercut our own produce markets.

(4) Because they are such nasty chemicals, **the body often does**

not have detox mechanisms to metabolize them. So as second best, they are stored in tissues just to get them out of the blood stream where they are more dangerous. Usually they are stored in the fat, where they slowly leak out to cause perpetual damage in some individuals.

(5) Once they are stored in the tissues, they are even more **difficult to detect and get rid of.** Sweating and weight loss (as in the healing phase of the macrobiotic diet where you diet off most of your fat) are the best ways, taking weeks at best. Meanwhile, the longer they persist, the more damage they do and the more they compromise detox nutrients and pathways.

(6) They can **mimic any symptom,** but the commonest target organs are the brain, gut, and nervous system. Headache, personality change, nausea, cramps, numbness and pain are common, and almost always accompanied by fatigue.

(7) The kinetics or chemistry can break many rules. For example, small doses can cause more **harm to the immune system** in some studies than large doses (Olson LJ, Erickson BJ, Hinsdill RD, Wyman JA, Porter WP, et al, Aldicarb immunomodulation in mice; and inverse dose-response to parts per billion levels in drinking water, ARCH ENVIRON CONTAM & TOXICOL, 16:433-439,1987).

(8) They can sit in hormone receptors of the body, as in estrogen receptors on cell surfaces and cause silent **infertility** (Choudhury C, Ray AK, Bhattachary6a S, Bhattacharya S, Non-lethal concentrations of pesticide impair ovarian function in the freshwater perch Anabas-testudineus. ENVIRON BIOL FISHES 36 (3): 319-324, 1993, and Cummings AM, Replacement of estrogen by methoxychlor in the artificially-incuced decidual cell response in the rat. LIFE SCI 52 (4):347-352, 1993.

(9) There is no question they are **carcinogenic**. A front page article in the WALL STREET JOURNAL told of one man, Mr. Latimer, who pesticided his lawn one day, mowed it the next, and had chronic symptoms for the next 6 years that no one could diagnose or treat. And within a few months of the pesticiding, he developed testicular cancer. A major problem was that he had also been on the stomach drug Tagamet at the time of the pesticide exposure. And this drug, as do many prescription drugs, ties up many of the enzymes that metabolize pesticides, thus increasing their toxicity dramatically. It is an example of how poorly appreciated the total load is (Allen FE, Lonely crusade. One man's suffering spurs doctors to probe pesticide-drug link,WSJ, CCXVIII, No. 74, pg 1, Oct 14, 1991).

(10) Pesticides can also cause **sudden death**, as the cover article of PEOPLE magazine reported. A young military official was home on leave, golfed on a newly pesticided course, came home and died. When lay publications start reporting this, you know we are in trouble.

(11) Pesticides **can damage enzymes that are necessary for absorption of nutrients**; for example, vitamin A absorption was inhibited after organophosphorus pesticide exposure. But organophosphorus pesticides are always marketed as "safer and relatively harmless" (Ember M, Mindszentry L, Rengei B, Gal G, Changes of vitamin A in blood and liver of organophosphorus poisoned suicides, RESEARCH COMMUNICATIONS IN CHEMICAL PATHOLOGY AND PHARMACOLOGY, 1:4, 561-571, Jul 1970).

(12) Pesticides do not have to be smelled or perceived in any way, but they do **drain the body of priceless detoxication nutrients.** For example, everytime you go in a supermarket with pesticiding, for every molecule of pesticide you silently

detoxify, you lose forever, a molecule of glutathione. And that glutathione cost you many minerals, energy and amino acids to make.

What can you do? **Prevention is the best.** Eat as organically as possible, filter your water, do not pesticide your home or lawn, use your right-to-know laws in terms of what exactly is sprayed at work and school. Often it is done on a contract basis, i.e., no bugs are seen, they just come in and do it for good measure. And fight area aerial spraying.

SHOULD I TAKE HORMONES ?

Hormone deficiencies are an often overlooked part of the total load. So let's look at some of the more common ones that can make a big difference.

THYROID

Most of the time regular thyroid functions are checked, but not all the necessary ones. For example, if you complain of fatigue, usually the T3 and T4 and a TSH are checked. This will show whether you have a gross thyroid lack. But the story does not end here. For example, some people make enough thyroid to make the blood tests look normal, but the thyroid that they make is not of good quality. They have what is called a **conversion defect**. So on paper they look normal; but feel tired all the time, have constipation, put on weight easily, and are always cold when everyone else is warm.

This is where a trial of thyroid comes in handy, because if you feel like you've been reborn once you take it, you obviously need it. Sometimes the need is only for a short while, as the nutrient deficiencies get corrected, for example. Then the gland starts making a better quality of thyroid again, and you no longer need it. But it serves to sort of jump-start the system.

Some chemically sensitive people make antibodies that attack their own thyroid. This makes it function erratically. One day you may feel hyperthyroid: nervous, edgey, like you want to jump out of your skin, aimlessly snapping at everyone, diarrhea, exhausted, and hot when everyone else is cold.

On another day when the thyroid is functioning below par, you have the exact opposite, with symptoms of hypothyroidism With hypothyroid function, you can be so tired it's a struggle to get out of bed, and you don't know how you are going to do anything once you do get out. Then on a day when you go the doctor's office, the thyroid function can swing back and be normal for a few days. It is enough to make everyone doubt your sanity, to be sure. But a measurement of **thyroid auto-antibodies** will pinpoint the problem.

And some who are known to be hypothyroid need predominantly T3 but they are on a prescription that is predominantly T4. Some, because of a copper deficiency, for example, cannot adequately convert T4 to T3. Others deserve a trial of thyroid regardless of tests, since it is rediculous to think we know it all.

So if you suspect thyroid problems, especially if there is a family history of it, be sure you are getting all the proper tests.

ADRENAL HORMONES

The adrenal gland makes a hormone, **cortisol**, whose lack can also make you very tired and more chemically sensitive, have difficulty with blood pressure control, and much more. The body does not store cortisol, however, but it must make it on demand. Obviously then, during times of stress to the body, mental or physical, more hormone synthesis is required. Surgery, chemical reactions, a stressful life and worry raise the demand, also.

The problem is that some people have a normal cortisol level on standard blood test, but the gland does not rally upon demand. In other words, in response to the stresses just mentioned, the adrenal is lazy and does not make enough of the extra hormone demanded. The result is the person feels wiped out by little things. The only way to diagnose this is with the cortisol stimulation test, and all the details and directions are in TIRED OR TOXIC ?

Another adrenal hormone deficiency that can also make one tired and more chemically reactive is **DHEA, or dehydroepiandrosterone.** The problem is that if someone does think to check it, often the wrong one is measured. You want an **unconjugated DHEA,** not the sulfated DHEA (one more arena **where you need to see the lab result yourself** to be sure the correct one was done). Then there are only a few pharmacies in the U.S. that carry it once you have identified the defect. This, too is often not needed forever. But as the body heals, the adrenal often heals as well, and starts making enough of its own.

DHEA prescriptions are available from Wellness Pharmacy 1-800-227-2627 and College Pharmacy 1-800-748-2263 and The Apothecary 1-800-869-9160.

TESTOSTERONE

This male hormone is made by the testicles and the adrenal gland. Many pesticides and other airborne chemicals experienced in daily life, as well as many prescription drugs like some antihistamines and anti-fungals can lower it. It, too can make a man fatigued, depressed, have poor libido or sex drive, as well as many other symptoms.

But because it is made in small amounts by the adrenal gland, you guessed it. Women also need it. You can have too little (poor libido) as well as too much (acne), as with any hormone.

ESTROGEN

Often women are advised to take estrogen to avoid post-menopausal osteoporosis. But by now you should be too smart to fall for that reasoning. For there are many people who suffer the increased risk of cancer by taking estrogen, only to end up with osteoporosis anyway. Likewise, there are many women who do not take it and never have osteoporosis. You will recall that **osteoporosis is a problem of not having the proper trace minerals in the system to hold the calcium in the bone.**

No one can pretend to treat osteoporosis without knowing the status of your intracellular (rbc) copper, chromium, manganese, zinc, molybdenum, etc. And you must have a magnesium loading test (directions in TIRED OR TOXIC? and the paper we published on it is in the back of THE CURE IS IN THE KITCHEN). For without proper levels of these minerals, the calcium you take cannot be incorporated into the bone. Instead it is put down in the arteries of the brain and heart and accelerates arteriosclerosis and aging.

If God had wanted us to take estrogen the rest of our lives, wouldn't He have implanted Premarin under our skin or something? What if you are poor, or live in a third world country? And yet if you are eating a diet of organic grains, greens and beans, grown on good soil, and following many of the healthful practices we have written about, your chances of getting osteoporosis should be vastly reduced.

I'm not saying there is no place for estrogen. That would be absurd. Some women are extremely depressed, exhausted, have a dry painful vagina, or wicked hot flashes, or a particularly scarey family history of severe osteoporosis. But never just take estrogen and consider the problem solved. Sometimes estrogen is prescribed daily forever. This I feel is wrong, since it is unphysiologic.

The reason it is unphysiologic (does not mimic the way our body chemistry is in nature) is that we do not have only estrogen in our bodies, but several types of estrogens, and progesterone as well to balance the estrogen. Just because a woman has had a hysterectomy is not good enough reason to not give progesterone to balance the estrogen. Many organs, including the brain have progesterone receptors. And more importantly, it is needed to balance out or neutralize the carcinogenic effects of estrogen.

The type of estrogen taken is important, as well. The number one prescribed estrogen is Premarin, which among its 14 ingredients is shellac. Do you need that? There is evidence that there are safer forms of estrogen to take, if you need it. Besides that, if you measure blood levels of a woman on the standard prescribed estrogen therapies, some of the levels are monstrously high. That's asking for trouble. Yet I rarely see a woman who has had levels measured after having been placed on it.

Another important point is that many environmental chemicals, like some pesticides, for example, can block the activity of estrogen, and be a cause of infertility or birth defects (Cummings AM, Replacement of estrogen by methoxychlor in the artificially-induced decidual cell response in the rat, LIFE SCI-

ENCES 52;347-352, 1993).

One place many women are missing the boat is by not putting estrogen on the target organ that could most benefit, rather than putting it in every cell in the body. The use of estrogen vaginal cream has been known for years to help the atrophied (shrivelled and dry) vaginal tissues, but no one puts it on the face. It does plump up the tissues and is worth evaluating if you feel you are prematurely aging visually since menopause. A trial of one month will tell you if it is advantageous. The estrogen is a prescription, but progesterone cream helps many, and that can be obtained in the form of Pro-gest (N.E.E.D.S.).

Punnonen R, Vaajalahti P, Teisala K. Local oestiol treatment improves the structure of elastic fibers in the skin of postmenopausal women, ANN CHIRURG GYNAECOL, Suppl [JC:51p] 202:39-41, 1987

Follingstad AH, Estriol, the forgotten estrogen?, JAMA, 239,1:29-30, Jan 2, 1978

Women's International Pharmacy 1-800-279-5708,
5708 Monona Dr.,
Madison WI 53716-3152

Cooper DS, Halpern R, et al, L-thyroxine therapy in subclinical hypothyroidism, ANN INT MED, 101:18-24, 1984

MELATONIN

We could write a whole book on any one of these hormones, but certainly one of the most interesting would be melatonin. It has strong anti-oxidant properties, anti-carcinogenic, anti-aging, it helps some with jet lag and insomnia, and much more. One important point is that the body makes melatonin in the pineal gland at the base of the brain, mainly when it is dark. In other words, if you sleep in a room that is too light, from a street light, for example, you may not make sufficient.

Pierpaoli W, Yi C, Dall'ara A, Aging-postponing effects of circadian melatonin: experimental evidence, significance and possible mechanisms, INTER J NEUROSCIENCE 51:339-340, 1990

Pierpaoli W, Maestroni GJM, Melatonin; a principal neuroimmunoregularity and anti-stress hormone: its anti-aging effects. IMMUNOLOGY LETTERS 16: 355-362, 1987.

Anonymous, Oxidation strongly linked to aging...but quenched by ubiquitous hormone, SCI NEWS, p 109, Aug 14, 1993

WHAT'S YOUR PASSION ?

The zest for life often stems from a person's passion. You need something that fills you with life, enthusiasm, and the will to survive. Something that when all else is going wrong, buoys you up just to think about it. It centers you, rescues you, relaxes you, focuses your energies, re-kindles your fire. If you don't have a passion, you are usually in trouble with depression, boredom, loneliness, and disease.

Now is a time for some serious soul-searching or even psychotherapy if there is not one thing that fuels you. Of course, your lack of enthusiasm could be biochemical, hormonal, etc. But barring that, take stock in what makes life worth living for you. It can be a hobby, your family, religion, occupation, etc., and the more you have, the better. Then make sure that you reserve proper time for it, for if you don't exercise that refueling, what good is it?

Along with lacking a passion or two, many are doomed for failure because they want to get healthy, but "do not have the time". If you do not have the time for some wellness, maybe you should ask yourself to write down some answers :

(1) What has your life been all about so far?
(2) Is that what you wanted? Still want? Has your goal changed?
(3) If you had 2 weeks, 3months, 6 months, one year, 2 years to live, what would you do differently within each of those time-frames? Is there any of that which you should be doing now?
(4) What was the greatest moment of your life that you would like to relive? What was the worst?
(5) What 3 changes in your life would make you the happiest?
(6) What fears keep you from this?
(7) Whom do you need to forgive? Yourself, as well?
(8) What do you need to do to make your life more complete?

Are you living or lingering? What are you going to do about it?

THE CANDIDA SOLUTION

How could you ever have a book on wellness without including Candida? Because the Candida syndrome is still a major problem for many people. In fact, 15 years after the problem was discovered, many people are still undiagnosed, many who are diagnosed are still not cured, and the majority of the medical profession thinks it is quackery. So let's see what can be done to solve all that, since it is a big part of the total load for many.

266

In 1978, a kind internist, Orion Truss, M.D., was covering for a colleague over the weekend. He was called in by a patient to treat a yeast symptom. A few days later, she called to ask what he had done? Why? Because her years of depression was gone!

He merely filed this away, until another opportunity presented itself. Instead of chaulking it up to two neurotic women, he reported his findings in a medical journal and in a book. But as you know, if it is not discovered by a big pharmaceutical firm or prestigious medical school, you can have the cure for cancer and you won't get anyone's attention.

But a few innovative physicians (you know the type, always looking for whatever it is that they still do not know, always questioning and looking for things that might help their patients) started investigating it and adding to the fund of information as well as making the condition more known to other physicians and patients. Foremost among these was William Crook, M.D., who has done more than any other single physician to spread the information about this condition.

Numerous books have been devoted to it. Physicians who do not know about it slough off patients who inquire by saying, there is no evidence for it. But that is not true. We described over 8 biochemical mechanisms of how it causes all the myriad of symptoms it does, and for the last 6 years, I have taught a 2 hour course (through the American Academy of Otolaryngic Allergy) on over a dozen biochemical mechanisms of the Candida syndrome.

Since there are numerous books on the subject, and because people interested in treating the more resistant cases of Candida are reading this and have most likely read all of the others, we won't reiterate how Candida, a supposedly harmless yeast, can cause just about any symptom you can think of, mimicing

267

diseases from food and chemical sensitivities, to depression, multiple sclerosis, lupus, chronic fatigue, and much more. Nor will we give any of the multitude of dramatic cases that have been turned around by merely treating this yeast. For it is the people who have done all the yeast- free, sugar-free diets, nystatin, Nizoral, Diflucan, etc., and still have the problem, that we are addressing here. But if you never heard of this, I urge you to read.

What causes resistant Candida? **A poor host.** What causes Candida in the first place? **A poor host.** Look at the thousands of people with poor diets sucking down cokes, coffee, donuts, and candy bars on their way to work. But they do not get Candida. Why? Their body chemistry is strong enough to resist it. So one of the major factors is what we call in medicine, **host resistance**, or how strong your body chemistry is to fight off this normally harmless yeast.

Some of the commonest symptoms of people who have recurrent resistant Candida symptoms are recurrent vaginitis, cystitis, colitis or irritable bowel, brain fog, depression, cravings, and chemical and food sensitivities. There are many others, but these are the most common.

First on the agenda of getting these victims well, is to be sure we have defined the problem. For example, many people who think they have recurrent yeast vaginitis, do not have yeast growing in the vagina. They have other organisms, including some very bizarre fungi. Most women have had many cultures and been told nothing is growing. We have solved that problem.

First be aware that all gynecologists, all doctors, and all hospitals, when culturing for yeasts, generally use Sabauroud's media in the petri dish. We published a paper a decade ago in the ANNALS OF ALLERGY showing that if you use a different media, you pick up 30% more fungi. Then we found another problem. When we would culture a body part and send the plate to the laboratory to have the fungus identified, they would have the report back to us in a week. But it takes 2-4 weeks for many of these slow-growing fungi to grow. Hence we have made available the special agar plus directions on how to do a culture and incubate it at home until the fungi are grown out. Then it can be sent to the local hospital laboratory for identification. These cultures may be made at home of the vagina, urine, stool, tongue, skin, etc, and are available to anyone.

And while we are on the subject of cultures, many do not clear their yeast vulnerability because there is too much mold and yeast in their various environments. You may send for these same petri dishes or mold plates and expose them in the bedroom and wherever you spend the rest of your time, return them in the mailer provided, and we will identify what fungi are present and to what extent. (The reason we no longer identify the body fungi is new rules regarding packaging of body fluids shipped through the mail would increase the cost too much.) So instead we show you how to obtain your specimen and incubate it at home. Then just have your local doctor write a prescription to have it analyzed at the local hospital. Furthermore, the reason some people never become strong enough to fight off Candida is they are too mold sensitive. To increase their resistance, they need to stimulate the body to make antibodies against not only Candida, but scores of other molds, some of which cross-react with Candida and which are in the everyday environment (more details in TIRED OR TOXIC?).

For others, the gut is actually full of other pathogens, not Candida. Or it does not have good digestion and assimilation of nutrients in order to make the gut mucosa more resistant. For example, **vitamin A** is essential for mucosal integrity and the ability to resist colonization by foreign pathogens or organisms. But if the **pancreatic and other digestive enzymes** are deficient, then one cannot absorb enough vitamin A. Likewise, if there is a **zinc deficiency**, they cannot convert the vitamin A to a useable form in the body. Here is where a **stool analysis** and pancreatic enzymes may do the trick. Some have such a gut full of yeast, that the Candida makes thiaminase, an enzyme that breaks down thiamine, vitamin B1, before it even gets absorbed. In these cases, a colon cleanse is useful.

For many, they are just not playing with a full deck. They have so many **nutrient deficiencies**, that the body has poor defenses in terms of resisting Candida. They need, bare minimum, the magnesium loading test, and rbc tests of manganese, copper, zinc, molybdenum, chromium, selenium, and potassium.

But when assessing minerals, be sure that plasma, serum and whole blood analyses are not done; for they will usually be falsely normal, due to homeostasis. As well, these people have deficiencies of **amino acids, essential fatty acids, vitamins, accessory nutrients** (like carnitine), and **hormones** (like DHEA). For example, if over-whelming **cravings** trigger symptoms, more than likely the person is **chromium and manganese deficient** for starters. Some need to fast to figure out that certain foods or chemicals trigger their symptoms, and all need the proper diet for their metabolic type. For those who have limited foods that are tolerated, food injections often save the day. For others, a lifestyle that encourages **eating out** frequently is what **keeps them from getting well.**

You are beginning to get the picture: **the total load is the only way to diagnose your way out of any 21st century disease** and to improve your host resistence. Common things I see that were overlooked were a home with too high a chemical overload, or a whole town, for example, where industrial exhausts and pesticides overload the individual too much to allow for recovery. For some the total load includes unhappy relationships, lack of a creative passion, dental amalgams, body burdens of pesticides, heavy metals, and other chemicals that are locked in the system and inhibiting wellness.

Some have used anti-fungal medications for so many years that they have fostered the growth of yeasts that are difficult to identify and resistant to anti-fungals. For these victims, the only way out is with the **total load: making the body so healthy, that it is able to fight off any organism.** The bottom line is, if you are spinning your wheels trying to rid your body of an incurable Candida condition, it is time to **forget about Candida and find what part of the total load is really missing.**

TOTAL LOAD CHECKLIST

Nobody in their right mind would presume to be able to make a comprehensive checklist for environmental controls, because we are constantly polluting ourselves, synthesizing new chemicals, and we are constantly learning. Likewise it would be impossible to make a totally comprehensive list for the total load. Because each person is highly individually unique, you never know what crucial and seemingly insignificant, little thing will make a big difference in unloading them and start to enable them to properly detoxify and heal.

It may be something as simple as taking **sodium alginate** for one week every month when they are off the vitamins to detoxify a heavy metal or making sure they do not sleep on a mattress that out-gasses formaldehyde, fire retardant and pesticide, etc. Every time we attempt to make a simple book

271

that addresses the needs of many, we end up with the same problem: explaining things for those who are the exceptions. Probably the reason is because I specialize in seeing the exceptions, the "rejects", the undiagnosable, the untreatable, the outlyers (from the bell-shaped curve of "normal"), the impossible to heal.

The strange thing about the total load is that each of the individual parts can seem too minor alone. I remember when I was totally unknowledgeable about the total load, I thought all the environmental controls(and especially any diet changes) were a waste of time and that I need not do them. I thought I only needed the major part of the program where I knew I had problems. But I cannot emphasize enough **that the more you pay attention to the total load of environmental triggers, the faster are your chances of healing. It is the sum of all this attention to detail that finally unloads the body enough to heal.**

I guess you could liken it to directing a symphony with scores of members in it. What difference would it make if just one player was off? Or what difference would it make if you removed just one member of the woodwind section, like the oboe? It would make all the difference in the world to the final performance. All of the rest of the members can be the best players possible, but with either of those too seemingly little errors, you change the whole nature of the result.

Or say you gash open your arm. Your urge is to get it sutured so that it can stop the bleeding and heal in the closed position. But if the surgeon does not take care of the total load and scrub the area, you could get such a rip-roaring infection that healing would leave a disastrously ugly scar or you could get a brain abscess from the infection. Or if you were not concerned with the total load, you might forget ice and elevation for the first

272

few hours, thus getting prolonged bleeding, maybe even a massive hematoma or blood clot. Or maybe a piece of the clot would float to another area of the body and choke off its blood supply. Or if the doctor forgot about the tetanus part of your total load, you could die from lockjaw. So you can see what trouble we can get into by forgetting parts of the total load even with more simple medical problems.

I must emphasize that even though the ideas in here will and have profitted many people who were at a diagnostic and therapeutic dead-end (including myself), there are some who will not be able to do some or any of these things, and a few for whom there is a worsening if they do them. Others will require very personal guidance and individualization, and/or additional modalities that are even too far out for this book, or have been uncovered since the writing of this book. So again, **consult a physician as your guide, and read, read, read.**

A very important point I would like to leave you with. Most people schedule an appointment with an agenda in mind, like going over laboratory results to see what vitamin and mineral levels are low and what should be prescribed. But there is a great deal of merit in periodically **scheduling an appointment to go over your entire program and chart together.** These **brainstorming sessions** are so logical, but are rarely done in medicine. One reason they are rarely done is because people have allowed insurance companies to set the guidelines for medical care that limit each session to problem and resultant drug treatment, with **no time for real thinking and brainstorming.**

But because there is constant new discovery, if you have a tough problem, you should periodically insist on it (and consider scheduling a double visit). Needless-to-say, these brain-storming sessions become proportionately more important with the severity of your illness, or the length of time that you have been at a plateau. For if you are in limbo or at a standstill in your progress, now is the time to take a fresh clean look at ALL the information that has been gathered regarding your system over the last few years. And often the most important information is not any lab test, but facts that come from your mouth, when the right questions are asked.

There is such a constant growth of information that rarely would all the known modalities be looked at for each person; but rather the most commonly beneficial things are looked at first. Most people will clear on specific limited programs and will never need to look further. And so it is cost effective to look at the most likely causes first and leave the more rare possibilities to the end. The problem is that there is such a huge array of possibilities.

But for the person who consistently falls through the cracks, who is not at the level of wellness he seeks, for whom many things do not work, this brainstorming is vital. For **the answer to all illness** lies somewhere in each person's specific **TOTAL LOAD.**

TOTAL LOAD CHECKLIST

I. MOLD

1. mold allergy, skin test for by serial dilution titration
2. expose mold plates
3. environmental controls for mold
4. avoid mold foods in diet
5. Candida program
6. injections for Candida and related molds to strengthen resistence to it.

II. FOOD

1. diagnostic or rare food diet
2. food testing; assess need for injections
3. trial of transitional(macrobiotic) vegetarian or transitional carnivore diet
4. definitely get off sugars and processed foods
5. whole organic foods
6. chemically clean water

III. CHEMICALS

1. test by injection method, or booth, or jar if unsure
2 read copiously
3. do environmental controls
4. assess nutrient levels in detox pathway
5. be sure rest of total load is as low as possible
6. test home and office objects with formaldehyde spot
7. check levels of chemicals and pesticides in blood and or tissues

IV.NUTRIENT DEFICIENCIES

1. check appropriate and select minerals, vitamins, aminoacids, essential fatty acids and accessory nutrients
2. check for heavy metals that can be displacing minerals

V. PSYCHOLOGICAL TOXICITIES AND SPIRITUAL DEFICIENCIES

VI. ELECTROMAGNETIC FIELD EFFECTS

VII.MEDICALCONDITIONS(neveroverlookhypoglycemia, leaky gut,thyroid conversion defects, DHEA deficiencies,

lazy adrenal, etc., etc.)

VIII. OTHER: This category will constantly grow as
we figure out more ways to poison ourselves

Just as there is no limit to the total load, there is no monopoly
on wellness. The techniques here are time-honored, safe,
inexpensive, and have scientific validation; many are natural
or God-given, and logical. Because they have never before
been collated and presented with evidence and explanation
makes this work unique. But there are many other therapies
that have been omitted that have great merit, for sure. I could
not even list them all, but probably chelation and sauna detox
programs would head the list, followed by homeopathy,
herbology, acupuncture, DMSO, H2O2, ozone, etc, etc.

HOW TO AVOID DYING IN THE HOSPITAL

With all you know now, you have guessed it, the hospital can
a dangerous place. Studies abound showing poor nutrient
quality foods and nutrient deficiencies galore. Other studies
you have learned show remarkable improvement in patients
who are supplemented versus those who are not. And as you
have seen referenced, it is often a matter of life and death.

Again, I will use magnesium as an example, because it is in over
300 enzymatic reactions, the 2nd most abundant intracellular
cation in the body (next to potassium), and the average person
gets less than 1/2 the recommended amount in a day.

**First, if you are sick enough to be in the hospital, you sure
ought to have a magnesium loading test.** First, it may be
therapeutic as well as diagnostic, and could even save your life!
Many studies of injections of magnesium (that were less than
the RDA) that were given to every other heart attack victim, left

a far greater number of those who received them on the opposite end of the grave than those who did not. Even a scant 54 mg of magnesium (less than 1/8th of that needed in a day) resulted in a 44% survival versus 33% in another group. And this was discovered quite by accident. You see, they were studying the effects of one 325 mg aspirin a day on its ability to ward off a heart attack by keeping the blood slightly anti-coagulated. But they could not figure out why the American study had an increased survival of 33% vs 44% for the British. The difference? The Americans were using a buffered aspirin....buffered with a puny 54 mg of magnesium.

There are no classic signs for magnesium deficiency, but surely you want to know your status BEFORE any cardiac surgery, since there is a high rate of fatality for post-operative arrhythmias, and most have a magnesium deficiency component. Certainly any complication, lung problem, respiratory distress, asthma, and heart complication like cardiomyopathy (which just means "we don't know what in blazes is wrong with the heart"), poor healing, depression, fatigue, cardiac failure, use of any medications and I.V.'s (since they all use magnesium in metabolizing them), pain, seizures, etc.

As one researcher said, there are so many blatantly positive double-blind studies, that it is "perverse to demand further placebo-controlled trials" (placebo trials are those in which some of the patients would get "dumby pills" or nothing, for comparison with the other trial patients who got the "real " thing that is being studied). And he is right. It is **unconscienable** to overlook magnesium deficiency in any patient in this day, with the preponderance of over 30 years' evidence. There were 25% fewer deaths in one month's time in one hospital study alone, and they were only giving one of 40 nutrients! Let's face it: it is malpractice not to assess magnesium status properly.

277

You may also want to know that you have the legal right to see your chart in the hospital. It is also a good idea to have a list of medications that were prescribed for you by your bedside. For $25, you can buy a PDR which lists all the side effects and decribes what the pills look like physically, in case you are given the wrong medication. It is no longer easy to be a patient, and it certainly should not be a passive ordeal, since **your life depends on your knowledge as well.**

I know you cannot be your own doctor, but there is a great deal you can do. By merely reading this, you know a myriad more facts than any other doctor you will encounter for a long time. For you now have entered the 21st century of molecular medicine where a cause is sought, rather than merely covering up symptoms with drugs. Never give up hope, just because someone in authority tells you to. And do not forget the total load. Any one (or multiple) part of the package could be the predominant cause of your problem.

Take for example, a 24 year old woman who had very intense chronic pain that had stumped her physicians. Another study found the same problem with 4 elderly patients. The cause (and treatment) of all their pain? A simple vitamin D deficiency. And these cases were published in 2 very prominent medical journals over 2 years ago, yet I have never seen a patient with chronic pain whose records showed that someone thought of ruling that cause out (Gloth MF, et al, Can vitamin D deficiency produce an unusual pain syndrome?, ARCH INTERN MED, 151:1662-1664, 1991; Chalmers J, Vitamin D deficiency in elderly people, BRIT MED J, 303:314-315,1991).

And do not let any surgeon touch you who does not at least, bare minimum, assess your rbc zinc and rbc copper. How does he know how well you will heal if even half the populus is low in at least one of these? And he should do a magnesium loading

278

test to be sure you don't die of an arrhythmia on the operating table.

And never forget that mood is part of the total load, as a study showed that laughter improved the cells in the immune system (Sakazar SA, et al, The immunologic effects of laughter, JOURNAL OF ALLERGY AND CLINICAL IMMUNOLOGY, 89:1, Part 2:267/abstract 489, 1992) The smarter move would be to consult a nutritionally-trained physician 4 months prior to elective surgery. Then you will have time to correct your deficiencies, and who knows, you may end up not even needing the surgery!

A mere smattering of the available evidence:

White RE, Hartzell HC, Magnesium ions in cardiac function: regulator of ion channels and second messengers. BIOCHEM PHAMACOL (1989) 38: 859-867

Woods KL, "Fletcher S, Roffe C, Haider Y, Intravenous magnesium sulphate in suspected acute myocardial infarction: results of the second Leicester Intravenous Magnesium Intervention Trial (LIMIT-2). LANCET (1992) 339: 1553-1558

Schwieger I, Kopel ME, Finlayson DC, Magnesium reduces the incidence of post-operative dysrhythmias in patients after cardiac surgery, ANESTHESIOLOGY (1989) 71: A1162. Abstract

Fanning WJ, Thomas CS, Roach A, Tomichek R, Alford WC, Stoney WS, Prophylaxis of atrial fibrillation with magnesium sulfate after coronary artery bypass grafting. ANN THOAC SURG 1991;52:529-533

Aglio LS, Stanford GG, Maddi R, Boyd JL, Nussbaum S, Chernow B, Hypo-magnesema is common following cardiac surgery, J CARDIOTHORAC ANES 1991;5:201-208

Hennekens CH, Peto R, Hutchison GB, Doll R, An overview of the British and American aspirin studies, NEW ENGL J MED 1988;318:9230923

Angomachalelis NJ, Titopoulos HS, Tsoungas MG, Gavrielides A, Red cell magnesium concentration in cor pulmonale: correlation with cardiopulmonary findings, CHEST, 103:3. 751-756, 1993

Webster PO, "Dyckner T, Magnesium in cardiac failure and diuretic treatment, MAGNESIUM (1986) 8:204-209

Angomachalelis JN, Titopoulos SH, Kazakou K, Panigyropoulou A, Spyridakis J, Red cell and plasma magnesium correlation with radionucleotide myocardial imaging of 'cardiomyopathy' in sarcoidosis. SARCOIDOSIS, 1989; 6(suppl 1):105

Zaloga GP, Chernow B, Pock A, Wood B, Zaritsky A. Hypomagnesemia is a common complication of aminoglycoside therapy. SURG GYNECOL OLSTET 1984; 12:146-147

Whang R, Oei TO, Watanabe A, Frequency of hypomagnesemia in hospitalized patients receiving digitalis, ARCH INTERN MED 1985; 145:655-656

Surawicz B, Is hypomagnesemia or magnesium deficiency arrhythmogenic? JACC, 1992; 268: 2395-23402

Altura BM, Altura BT, Carella A, Gebrewold A, Murakawa T,

Nishio A, [Mg.sup.2+]-[Ca.sup.2+] interaction in contractility of vascular smooth muscle: [Mg.sup.2+] versus organic calcium channel blockers on myogenic tone and agonist-induced responsiveness of blood vessels. CAN J PHYSIOL PHARMACOL 1987: 65: 729-745

RESOURCES:

Books about Candida:

Crook WG, CHRONIC FATIGUE SYNDROME AND THE YEAST CONNECTION, Professional Books, Inc., Box 3246, Jackson, TN 38301 1992, ph 901-423-8366

Also Dr. Crook's foundation has a wealth of resources: International Health Foundation, Inc., Box 3494, Jackson TN 38303

Rogers, SA, THE E.I. SYNDROME, 1986, Prestige Publ, Box 3161, Syracuse, NY 13220, 1-800-846-ONUS

Rogers SA, TIRED OR TOXIC?, 1990, ibid.

Laboratory for tests of intestinal dysbiosis and the leaky gut: Great Smokies Diagnostic Laboratory
    18A Regent Park Boulevard
    Asheville, NC 28806
    1-800-522-4762

Source for special mold plates for home and body culture: Also use this address for the formaldehyde spot test (one $40 vial tests over 100 objects in home and office for excessive formaldehyde out-gassing):

Mold Survey Service
Box 2716
Syracuse NY 13220-2716

For an excellent television quality video on chemical sensitivity, suitable for PTA, church, business, and groups:

write: Robin Kormos   (212)460-8921
      149 Avenue A
      NY,NY 10009 $17 (includes S +H+Tax)

For the Central New York HEAL group newsletter or help with environmental illness: Eleanor Hathaway
                      Dorthy Drive
                      Syracuse, NY 13215
                      (315)492-0091

For Dr. Wm J. Rea's catalogue of products for chemical sensitivity: American Environmental Health Foundation, Inc.
      8345 Walnut Hill Ln
      Suite 225
      Dallas Tx 75231
      1-800-428-2343 or (214) 361-9515
      Fax (214) 691-8432

Other books and articles of interest:

Hunter BT, CONSUMER BEWARE, YOUR FOOD AND WHAT'S BEEN DONE TO IT, Simun & Schuster, Rockefeller Center, 1230 Avenue of the Americas, NY NY 10020 (1971)

Hunter BT, THE MIRAGE OF SAFETY: FOOD ADDITIVES AND FEDERAL POLICY, The Stephen Greene Press, Fessenden Rd., Brattleboro VT 05301, 1975

Rea WJ, Liang HC, Effects of pesticides on the immune system, J NUTRIT MED 2:399-410, 1991

Rea WJ, CHEMICAL SENSITIVITY, Lewis Publ., CRC Press, Boca Raton FL, 1992

Walker M, Frankenstein food, TOWNSEND LETTER FOR DOCTORS, 118:422-425. May 1993

Tate G, Mandell BF, et al, Suppression of acute and chronic inflammation by dietary gamma linolenic acid, J RHEUMATOL 16:729-733, 1989

Arlien-Soberg P, SOLVENT NEUROTOXICITY, CRC Press, Boca Raton FL, 1992

Manhattan SE, TOXICOLOGICAL CHEMISTRY, 2nd Ed., Lewis Publ., 121 S. Main St, Chelsea MI 48118, 1992

Kaloyanova FP, El Batawi MA, HUMAN TOXICOLOGY OF PESTICIDES, CRC Press, Boca Raton FL, 1991

Sullivan JB, Kriger GR, HAZARDOUS MATERIALS TOXICOLOGY, Williams and Wilkins, Baltimore, 1992

Di Fabio A, THE ART OF GETTING WELL. RHEUMATOID ARTHRITIS CURED AT LAST!, The Rheumatoid Disease Foundation, PO Box 360, Fairview TN 37062, 1988.

Chapter 7
THE FAITH FACTOR
Spirituality

Have you noticed? There is something pretty scarey going on in the world. Murders are no longer the exclusive property of gangsters, mobsters, muggers, thieves, gilted lovers and residents of Cabot Cove. Murders of innocent people are becoming epidemic. I picked up one Sunday paper at random. It reported 8 murders of innocent people in the last week in public places where you would never dream of seeing someone with a gun, much less being killed yourself: restaurants, courthouses, movie theaters, hospitals, real estate and doctors' offices.

But this is exactly what we should see, given that the brain is the number one target organ to suffer:

(1) We have more nutrient deficiencies than ever before, due to food selection and processing.

(2) We have people hyped up on coffee, sugar, Nutrasweet or Equal, and dyes in sodas and fast foods.

(3) We prescribe anti-depressants, tranquilizers, amphetamines (Ritalin), and mood elevators that have abnormal effects in the brains of some people,

(4) We are exposed to more mind-altering chemicals in our air than at any other time in history, and

(5) These serve to further lower nutrient levels, leading to increased alterations of mood, thought, personality, and actions.

(6) In an era where we have an overwhelming amount of

scientific data on undetected nutritent deficiencies as being part of the cause of many illnesses, plus the indisputable loss of nutrients with the use of medications,still medicine does not routinely search for them. Needless-to-say, they have a bearing on the function of the brain.

(7) And we are daily exposed to numerous chemicals, many of which are lipid soluble, which means they make a bee-line for the brain. And many victims do not possess as healthy detox systems as they need to metabolize these chemicals and remove them from the brain in a timely fashion.

If this were not enough, we no longer discipline children in schools, and worse, we have undervalued religion by removing the right to even pray in school. Without religion, there is no accountability. As teachers tell me, kids intentionally break rules, only to defiantly tower over the teacher with hands on hips, asking, "And what are you going to do about it?"

You know the world is feeling the pressure when in one month, 3 of the books on the best seller list (for the first time I can ever recall) deal with these issues: Thomas Moore's CARE OF THE SOUL, Bill Moyers' HEALING OF THE MIND, and C. Scott Peck's A WORLD WAITING TO BE BORN; CIVILITY DISCOVERED.

And religion and spirituality are certainly among the last subjects I ever thought I would get involved in. My childhood background in them, as typical as it may be, is pretty sparse.

My Daddy made us 7 children gather around the table after dinner at night and memorize the 23RD PSALM. We went to Sunday school occassionally as kids, but I don't remember learning a great deal. In high school, because of my gift of a coloratura voice, I went to church to sing in the choir. Then after

I got married I didn't set foot in a church again for 23 years until we were at the christening of a friend's child and we were the God parents. That doesn't mean that I am not religious, in fact, I don't know how anyone could be agnostic if they knew anything about science. Just look at any part of the body.

Look at the intricacy of the genetic structure of the DNA helix and you know there is a power with infinite wisdom and planning, or look at our detox pathways that we are struggling to research, understand and explain. Somebody up there knew we were going to poison ourselves in the 21st century and so He had a mechanism in us to detoxify chemicals that were just synthesized yesterday!

Aside from that, when I had severe brain fog with my severe chemical sensitivity, I totaled 5 cars. Each time I heard people ask as they surveyed the wreckage, "Did anyone live?" I literally walked away from each one unscathed. In addition, numerous other times throughout my life I felt the hand of God reach down and gently rescue me by the scruff of my neck.

A decade ago, a few days before doing a television show on formaldehyde, I was coming up a blind hill on a curve on a busy main two-lane highway. Suddenly my truck took wings on the wet October leaves during the first snowfall. It spun around, flipped, and landed upside down in the culvert, never to be driven again. I squeezed out the window and walked away without a scratch. And those of you who have followed the other 5 books know what my truly greatest gift of all from God has been through all of these years (Luscious).

But there were several circumstances within the last few years that ignited my quest for more knowledge about God, and brought me to a spiritual level that I have never before experienced. One day my attorney girlfriend, who had become Born

Again, turned to me and said "Granted you and I struggled a lot to pull me out of trouble twice when the oncologists said there was no hope. Twice you turned off my disease, once when I was given 3 months and again when I was given 48 hours to live. But now that I am free of disease, do you truly think that it was all totally the programs? Don't you think that God had a major part in this as well?" As usual, she gave me a lot to think about. And, as I filed it away in the back of my mind, it kept playing over and over in my head when I least expected it.

Then another one came along. I saw a patient one day reading a book, A SCIENTIFIC APPROACH TO CHRISTIANITY by Faid. That book just seemed to call out to me, so I called Sacred Melody bookstore and had them mail me a copy. It turns out it was a true story by an agnostic scientist in his forties who had developed cancer. He was told by his doctors that there was no effective treatment for this type of cancer and it was known to be aggressive and fast growing. His wife, who was a devout Christian, went off and prayed for him with her friends for several days.

After that, the scientist's physician came into his hospital room one morning and announced "I am totally embarrassed. I don't know how to explain it; don't ask me any questions, but your cancer is gone. You may go home". This was enough to pique the curiosity of the scientist. He reasoned that if God were that powerful, there should be enough scientific proof of His existence. And in this book I think he did a splendid job in doing just that, proving the existence of God.

Like he says, once we know that it is not a fairy tale, it is not just a comfortable myth, then it truly becomes the most important thing in life. It takes precedence over all else, and it dramatically shifts all priorities and perspectives. It becomes totally

287

logical that the top priority should be to read the BIBLE and to learn of God's spoken word.

At the same time I read Charles Coleson's BORN AGAIN. As you recall he was the attorney who was President Nixon's right hand man. Those books started me on an intensive quest for knowledge as I read through C.S. Lewis' books, the BIBLE, Billy Graham's books, as well as several other books about the evidence for God. When I had read the rest of Colson's books, scores of others of diverse nature followed.

I realized I had a tremendous lack of knowledge, and was determined to do something about it. I also had a million and one questions as well as a basket of arguements. But having been in private practice for over 23 years, I can emphatically state that I have seen many medical miracles through prayer. When you have something that is a serious illness that is interfering with your life, it certainly makes sense to try to find out what message is to be gained by this and to tap into the infinite healing powers of God's universe.

I admit, I had a tough time relating to the BIBLE for a long time and it just did not make sense. However, my wonderful attorney girlfriend saw the need that I had to understand, and she bought me a student BIBLE which has explanations scattered throughout. Later on, for a Christmas present she gave me the BIBLE on audio-tape, which also helped. Then we explored the Christian book stores together, and found numerous books that go into further discussions of the various books of the BIBLE, and we would spend hours there.

As well, there are many fellowship groups, most likely your church has one, where people learn together about the word of God and grow as they help one another understand the language and to interpret what was really meant. In this day when we have strayed so far, explanations are more necessary.

Having spent many years studying various types of psychology and psychiatry in medicine, it appears to me as a physician that the best psychological system in the universe is a strong spirituality. It is the most clever psychological system I have ever witnessed, for it provides an answer for everything. And oddly enough, the longer one absorbs oneself in it, the more that is learned, and the more irrefutable it becomes.

As for myself, the more I learned, the more appalled I was that I had been so ignorant for so long. And naturally, my perspective on those who had been more knowledgeable has made a 180 degree change. No small wonder that our whole existence, even down to our calendar, holidays and money reflect that God should be first and foremost in our thoughts, guiding us in the most fundamental as well as perplex aspects of our lives. And even if it were not true, it provides the best guidelines for living; so it is actually is a win-win situation. But in this era, with so much emphasis on tangible acquisitions, it is very difficult for many yet to appreciate the far greater spiritual gifts.

By now you all know how paranoid a doctor gets about not having the scientific evidence to convince his or her colleagues that a particular therapy has been proven in the medical literature. So you can imagine my glee at finding this one in Dr. Pearsall's excellent book!   In 1988 a cardiologist, Dr. Randolph **Byrd**, did a clever, and very well- thought out study that was fault-free, in a coronary care unit in a San Francisco hospital.

One group of 192 patients were prayed for by Roman Catholic and Protestant groups, while the other group of 201 patients was not. Neither the patients, doctors, nurses, nor the families of the patients knew who was in which group.

The results showed that the prayer recipients required five times fewer antibiotics, and had three times fewer complications, and none of the prayer group required a life- support system (Randolph C. Byrd, Positive therapeutic effects of intercessory prayer in a coronary care unit population, SOUTHERN MEDICAL JOURNAL, 81:7, 826-829, 1988).

There are other impressive studies in the literature showing the improved growth of plants that were prayed over versus the relatively stunted growth, or that were fed water that healing hands had impacted. And later I was to discover a whole book of evidence collated by two medical doctors (see Mattews and Larson ref.) They collected numerous papers in the medical literature showing the power of prayer in accelerating or promoting healing.

But anyone will immediately see the value of spirituality in healing when he thinks of the physiology of healing. **The autonomic nervous system** could be thought of as the **automatic nervous system**. For it takes care of many body functions automatically so we do not have to think of them. It regulates the heart rate, breathing rate, the secretion of glands, the blood pressure, and much, much more. It is divided into two types of control known as the **sympathetic nervous system** and the **parasympathetic.**

Like the yin and yang of life, neither is good or bad, but rather it is the balance or imbalance between the two that makes good or bad. Basically the sympathetic prepares us for fight or flight, while the parasympthetic is the relaxing and digestive mode. It is much more complicated than that with lots of overlap, and I have very much over-simplified it. When you are fearful (or angry, anxious, or full of panic), your sympathetic nervous system is in control. One of the things it does is pool much of the blood in the muscles for the "flight or fight reaction". This shunts blood away from the vital organs of digestion and away from many many glandular functions that are so necessary for healing.That's why people heal most in bed?

But when you have a strong spirituality, express gratitude for your blessings, and stop feeling anger for your misfortunes, you relax and shift into parasympathetic dominance. When that part of the nervous system takes over, the glands are secreting, digestion takes place, and healing is facilitated. (Holtman G, Singer MV, et al, Differential effects of acute mental stress on interdigestive secretion of gastric acid, pancreatic enzymes and gastroduodenal motility, DIG DIS & SCI, 34:1, 1701-1707, 1989.

Remember Norman Cousins, former editor of the SATURDAY EVENING POST who healed "incurable" (and genetically determined) ankylosing spondylitis (and it still is taught to be incurable) with, among other things, laughter and happy thoughts to boost the healing endorphins (ANATOMY OF AN ILLNESS). The body has to relax and be in a happy and serene mode and conserve its energy for maximum healing. This principle is merely an extension of the total load. But it also illustrates why outlook and state of mind are so crucial to healing.

FOR GOD'S SAKE DON'T MENTION
RELIGION IN YOUR BOOK!

Now I realize that I am treading on thin ice to mention religion. But by now you must realize that I merely spend the majority of my life searching for more ways for people to get healed. And when I find things that work, no matter how much flak I may receive for stating them, I feel bound to let the secrets out. Hence, regardless of over a decade of denigrating remarks being hurled at me by medical colleagues, I was compelled by the struggles of thousands of people (including myself) to find wellness.

So decades ago I squared my shoulders for the attack and incorporated into my practice chemical sensitivity, then macrobiotics, nutritional medicine, etc. And, with time and much effort, they have all become progressively more understood by the world at large. In fact not one thing has ever been disproven. In fact, as they have all become better understood, they have all gradually become embraced by mainstream, reproven, and thus accepted as their own discoveries.

Anyway, well-meaning friends told me emphatically not to mention religion in this book, but I made a promise to my attorney girlfriend that I would. Just because I am a Christian does not in one way detract from Jewish friends of mine, like Elaine Nussbaum, who cleared her cancer against all odds with macro, her family and her religion. There are multiple religions among just my own friends that I know nothing about. But the important thing is that I have observed that one's spirituality has a beneficial effect on one's healing. And as with other aspects of healing, we cannot ignore something good just because we cannot fully explain how it works. Why even the mechanism of action of over half the prescribed drugs is not even known. But no one seems to care.

And although I have explored numerous books on comparative religion, I now have more questions than I do answers. Look at all the wonderful people throughout the world who are inspired by their religions, whether they be Jewish, Christian, Moslem, Buddhist or any other. I don't even know how many systems there are. But I do know that far too many people attribute a major part of their improvement to their religion or spirituality for me to ignore mentioning it. I think it would be dishonest to omit this. I am only familiar with basically one, my own. And I'm not really knowledgeable about that. So you can imagine my trepidation and humility in writing about it in the face of all these adamant warnings.

One big problem, however that turns many away from religion, I think, is that each religious group thinks they are the only ones pleasing God. WE CANNOT REDUCE GOD TO SOMETHING SO PETTY("the same Lord is Lord of all", **ROMANS** 10:12 **NIV**). In the August 23, 1992 Sunday PARADE magazine (page 8), they stated that 137 million or 55.1% of Americans are Judeo-Christians. Roman Catholics numbered 53,385,998, Southern Baptists 18,940,682, United Methodists 11,091,032,, Black Baptists 8,737,667, Jewish 5,982,529, Evangelical Lutherans 5,226,798, Presbyterians 3,553,335, etc. Do we need to be so divided?

It seems to me that one of the impediments to peace and one of the greatest sins of all of us is to not take steps to draw us all closer as a family. We are all God's children; we all sin, we sorrow, we love, and struggle. It is the sincerity of our faith and works that counts. **The proof of the pudding is how we conduct ourselves in regard to our fellow man.** And in view of our failings, it becomes evident why it is a premiere urging.

Other friends said that religion is a ply to control the masses (I wish I could get them to read Colson, Elliot, and Robertson so they could learn all the evidence to the exact contrary). For on the contrary, without a strong personal religion, I am not sure if we would have the fortitude to resist the idiocy that is constantly thrust upon us by those who really do strive to control the masses. For details of this, I suggest you read Pat Robertson's THE NEW WORLD ORDER.

Not a solitary one of us was put here perfect, much less all-knowing. But in far too many patients, I have witnessed the healing power that a strong spirituality has brought too many times to ignore it. And on the opposite side of the spectrum, I have witnessed some people struggling with all their might to get well, but somehow lacking something. And even when I sensed that a renewed and expanded spirituality might be the turning point for them, I was uncertain how to convey this.

Many people have negative ideas about God, and as a result, they are in emotional and spiritual imprisonment. Others, if I have mentioned it, cavalierly say, "Oh, I'm all set in that department." But are we ever? That is like the doctor that tells you he does not have time to read an article pertaining to your symptoms. He is in essence saying "What you see is what you get. I do not have time for further growth. Since I do not have time to read, I'm as smart as I'm ever going to be". Likewise, **spirituality is a growth process**, not a static entity. There comes a time to bring it to new levels of awareness and application. But that takes study. If spirituality is something that you think would benefit you, or if you feel stuck, please pursue some of the references on your own.

For I am not the only one observing that there is a tremendous connection between spirituality and healing. Even many psychiatrists and psychologists are now incorporating it into their therapies (Williams G, Mind, body spirit, $90-an- hour religion? The trend toward spiritual psychotherapy, LONGEVITY magazine, Oct 1992).

Dr. Bernie Siegel, a cancer surgeon, has done a great deal to help bring the mental and spiritual aspects of healing into play. He has shown how they can be a crucial part of the total load in his book, LOVE, MEDICINE, AND MIRACLES. Likewise, LeShan, in his CANCER AS A TURNING POINT, shows how necessary a passion in life is. And one passion could be to learn more about your own chosen path of spirituality.

FACILITATED HEALING

This brings to mind the studies of healing hands, such those published by Dr. Delores Krieger, Ph.D., R.N. (THE THERAPEUTIC TOUCH, 1979, Prentiss Hall Inc., Englewood Cliffs, NJ 07632). She showed statistically significant changes in the hemoglobin (amounts of red blood cells) of patients receiving hands-on healing touch, as compared with those not receiving it. This suggests it appears foolish not to tap into the universal healing source of energy and utilize it. But to tap into this requires a profound belief. And unfortunatly, as medicine becomes more high tech, it becomes less hands-on. I am very lucky, for in addition to being able to give occassional hugs, I receive hugs throughout the day from patients. I can't tell you how important this is. And I cry with them.

In medicine, in the late 1980's, a new field emerged, **psychoneuroimmunology.** Basically, it rediscovered what your grandmother already knew; that the mind is part of the body and therefore, can influence the functions, and hence the health of the individual. There were all sorts of documented studies showing, for example, that when people are grieving over the death of a spouse, their (immune) T-cells were so adversely affected that these people were ripe for any illness——a heart attack, cancer, whatever. The bottom line is that **what you think profoundly affects your health.**

It is logical, then, that in the face of a life-threatening illness, that the mind should be able to optimize functions as opposed to minimizing them, in order to facilitate healing. So regardless of your chosen religion or spirituality, to develop a solid belief that can lead you to generate beneficial chemistry certainly seems prudent. Consider tapping in to that UNIVERSAL HEALING POWER.

Stress can adversely affect the immune system And when one's life situations exceed one's resources to deal with stress, you can get disease. We have all seen it, for example, in the death of a healthy person shortly after the death of their spouse. But if you have God in your heart, you can have unlimited resources. And neutralizing or balancing that stress can be a major part of healing.

SPIRITUALITY AND E.I. HAVE MUCH IN COMMON

As I think of it, the BIBLE is a great deal like E.I. It is impossible to comprehend for the person who has not invested time to learn it. Look at all the denigrators of E.I. who haven't the faintest glimmer or knowledge of the biochemistry of xenobiotic detoxication. I have a literal box of published medical papers by prominent men and women in medicine who in their slamming comments about E.I. unknowingly demonstrate that they are totally uneducated about this biochemistry. In their defense of their position that there is no such thing as chemical sensitivity, or that most of the symptoms are psychological, they have innocently demonstrated that their lack of knowledge is unfathomable. We may never be on the same wavelength. It would be like trying to teach a 3 year old quantum physics.

The same with the BIBLE. I was just as guilty as the next person, always saying how impossible it was to understand and that I got nothing out of reading it. More than once I foolishly started with good intentions with GENESIS. Of course by the time I reached all the lineage about who begat whom, I was bored and lost and abandoned the project for another few years. It wasn't until recently that I learned that that is comparable to trying to get the best use out of the dictionary by reading it cover to cover.

It isn't until one makes a serious effort to understand anything that he then can benefit from whatever it has to offer. Now I learn something new everytime I read, even parts I've read 3 and 4 times before. Like E.I., it appears to me that we are only ready to assimilate a specific amount and at a specific level at any one time in our development. Likewise, it has vastly changed my perspective of many people, as I understand (and share) their perspective.

Nowadays, if something particularly upsetting occurs, rather than brood over it, I open the BIBLE and just start reading. Often at some unexpected moment within the next 48 hours, tears turn to laughter at three a.m. as it suddenly hits me why this bad or aggravating thing was actually a tremendous gift. I can finally see how searching can lead to a totally opposite and usually healthier outlook.

Man is frightfully limited in his understanding of things in God's universe. And it is so easy to get thoroughly immersed in the materialistic world that is becomes easy to see why so many doubt the mere existance of God, or give spirituality a backseat in their lives. But again, it is so much like environmental illness and chemical sensitivity.

For example, when I first see a person with severe brain fog, he usually has never heard of brain fog. And though he has spent thousands of dollars trying to get well, the thought never crossed his mind that what he eats and the molds he breathes and the chemicals in his environment have a direct cause for many of his symptoms. As he reads and tests and becomes progressively more knowledgeable, he starts to become more aware of the cause and effect.

In a few weeks, he is back in the office exclaiming "I can't believe how much better I feel. And I can't believe how much control I have over how I feel. I have identified so many triggers for the symptoms that I was told I would have to learn to live with. I found that the gas stove gives me severe backache, gassing my car gives me depression, the copier at work fogs me out, and sugar and wheat do the same."

What has happened is that now that he has an **awareness** and **knowledge** about chemical sensitivity and food and mold allergy, it opens up a whole new world of control for him. He realizes **everything has a cause**. And as time goes by and he is learning more, he gets even better at it and hence, happier. He is **no longer a victim** of the world, not knowing when symptoms will attack and leave him debilitated. There is an awareness and control that was not there before.

Likewise, as a person studies the word of God and learns more about of what He expects of us, how He thinks, and how to relate to Him, his world no longer seems so random and unpredictable. And his emotions are not as easily thwarted by the least little adversity. Because here too, there is an awareness that was not there before. And it becomes more pronounced with further education. It changes your whole modus operandi.

But, if a person is unknowledgeable about chemical sensitivity, he thinks it is ludicrous when he hears people say they cannot concentrate (classic brain fog) when they smell certain perfumes. Likewise, when someone with minimal knowledge of God hears someone talk of Him, it sounds strange to him and he brands him as a Bible-toting weirdo. But both are examples of how people can be totally misbranded for severe lack of knowledge on the part of the person doing the branding.

And there have always been those with angry cruel minds like a steel bear trap, with vicious tactics who cannot rest until they destroy the truth and goodness that they see as obstacles to their own agendas. When at a loss, their favorite tool is character assassination, which they are particularly adept at since they have extensive power over the press at many levels. You have seen it many times in many arenas of life. For you can readily recognize some of the pioneers in any field......they are the ones with arrows in their backs.

It brings to mind an article I recently read in a cancer journal reporting on Mexican facilities where some of the techniques in this book are used. They have good track records with serious cancers and other diseases, because they use all of these techniques. And because they are in Mexico, they are not ruled by the FDA and AMA, which in part are manipulated by the powerful lobbyists of the pharmaceutical industry (If you find this hard to believe look at the drugs that have been released "after years of study" only to be found to cause serious liver abnormalities in 6 weeks. Or look at the safety record of supplements, yet the push to make them prescription or off the market).

Anyway, since the Mexican cancer clinics are not under FDA control they use no chemotherapy. They believe in strengthening the system, not poisoning it into temporary submission. So instead, they use juicing, enzymes, coffee enemas, etc.

Well, apparently some doctors went there to see what was going on. As a result, they wrote an article explaining the whole program. Not being very solid characters, apparently, they wrote it anonymously (can you imagine my chances of ever getting an anonymous article published?).

But the real irony of the whole thing was that after they finished relating all the different treatments, they never once addressed the fact that people healed "incurable" conditions that they had been powerless to heal in the states. That part was irrelevant. Whether or not the patient recovered against all odds was not germane to their paper.

They merely related the treatments they observed, stated that there was no evidence for the rationale of using these treatments (hmmm...they must not have done their homework and read the scores of journals cited here), and that these patients were being denied the opportunity of having chemotherapy and treatments by oncologists (Anonymous, Questionable cancer practices in Tiajuana and other Mexican border clinics, CA-A CANCER JOURNAL FOR CLINICIANS, 41: 5:310-319, 1991).

Where do they get the audacity to call themselves scientists and write anonymously? And not to address the most important question of all: Did the treatments work? Their only conclusion was that they were taking money away from people that should be spent on "legitimate" chemotherapy and irradiation. I wouldn't have believed that "scientists" could behave that way if I had not just finished witnessing the same thing happen in my field for the last two decades. The literature contains many articles by allergists saying, do not go to clinical ecologists. The articles do not address the fact of track record, just political bias. They do not mention a thing about getting people back to work, saving money by finding causes, getting them off a lifetime of medications, etc. And yet they blackball our papers, refusing even to print our referenced rebuttals to such rubbish.

Similar and worse atrocities have been carried out against religion. History seems to reflect that the more unknowledgeable someone is about any subject, the more negative things they have to say about it, and with a great air of authority. But if you want to be fair to yourself, learn the historical evidence. For in the words of Pastor Robert Cough of First Baptist Church, Three Mile Bay, New York, HISTORY is HIS STORY.

THE CORROSION AND COLLAPSE OF CHARACTER

As Americans I'm afraid we are standing back and allowing far too many deceptions and atrocities. Many of us have lost our guts; lost the fighting spirit upon which this nation was founded. You can do anything to us and we won't even so much as flinch. We are progressively more spineless, and are losing our spirituality.

You can take away the right to pray in schools, but require grade-school children to watch sex education movies in school that condone homosexuality and condoms. Kids don't have to salute the flag; they can gun down other students, and knife the teacher, but discipline is "old-fashioned".

And when it comes to health, many Americans have been stripped of their health-care freedom without so much as a whimper. 60 Minutes television show (CBS) aired an exposee' on health insurance (November 11, 1990 transcripts available). They gave an example of 2 young people, both under 45, with no prior illnesses who precipitously got cancer. When their health insurances suddenly dumped them, their physicians at a prestigious medical school went to bat for them.

When an all-out legal attack was mounted in their defense, the real tragedy reared its ugly head. It seems that years ago the powerful insurance lobbyists silently got some last- minute legislation passed. What it says is that if you take an insurance company to court for reneging on their promises, and if by some miracle you win (they can afford a stableful of expensive lawyers), you have won nothing. Because what the legislation says is that they owe you no more than they would have originally paid when they started arbitraily and capriciously denying payments ump-teen years prior. They owe no dam-

301

ages, even if you go blind or die as a result of their delay; they owe no interest for holding onto your money all those years, they owe nothing for the court costs, **nothing.**

So it behooves them to jerk everyone around as long as they want. Many will give up, and if you do take them to court, so what! They pay what they should have, but in the meantime they had your money. Anyone who has followed the insurance company performances for the last few decades knows that in general they pay for less and less as their premiums cost more and more. And the magical decisions as to what constitutes science, and what types of treatments should be paid for and which should not, are devoid of basic knowledge of the medical literature and biochemistry. In fact many expensive treatments that are covered have not been adequately studied, and are far from proven, for they have an abyssmal track record. And this includes many forms of chemotherapy.

Meanwhile they cover many expensive drugs, few for which the mechanism of action is known. If you don't believe it, look in the PDR (PHYSICIANS' DESK REFERENCE). It is a book that explains all the prescription drugs. When it comes to how the drug works in the body, the vast majority say "the mechanism of action is unknown".

In the meantime, efforts are still active to remove the nutrients from the market, even though
[1] the need for them is essential to life,
[2] they are depleted by the daily work of detoxication,
[3] they have no side effects if used correctly,
[4] they have been removed from many of the foods, and
[5] there have been no deaths from their normal use, as opposed to many recorded deaths from prescription drugs.

And any nutrient deficiency can serve as an example of how

disease begins. For example, our genetic structure is determined by the order of amino acids on a ladder-type helix. Of course, they get old and worn out, so the body breaks them down periodically to replace old parts and replace them with new. But if, as you have learned, the enzyme that puts the pieces back together appropriately, DNA polymerase, is lacking in zinc, a mistake can be made and a new genetic message can be initiated, like start prostatic cancer developing, or chemical sensitivity, or multiple sclerosis.

Likewise, besides nutrient deficiencies, errors in this process can occur when an inhaled chemical that happens to be in the blood stream at that time interferes with the rebuilding process that day. And indeed, this is how a lot of **chemicals cause cancers** to start developing.

It is known that a mutation or change in the genetics in just one tiny spot can cause diabetes (Reardon W, et al, Diabetes mellitus associated with a pathogenic point mutation in mitochondrial DNA, LANCET, 340:1376-1379, 1992). Likewise, a point mutation from a single exposure to a chemical can cause a defect in the cell that initiates chronic fatigue and poor energy metabolism (Coates PM, Tanaka K, Molecular basis of mitochondrial fatty acid oxidation defects, J LIPID RES : 1099-1110, 1992). I mean we do not have room in one book to put all the evidence and facts.

And did you ever wonder how they get animals, for example, on which to test their cancer drugs? They give many of them only ONE, yes **ONE dose of a chemical to cause the cancer** (O'Connor TP, et al, Effect of dietary intake of fish oil and fish protein on the development of L-azaserine-induced preneoplastic lesions in the rat pancreas, JOURNAL OF THE NATIONAL CANCER INSTITUTE, 75:959-962, 1985). **One dose of a chemical is enough to cause cancer**, but all the chemicals that abound in your food, air, water and medications are fine for you, and certainly have no bearing on your health. At least that is what the AMA would have us believe, as the December 1992 official position of chemical sensitivity is that there is not yet enough evidence for it. And more importantly, it is the repleteness of the nutrients that in large part determines how vulnerable an organism is to any chemical.

Most Americans have lost considerable health freedom, and they do not even know it. They allow their insurance companies to tell them what diseases they can have, how long they can have them, and what treatments they can have. As a physician who specializes in treating the medical problems that have fallen through the cracks, cases that are some of the most difficult to diagnose or treat, I've repeatedly witnessed companies fully reimbursing patients for wrong diagnoses and treatments that had nothing to do with what was wrong with them. But then refuse to reimburse them for the treatment that not only made them well, but continues to keep them well, and gets them back to work for the first time.

Naturally, these erroneous treatments did not help the patients, and often made them worse. But all was paid for with no questions. But when they got well with non-drug therapies, they had to fight like mad to be reimbursed, often unsuccessfully. And here the treatment was less expensive and they were able to work again and pay their premiums!

An example of some of the desperate treatments, one asthmatic was so severe that the board certified allergist treating him prescribed a couple of months of intravenous gamma globulin injections at home to the tune of $27,000. Another gentleman had obvious E.I., but when he went to a doc who specializes in Lyme's disease, he was prescribed 17 weeks of intravenous antibiotics, for the bargain price of $40,000. Neither of these monstrously expensive treatments helped. And those of you who are students of environmental medicine know what the antiobiotics did to the 2nd gentleman's Candida status and his chemical sensitivity and food intolerances. And we all pay for this. Don't ever delude yourself that you don't.

On tonight's news, they tell us the national debt is so high, that it could only be wiped out by having every single family in the U.S. donate $70,000. In the meantime, it increases by $12,000 every second! And without people taking responsibility for health and moral fiber, you know where we are headed. Many have health plans that allow them unquestioningly to have a prescription for a new antihistamine that costs $190 per one hundred capsules, but not for allergy injections that would train the body to make antibodies to turn off the allergy and eventually not need medications (with all their side effects) or injections. And antihistamines do nothing for the allergic fatigue, but injections usually clear it.

DRUG TO "PREVENT" BREAST CANCER
CAN CAUSE LEUKEMIA AND BLINDNESS

There is no limit to what Americans will put up with it appears: The U.S. government is using ten million of your dollars to fund a study on **tamoxifen**, to see if it will prevent breast cancer. It is a form of **chemotherapy** that is being given to over 16,000 women throughout the U.S. in over 270 medical schools. These women have volunteered, and only have to be between the ages of 25 and 65 and have a blood relative who had breast cancer.

There are many problems with this study, however. First, (1) the study ignores the true risk reducing factors like diet, for which there are over 100 articles in the scientific literature just in the last 2 years alone. And second, (2) like all chemotherapy, **tomoxifen actually can cause cancer** itself in a few years.

If you have even the remotest idea of participating, please read SCIENCE NEWS 4/25/92, p.259, and 5/9/92, p.309 first. The article outlines all the other types of cancers that the drug tomoxifen causes, like leukemia, bowel and uterine cancers. And it can **cause** breast cancer itself. It is common knowledge that **all chemotherapy eventually causes cancer** by itself, because of the chemical nature of these drugs being cell poisons and free radical initiators (the process behind all cancers and many other diseases).

You might also like to know that there are studies in the ANNALS OF OPHTHALMOLOGY (21:420-423, 1989) on severe eye toxicity from the drug. On the basis of this, it is calculated that at least **25 healthy women should go blind** from this one side effect of the drug alone. Remember this is 25 healthy women who have nothing wrong with them who are going to go blind, just because they participated in this study.

And this number is an under-estimate, since it is based on the original 113 centers that were going to participate in the study. After it had been under way for less than a year, it expanded to 270 medical centers. I wonder how many of the researchers and doctors administering the study have their wives and daughters use the drug? (SCIENCE NEWS, Vol. 142, 7/4/92, pg. 12)

I had to laugh. They came out with a new 24 hour antihistamine last year, yet there are over 35 of them in the PDR already. It is not like we are desperate for another, but nevertheless, being that the drug industry is the number one profit making industry in the U.S., this drug made the front page of USA TODAY newspaper in August of 1992. When I read the PDR fine print on adverse side effects, it said the side effects of the drug included a significant increase in liver cancer and infertility. And the drug was a mere $190 for a bottle of 100. It is as though we are supposed to think it is worth it. But many have paid prescriptions (with a deductible like $1-5) so they never get to even know what the drug costs. Others have plans that almost force them to buy 3 months' worth at a time, even if they know they probably will only use it for a few weeks in the height of ragweed season, for example.

There is something very rotten in medicine, and it needs to be fixed before more **people needlessly suffer physically and financially.** Prescription drugs released by the FDA are supposed to have years of testing. One of the simplest things to monitor is the inexpensive liver function profile. Yet in the last decade there have been several drugs that came off the market within 6 months of being released because of severe liver problems.

But look at the drugs that had serious side effects that were not removed. Just look in TIRED OR TOXIC? at the nutrasweet story. It is really interesting how a substance that is not only metabolized into methanol (an alcohol that can cause blindness and liver damage), but is also metabolized into formaldehyde (which can potentiate chemical sensitivity and cancer) can become a common ingredient throughout the processed foods industry.

Yet when a Japanese manufacturer of **tryptophan** (through genetic engineering) skipped one important step to save time and money, the result caused a toxic aldehyde to be formed in the bodies of susceptible individuals which caused the eosinophilic myalgia syndrome. Some individuals died. But, once the problem was identified, tryptophan was never returned to the market. And tryptophan is an essential amino acid, in other words it is one that the body cannot live without. It is the precursor to serotonin needed to ward off depression and insomnia. It is also useful in some cases of hyperactivity and much more. And the mechanism of action is known for tryptophan, which is a lot more than can be said for the majority of prescription medications.

Currently, in fact, there are government officials who are working to take supplements off the market. No one knows if they would be prescription then (and cost 10 times more), or if synthetic substitutes (as you read of for vitamin A) would be the only modality available. That means that the natural form would no longer be available, plus you can be sure it would be at least 10 times more expensive. Right now vitamins and minerals have reportedly gone prescription in one northern European country and $3 worth of zinc is now around $50, exclusive of the doctor's visit.

And you have learned in the other works how each year the laboratory value for the lowest acceptable level for nutrients in the blood goes down! And when I called the lab several times to ask how they set the new standard at a lower level, they said they just used the blood they had accumulated in the laboratory (from sick people) to establish the new and lower norms. Yes, we doctors get a yearly notice, for example, saying, by the way, the normal for B12 is no longer 200-900. It is now 160. I called up and asked how they got it. They said they just pooled a bunch of bloods they had lying around and got the new cut-off. When I said, "You mean from sick people ?!?", they saw nothing wrong with it.

Additionally, the scientific governing board that establishes the recommended daily intakes for all the supplements appears to be unaware of a vast body of scientific data. Because, they too, often lower the requirements of certain nutrients, which saves money for the food manufacturing industry (which happens to have powerful lobbyists). The recommended daily need for most nutrients is vastly below what the data indicates, and it is only common sense that most people need more with progressively more food processing and increasing loss from chemical exposures to detoxify. But many levels remain at the inadequate levels recommended years ago, and some have been lowered.

There is no question that there is a serious erosion of health care freedom and consciousness in the U.S. It is under the control of big business, primarily the chemical, pharmaceutical and processed foods industries, which have expensive lobbiests. In many areas, health care is not remotely related to healing, but merely the masking of symptoms with expensive drugs, which must by their very nature promote illness as the neglected cause of symptoms is swept under the rug, only to later surface in another doctor's specialty. In other words it is a system that guarantees that THE SICK GET SICKER, QUICKER (see chapter 5).

It is getting scarey how far from reality and morality we can drift. As we become more complacent and fail to educate ourselves and take responsibility for our health and spiritual growth, we relinquish control to government agencies. Less and less do we stand up for what is right. As Colson and C.S. Lewis have written, without a higher power to obey, there is no accountability for man. And that is what we are witnessing in the "Me" generation. Our forefathers fought for their religious freedom. But you just let them tell you that your kid can't pray in school. This serves to tell your child that what you are teaching at home has no real value. Religion serves to provide a sense of responsibility, accountability, and a strong moral code. You just gave part of that away with hardly a word. And now you are giving away your right to select your own health care, even when you are armed with scientific evidence.

In essence, we need to stop worshipping the false gods of medicine and realize that the **acute care system** that we have is the best in the world. But in terms of **chronic care, we do not know that health comes from the individual taking responsibility, becoming knowledgeable, and taking charge of his diet and environment, which have a major bearing on his health.** And that greater health and economy comes from eating more from God's bounty than from the factory; whole foods as opposed to processed, chemicalized foods.

And this is analagous to our spiritual growth. You know that to be maximally healthy, you cannot turn your care completely over to you doctor, without a care of what you eat or your environment, and hope to get well. Likewise, you cannot just go to church, mosque, temple, synagogue, or whatever, and expect to grow spiritually. It takes reading and a concerted effort. But the pay-offs are tremendous.

In fact, if you are not growing each time you read about the word of God, most likely, you may not be tuned in or really trying. It is analogous to the person who is not tuned in to what effect his diet and environment have on his symptoms. Without really trying, he is oblivious and can see no relavency to his life.

I certainly do not profess to have the answers, nor to tell anyone how they should believe. Heavens! I have too many questions of my own. I can merely relate what many loving patients have taught me: that a strong belief has helped many an individual whether they be Christian, Jewish, Moslem, Buddhist, or any thing else, overcome illness. And there appears to be an urgent need to extend this moral strength to correct our social and medical system ills as well.

WHAT DO WE CALL THIS PROGRAM?

We've noticed that often doctors have egotistically labeled all sorts of programs for themselves. I don't think this program should be any one man's (or woman's) name. Much of this program is God-given. We are returning to common sense, whole foods, organic foods, an awareness of the effects of our environment, clean air and water, and an intensive revitalization as well as detoxification of the body so that it can heal itself. For after all, healing only occurs through nature (which is really God). We are merely returning to more humble means and allowing the body to take over.

Many people can ironically deal with the word nature, but not God. But NATURE IS GOD. In the 1920's, the physicians supporting this type of medicine called it natural hygiene, which is what it is. And since these therapies derive from humble origins, and God-given inexpensive remedies, I would call this program "Humble Healing". Many of these programs in here originated with these pioneer physicians in the 20's and even earlier. Why Hippocrates in 500 B.C. even said "LET THY

311

FOOD BE THY MEDICINE". Where did we go wrong that we stopped listening to wisdom and logic?

Probably the only reason we need to resort to sophisticated, biochemical assays of nutrient levels and correction of those with physicians who are well-versed in biochemistry, is because we have so damaged and depleted man and his environment and food. We have made two glaring errors in this century. We're the first generation to process so many foods and strip them of the vital nutrients that are protective against cancer and disease, and we're also the first generation to force everyone to detoxify so many chemicals. The average person detoxifies in excess of 500 different chemicals in a day. There are over 500 chemicals in the average city water, and the average home. This process of detoxification also accelerates the loss, or using up of precious nutrients.

Those gentlemen who wrote about natural hygiene lived in simpler times, before the drug industry grew to be the number one largest for profit business in the U.S. that it is today (according to the WALL STREET JOURNAL). They lived before 95% of the ingested food was processed, water heavily chlorinated, foods grown predominantly with synthetic fertilizers, hormones, pesticides and herbicides, then altered through genetic engineering and irradiation. And before high tech medicine where anything in the body that is unwanted is cut out or burned out, where there is no time wasted in healing.

If the body is a temple, if each of us must seek to find out what is God's planned work for us, if we are to help our fellow man, we had better be healthy first. For what we eat determines not only our body health, but our mental and spiritual health. And from that emerges our moral fiber and the strength to stand up for what is right. On simple diets, people are more intuitive, spiritual, rationale and kind. The more you hype them up with processed foods with dyes, additives, and other chemicals, the more you compromise the function of the brain (Rapp DJ, IS THIS YOUR CHILD?, Random House, NY).

It is known that it is criminal to prescribe Ritalin for hyperactive children without first being sure that there are no hidden food, chemical and mold sensitivities that are causing the symptoms. For a child should not be on an amphetamine that is directly related to illegal street "uppers" unless everything has been ruled out. However, there are influential circles in medicine where there is never a concern for cause, and Ritalin is prescribed automatically.

The world is losing contact with reality so fast, that a 1992 WALL STREET JOURNAL front page article told how some doctors have now decided that adult underachievers at work may represent the adult counterpart to the learning disabled or attention deficit child, and that perhaps they should be on Ritalin as well. Can you imagine being on the same highway as the harried executive who is striving to climb the corporate ladder and convinces his doc to prescribe this?

You'll be face to face with a person who revs himself up with several cups of coffee, maybe a few donuts to get his sugar kick, then his Ritalin. Add a few cigarettes to get his nicotine level up and a day of stress in the corporate jungle, then a few martinis on the way home. And they think they had problems with guys driving pick-up trucks into Big Mac and blowing a few heads off with a rifle? They ain't seen nothing yet!

When the youth of today are raised on a diet of over 30% sugar, demand running shoes that cost more than some laborers make in a week, and they don't even have any place to run to, we had better check our priorities. Better to buy them a child's BIBLE early and teach them some values they can grow with.

313

****

After my dear friend turned her cancer around for the second time, with a different therapy, having a high intellect and strong will, she got bored. After all, she had had two doctors at one point telling her that there was no way in the universe that she could live more than 48 hours. She rallied from that just as she had when 6 doctors and three major medical centers had told her she only had 3 months to live earlier.

So being bored, she adamantly abandoned the program for an exhausting campaign to run for judge, reasoning that now that it was so easy to TURN HER CANCER ON AND OFF, she could do it any time she needed to. Her cancer came back, and try as she might, she could not rally a third time, partly because the white count went to an all-time high and choked the life out of crucial organs. I must add that she was forever trying to convince me to become born again, but at that point I could really not appreciate what it meant. Likewise many other friends told me that they, too, were praying that I would evolve.

Anyway, two days before she died, 3000 miles away, I was standing in church, just having finished singing in the choir (one of her many accomplishments with me was to get me to go to church for the first time since my teens, even though it was only while on vacation).

Suddenly I felt as though my body had been hollowed out from the top of my head to the soles of my feet, creating a hollow core a foot in diameter. At the same instant it felt as though lightning had been poured through me. It was not painful, nor was I frightened. It was not hypoglycemia or a transient ischemic attack or syncope or vasospasm. I had had my normal breakfast, and was, of course, on no drugs; there was no medical explanation for it. It was the most powerful force I have ever felt, ten times more powerful than touching my electric horse fence, for example, but it did not cause me to lose my balance or fall.

And there was absolutely no disagreeable sensation associated with it. It was more like something wonderfully kind trying to get a very dumb person's attention. I immediately burst into profound, uncontrollable tears, yet I was not sad. I could not stop crying, and yet I had nothing to cry about. I have never experienced such a supernatural feeling in my life, nor have I heard of such. Although I had no way of knowing then, I now think her strong and loving spirit reached me over the miles through God.

But why me? I know thousands of people who would literally give their right arm to get a sign from God, to "feel" something. I never asked for verification (it never occured to me to); but now I wonder what I am supposed to do with this awesome gift? I think I have already been given enough gifts. Now I wonder what I am supposed to do with this one. When I got terribly ill years ago with the many aspects of E.I. and then got well, I should have picked up my life and gotten on with it. Instead I felt overwhelmingly grateful to have been given the brain and the resources to get well. How many others could have had so many maladies that were "undiagnosable and untreatable", yet still have the fortitude to continue working and research biochemistry night and day? On top of that I was able to travel to learn and lecture. I felt beholding to other victims of E.I. to teach them how to accomplish the same or better, hence the previous 5 books and my practice.

But during that time of intense struggle, I would go to bed nightly in tears, asking "Why me? Why isn't what I have in all my thousands of dollars worth of medical books? What good

315

was my medical school education if it does not even help me figure out what is wrong, much less how to cure it?" Now of course, I know why. But I am still at a loss for what to do with this more recent unfathonable treasure.

Meanwhile, upon learning of my friend's death, I wanted to throw my computer in the sea. But she made me promise many times to make this information, which she and I had so agonizingly and lovingly gathered, available to others, so that her suffering would not be for naught. I have a thousand painful questions for God, as does anyone who loses someone they love. But I will have to be satiated with her many gifts.

RESOURCES

Matthews DA, Larson DB, Barry CP, THE FAITH FACTOR; AN ANNOTATED BIBLIOGRAPHY OF CLINICAL RESEARCH ON SPIRITUAL SUBJECTS, National Institute for Healthcare Research, 2111 Wilson Blvd, Ste 1130 Arlington VA, 22201 (Ph (703) 527-NIHR), July 1993

Any and all books in this section can be obtained from Sacred Melody Bookstore, Syracuse, NY, phone 1-800-234-2211 or (315) 437-1095

Kohlenberger JR, THE ONE MINUTE BIBLE, Gaborg's, Bloomington, MN 55422, 1992

Pearsall P, MAKING MIRACLES, Avon Books, Dept FP, 1350 Avenue of the Americas, New York, NY 10019, 1-800-238-0658

Sheldon CM, IN HIS STEPS, Fleming Revell, Baker Book House, Grand Rapids MI 49506, 1984

Faid RW, A SCIENTIFIC APPROACH TO CHRISTIANITY, New Leaf Press, P.O.Box 311, Green Forest AR 72638, 1982

McDowell J, EVIDENCE THAT DEMANDS A VERDICT, Here's Life Publ, San Bernardino, CA, 92402, 1989

Keller W, THE BIBLE AS HISTORY, Wm Morrow & Co., NY, 1964

Martin W, THE KINGDOM OF THE CULTS, Bethany House Publ, Minn, MN, 55438, 1965

Colson C, LOVING GOD, Harper Paperbacks, 10 East 53rd St. NY, NY 10022, 1987

Colson C, THE BODY, Word Publishing, Dallas 1992.

Keller WP, A SHEPHERD LOOKS AT PSALM 23, 1970, Daybreak Books, Zonervan Publ, 1415 Lake Drive, S.E., Grand Rapids, MI 49506

Keller WP, STRENGTH OF SOUL, Kregel Publ, Grand Rapids MI, 49501, 1993

Williamson M, A RETURN TO LOVE, Harper Collins Publ., NY, 1992

Keller WP, A LAYMAN LOOKS AT THE LORD'S PRAYER, Moody Press, Chicago, 1976

Chapin A, 365 BIBLE PROMISES FOR BUSY PEOPLE, Tyndale House Publ, 351 Executive Dr., Box 80, Wheaton IL 60189-0080, 1992 HOLY BIBLE

Colson C, AGAINST THE NIGHT, Servant Publ, Box 8617,

Ann Arbor MI 48107, 1989

Robertson P, THE NEW WORLD ORDER, Word Publ, Dallas, 1991

Colson C, KINGDOMS IN CONFLICT, Harper & Row, 10 E 53rd St., New York, NY 10022, 1987

Kushi M, Jack A, THE GOSPEL OF PEACE. JESUS' TEACHINGS OF ETERNAL TRUTH, Japan Publ., Kodansha , 19 Union Sq W, NY NY 10003, 1992

Colson C, THE GOD OF STONES AND SPIDERS, Good News Publ, Wheaton IL 60187, 1990

Limbaugh R, THE WAY THINGS OUGHT TO BE, Pocket Books, Simon & Schuster, 1230 Avenue of the Americas, NY, NY 10020, 1992

Choate P, AGENTS OF INFLUENCE, Touchstone, Simon & Schuster, NY, 1990

Lewis, CS, MIRACLES, Collier Books of Macmillan Publ. Co., 1947

Lewis CS, THE SCREWTAPE LETTERS, ibid, 1961

Lewis CS, THE CASE FOR CHRISTIANITY, ibid,1943

Macartney CE, TWELVE GREAT QUESTIONS ABOUT CHRIST, Kregel Publ, Grand Rapids MI 49501, 1993

Cox JW, ed, THE MINISTERS MANUAL, Harper Collins Publ, 10 E. 53rd St., NY, NY 10022, 1993

Lewis CS, MERE CHRISTIANITY, ibid, 1943

Lewis CS, SURPRISED BY JOY, Harvest Books of Harcourt Brace Jovanovich, Publ, NY, 1956

Swindoll CR, LAUGH AGAIN, Word Publ., Dallas, 1992

Graham B, HOW TO BE BORN AGAIN, ibid, 1977

Girzone JF, THE SHEPHERD, Macmillan Publ Co, 866 Third Ave, NY 10022, 1990 (1800 323-7445)

Girzone JF, JOSHUA, ibid, 1987

Girzone JF, JOSHUA IN THE HOLY LAND, ibid

Colson C, Eckerd J, WHY AMERICA DOESN'T WORK, Word Publ, Dallas, 1991

Colson, C, WHO SPEAKS FOR GOD?, Good news Publ, 1300 Crescent St, Wheaton Il 60187, 1985

Stanley C, HOW TO LISTEN TO GOD, Thomas Nelson Publ, Nashville, 1985

Strauss RL, THE JOY OF KNOWING GOD, Loizeaux Bro Inc, Neptune NJ, 1986

Henry M, GREAT THEMES OF THE BIBLE, Kregel Publ, PO Box 2607 Grand Rapids MI 49501 1993

Krieger D, ACCEPTING YOUR POWER TO HEAL, Bear & Co., (1993) Santa Fe, NM 87504-2860

If you need BIBLE study and cannot go to church, there is an excellent set of 4 tiny booklets (MILK, MEAT, BREAD, FISH) from

PROSACT
P.O. Box 1948
Rocky Mount, NC 27802-1948

Chapter 8
HUMBLE HEALING

How Not To Die From Labelitis

Every moment people are dying all over the world from **labelitis.** You won't find it in any medical books, but it is a **primary cause of illness and death.** Medicine functions in a rather predictable way, when you understand in contrast how much we know about the mechanisms of disease. In medicine we listen to the story, that's called taking a history; we do a physical exam, we do laboratory tests, X-rays, biopsies, EEG's, nerve conduction studies, etc. and put a label on the patient. Once the patient has a diagnosis or a label, then we are happy. Then we go to our magical computer and it says for this **label** or this **diagnosis** these are the only accepted treatments; anything else is unproven, quackery, etc. Hence most disease states come out looking like a deficiency of medications.

Even the most politically naiive persons now know that lobbyists run this country. And many know that the chemical industry is the most powerful industry, and is also the father of the pharmaceutical industry. So it should not be difficult to understand that medicine is ruled by the drug industry. Hence, the message has been bought by medicine and lay alike without any questioning. It is accepted that most disease states come out looking like a deficiency of prescription medication.

For example, **a headache is a Darvon deficiency** or an aspirin deficiency. Arthritis is a Motrin, Advil or ibuprophen deficiency. Cancer is a deficiency of cellular poisons like chemotherapy and irradiation. Don't get me wrong, sometimes these are needed for the person to live long enough to allow healing therapies to work. But on the whole, these do not take into account the mechanism of healing, only the destruction of

321

reacting parts or covering up and masking of symptoms. In view of the overwhelming evidence, these limited protocols fall way too short of what could be done to bring about greater wellness for a large majority, and for far less money.

CASE EXAMPLE

I recently saw a young attorney from the mid-west in my office. He had been to several of the top medical facilities in the U.S. to see why at 48, he was having life-threatening arrhythmias (abnormal beats of the heart). He had gone to the premiere prestigious cardiac diagnostic center in the world (in the U.S.) for weeks of tests and a $10,000 workup. As we were going through his voluminous medical records I saw that two reports showed a pericardial effusion.

This means that there was an inflamatory reaction in the sac that lines the heart, and it was filling up with fluid. The startling point of this whole thing is that it is a perfect reflection of where medicine is headed. For he was told, just as it was stated on the reports, that the pericardial effusion was "insignificant".

What? The heart sac is reacting to itself and filling up with fluid and that's insignificant? That's like insignificant cancer or insignificant pregnancy. Either it is or it isn't. But insignificant?

Since no one in their right mind should believe that a reaction of the heart tissue, the organ that is exhibiting life-threatening symptoms, is insignificant, I suddenly realized how to interpret this common scenario. What they meant by "insignificant" is that the reaction is not yet large enough to merit the use of life-threatening drugs, and it is not yet large enough to enable the insertion of a needle by x-ray guidance in order to drain off the fluid. Never a word was uttered, even though he asked, about the possible **causes** of this fluid or what might be done to get rid of it or at least stop its progression. It was the old, "Come back an see me when it is worse," routine.

It is analogous to the scenario when you go to the doctor complaining of some symptom like fatigue. Since nothing shows on physical, blood tests, or x-ray, you are told to come back in 3 to 6 months, or if the problem worsens, sooner. In other words, it has to be bad enough to warrant drugs that have adverse side effects, or it must reach a point where it is a full-blown disease with a recognizable label, like multiple sclerosis.

By identifying his hidden allergens and environmental triggers and correcting numerous nutrient deficiencies, he was well for the first time in years in just **two months**. But guess what? The insurance company paid all of the $10,000 of tests done by the medical center, even though they did not do one thing to improve his health. They did not even have a diagnosis, much less an explanation of what was wrong with him and why he had over 12 symptoms, one of which was immediately life-threatening. But because it was this prestigious center, no questions were asked.

But when this attorney sent in the bills for the laboratory tests for the mineral deficiencies that were life- threateningly deficient, the company said they would not pay them. And this treatment made the person well, but that was irrelevant. The reason? These tests were **not done routinely** by the rest of the medical community. In fact they were indeed not done by the medical center which is called the most prestigious center for cardiac problems in the world!

Whoa! Do you know what this translates to? They now have decided to only pay for simple things that every doctor knows how to treat. This means your care, in order to be reimbursed, has to be at the lowest denominator, or what the average physician knows. That includes the fellow who when his patient asks him to read about a magnesium loading test, for example, says he does not have time, or if it were important he would have read about it in the NEW ENGLAND JOURNAL OF MEDICINE.

Heaven forbid you should have a problem that no one can figure out. If you have a difficult problem and use therapies that look for the actual cause and cure like nutrient deficiencies, then you are out of luck. And results are inconsequential. It does not matter one iota who or what gets you well. That is scarey, considering the increasing number of modern day plagues that are continually appearing. And the bottom line is that it translates into bigger profits for the pharmaceutical industry.

For as people get more desperate for help, they demand that drugs be released before proper testing. Therefore, millions of dollars are saved (by having demand for these drugs supercede the need to do adequate testing), yet high prices are still charged for these experimental therapies.

Remember the(6\13\90) JOURNAL OF THE AMERICAN MEDICAL ASSOCIATION showed that 90% of physicians never even thought of looking for a magnesium level in patients who were so sick as to be hospitalized? And some of them died from it. Yes, over 54% of these 1033 hospitalized patients were low in magnesium, and 90% did not have doctors knowledgeable enough to check for this as one of the causes of their sickness. And because that is the norm, you must be penalized? This is in spite of a plethora of articles (over 100 on my desk just from 1993 and the year is only half over) showing how serious and common the deficiency is. And I won't even tell you the cost of all the drugs they used in trying to treat these people without correcting the cause.

So you are penalized for their playing golf instead of reading the current scientific literature. It is as illogical as removing the right to say a prayer in school. I think Pat Robertson's THE NEW WORLD ORDER has hit the nail on the head. Some group is mighty power hungry to control the masses and will stop at nothing. And they seeem to have us sufficiently snafooed that no one even blinks an eyelash, much less musters up the good old American fighting spirit that founded this great nation.

At this moment, in spite of numerous articles right in the rheumatology journals about food allergies, I have not yet met or heard of a rheumatologist who puts patients on a diet to see if hidden food sensitivity might be the cause of their pain. But I will tell you, I would be in an insane asylum from the pain that I had, as would hundreds of my patients, had they not cleared their rheumatoid arthritis, osteoarthritis, degenerative arthritis, traumatic arthritis, lupus arthritis, and many other forms by identifying what foods and chemicals they were reacting to, and what nutrient deficiencies were keeping us in a constant state of muscle spasm and unrelenting pain.

I have even had patients go back to the rheumatologist and tell them "Doctor, you have worked so hard to help me with my arthritis, even prescribing narcotics and chemotherapeutic agents for the pain, I thought you would like to know it was due to certain foods". They have reported that the doctor just looked at them as if they had just dropped their drawers and said "There's no evidence for that you know."

Likewise, other diseases such as multiple sclerosis are supposed to have no known cause or cure and anyone who says they can change those diseases is automatically labeled a quack. Yet I have seen many halt or reverse it. For cancer, it appears that the only acceptable treatments are the various protocols of chemotherapy, radiation, surgery and transplants, which in many cases at best only give the sufferer a few extra years. Yet there are numerous books, for example, of people who have done the impossible and cleared their cancers with natural remedies: HOW I CURED CANCER NATURALLY, CANCER FREE, THIRTY WHO TRIUMPHED OVER CANCER NATURALLY, RECOVERY, RECALLED BY LIFE, PHYSICIAN HEAL THYSELF, and many others quickly come to mind.

Dr. Vivien Newbold, an emergency room physician, cleared her husband's cancer of the colon with macro in 1983. When she notified the American Cancer Society that she would be happy to teach them about it, she was told they were not interested (OPTIONS: THE ALTERNATIVE CANCER THERAPY BOOK, p 163, available from MACRO NEWS, 234 Dickinson St., Philadelphia, PA 19147).

And don't forget the evidence in medical journals shows that diet heals the impossible where high-tech drugs and surgery fail. Ornish (LANCET 336;129, 1990) showed that with macro people reversed their arteriosclerosis in the coronary arteries when surgery and cholesterol-lowering drugs were powerless. And Carter, et al (J AM COLL NUTR 12;3, 209-226, 1993) took two of the deadliest cancers and showed how healing a macrobiotic diet was. When you do everything medicine has to offer for cancer of the pancreas, at the end of one year, less than 9% of the people are still alive. But if they did even 3 months of macro, over 54% were alive!

And the evidence goes on. Cancer of the prostate is another cancer with poor survival. The median survival if you do everything medicine has to offer is 72 months. But if people did any form of macro 3 months or longer, it increased to 228; that is 6 years versus 19 years! So in essence **scientific studies show that a macrobiotic diet reverses arteriosclerosis and more than triples the survival of cancers of the pancreas and prostate.**

It makes so much sense that a **truly healthy body can clear anything. So don't be stuck with your label.** Often times people will say "Well, do you have a cure for this or that disease"? **It really doesn't matter what you have.** When someone presents in our office we don't care what they have; old age spots on the back of their hands, high blood pressure, high cholesterol, a history of three heart attacks, asthma, eczema, migraines, colitis, rheumatoid arthritis, eczema, attention deficit disorder, autism, prostatitis, neuritis, lupus, multiple sclerosis, chronic alcoholism, depression, schizophrenia or cancer. Many do not even have a label, they are so "hopeless" and "undiagnosable".

They have bizarre symptoms that are not in the medical books, and why would they be when we keep poisoning ourselves with new chemicals; while in the meantime, medicine has not yet embraced environmental medicine, even though it has been known for over 40 years. On the flip side, there are groups in medicine that have tacked "environmental medicine" on their title in this decade, but scores of patients have reported that when they see these docs and ask about allergies, they tell them that has nothing to do with chemical sensitivities. A fine state of affairs when the patient knows more than the specialist. I could have guessed this anyway since their journal articles reflect the same; no mention of allergy and no mention of xenobiotic detoxication pathway nutrients. And it goes without saying, no appreciation of the total load.

Suffice it to say, **it doesn't matter what your label is.** What matters is whether you can get your whole being well enough **mentally, physically and spiritually** so that it can overcome and clear your symptoms and disease. If you want to live in spite of medicine, if you want to live when all else has failed, I suggest you start reading and learning and you may very well be one of the "miraculous" survivors that we have all seen and read about.

THE MOST COMMMON BLUNDERS OF MEDICINE

Now that you know so much, you can begin to appreciate that there are numerous deficits in "modern" medicine. Let's just take a quick run through the many specialties and see what they could do tomorrow to begin to bring themselves into the 21st century.

The **pediatricians** could cut way down on recurrent ear, throat, and sinus and chest infections in kids by just teaching mothers the diagnostic diet (THE E.I. SYNDROME, TIRED OR TOXIC?). Many kids have a marked reduction in phlegm just omitting milk (and if you find yourself asking, "Then what do we do for the calcium for growing bones?", you missed some important concepts and need to read).

The **internists and cardiologists** could begin to do the magnesium loading test on all hypertensives, arrhythmias, angina, and just empirically give a shot of magnesium to anyone who has just had a heart attack or is suspected of having one. They can drop the death rates precipitously. And when they get fancier and more sophisticated in their knowledge, they can check the high cholesterol patients for rbc chromium, manganese, magnesium, copper, and the many other nutrients that have a bearing on how efficiently the body is able to metabolize cholesterol. And they can stop recommending margarines, poly unsaturated hydrogenated oils and processed foods which actually promote business.

The **rheumatologists** could start by prescribing the diagnostic diet so people could identify some of the possible causes of their arthritis and fibromyalgia. They could help a vast number of people by just learning the nightshade-free diet we described in Chapter 2.

The **gastroenterologists** could learn how to put people on the diagnostic diet and learn about intestinal dysbiosis, and stop poisoning people with aluminum antacids. The **pulmonologists** should learn some allergy for starters, while the **allergists** could learn some environmental medicine, and begin with the diagnostic diet to rule out food-induced symptoms. The **occupational medicine** people obviously will never clear chemical sensitivity until they actually learn some environmental medicine. Why they could even start by not wearing aftershave, so they don't fog-out their patients with chemical sensitivity or trigger asthma in the asthmatics.

The **surgeons** should learn to at least assess an rbc zinc, rbc copper, and a magnesium loading test. I'd sure not want to operate on anyone who has a poor chance of healing well. And they should call in a specialist in environmental medicine whenever a patient is going downhill after trauma. Some people mysteriously go downhill after a particular accident, surgery, or illness, and die needlessly. In some cases it is just because the accident brought their nutrient reserve down to a critical level. Then I.V.'s, hospital food, and a barage of drugs, finished the job.

And the **orthopedists** could learn to do the magnesium loading test and diagnostic diet for all those chronic backs. And remember that article of 80 year olds who were on the orthopedic floor with fractured hips? The ones who had nutrients had **half the complications** and **half the death rate** compared with a comparable group that received no supplements! In other words they doubled the survival with a simple vitamin supplement.

The **neurologists** could start by having all the migraines do the diagnostic diet and a magnesium loading test; the **endocrinologists** could begin by looking at the unconjugated DHEA in fatigued patients, and later on learn to do nutritional and environmental assessments to learn why the glands are hypofunctioning in the first place.

The **gynecologists** should, of course learn to do the yeast program, and then to do the nutrient assessments that have enabled so many to reverse their cervical dysplasias without laser or conization. The **urologists** could learn that food sensitivity is a common cause for chronic non-specific urethritis (complaints but no bugs), and the **oncologists** should be experts on everything in this book and more.

It does not mean to say that the above examples are the only causes of the symptoms, but that they are so fantastically common, and there is so much scientific evidence for them, that it is poor medicine to not do them. And once a doctor sees how many of his "chronic", medication-dependent patients suddenly get relief, he'll hopefully be motivated to learn more. For surely this small smattering of suggestions for starters will turn the tide for physicians who are still thinkers. Once they see the results they will, like the rest of us, never be able to return to "drugs-only" type of medicine, which rarely cures. Drugs merely cover up symptoms, but the underlying problem eventually rears its ugly head again, but usually in a different target organ.

For the division of medicine into specialties is idiotic in this era. **It matters not what the label is. The only thing that counts is what is causing the symptoms.** Specialists should be reserved for the person for whom an environmental trigger and bio-chemical defect cannot be found, or for the lazy or less intelligent person who just wants a quick fix. He just wants medication and to get on with it. He doesn't give a hoot about cause, and he certainly does not want to have to do anything himself for his health, much less a diet change, etc.

NO ONE HAS MORE POWER OVER YOUR HEALTH THAN THE PERSON WHO PREPARES YOUR FOOD

Anyone who thinks their doctor has the biggest influence on their health and is a major factor in their longevity and freedom from disease is wrong. Rather, the one who has the greatest influence over your health is **the person who shops for, plans, and prepares your meals.** When we look at how all these people did the impossible, cleared cancers, MS, rheumatoid arthritis, chronic fatigue syndrome, chemical sensitivity, etc., they did it with humble, natural, God- given things. They did it with things that do not support the drug industry, but are within the reach of every human being. And do not misinterpret me. There is great benefit in **drug- and surgery-oriented medicine.** It can allow the person to live long enough to make **a natural and thinking therapy** work. It is only inappropriate when the patient is condemned to a lifetime of drugs without the benefit of a workup to determine if cause and cure can be found. Likewise it can be a marvelous adjuct or addition to a program for which only some of the causes can be found.

I have a vision of receiving stories from people around the world with medical documentation (copies of doctors' summaries, pathology reports and/or x-rays and blood tests, and permission for me to use it) demonstrating the presence of a

331

cancer, then the same reports months or years later demonstrating that the cancer was gone. I already have quite a collection of these. I would like to write a further book and include all of these people in it, because it would give hope to all of those who dare not venture out into unchartered waters. For from what I have witnessed, and from my belief of how the universe is designed, it makes more sense to me that healing by humble means is what the great Master Planner had in mind, not making us all dependent upon the drug industry.

And if chemotherapy or surgery is the chosen mode of treatment for a particular problem, it still makes more sense to incorporate some of this knowledge about healing into those programs to improve the odds as well as improve the quality of life for the patient. An obvious example is the use of coffee enemas for the discomfort and potential death of chemotherapy.

Whatever level of wellness you have, I hope you will never take it for granted, for it can be snatched from you at any moment. I hope you will make time in your busy 21st century life for some humble healing. For even if you have nothing you want to heal right now, there are parts here you can use to improve the quality and longevity of your good health. For example, you could include more whole grains, beans, and fresh vegetables in your daily diet, or purchase a water filter, or have your key anti-oxidant nutrient levels prophylactically checked, periodically.

When I broke my shoulder a few years ago it gave me a renewed appreciation like I had never had before of how much time is actually involved in real healing. Real healing of a bone or ligament, for example, takes about a year and a half. Sure, you can be using it without problem a lot sooner, but there are many evidences that the process is incomplete. Skin heals very

332

quickly, but nerve growth, for example, takes years. Obviously more serious conditions take longer. We are so accustomed to a quick fix with drugs that we forget that real healing takes months and years. Sometimes when someone has healed a cancer in two or three years with macro, Gerson, or Kelly, we'll learn that they went off the program. They then become very ill and get the cancer back quite easily. It appears to happen more quickly and predictably if they had not first taken seven years or greater to rid the body of the condition.

ALCOHOLISM AS A MULTI-FACETED DISEASE

Some labels are more devastating than others, for example that of alcoholism. A real disservice is done whenever anyone thinks that it is a disease of poor moral fiber, for it is a disease of abnormal biochemistry and allergy, just like most other problems.

These people usually have allergic family histories, they always have multiple nutrient deficiencies (often chromium, magnesium, zinc, and manganese which make them crave more alcohol which can make them very irritable, edgy and have insomnia, etc.). (You are a fast learner! Yes, the **zinc was used up or lost** by the extra work of the zinc-dependent alcohol dehydrogenase enzyme, as well as being deficient because of the missed meals and vomiting).

As well, the alcoholic usually has multiple allergies to mold, especially Candida, and many foods which actually drive their cravings. Wheat, sugar, milk and ferments are some of the more common foods. Also, they have amino acid deficiencies, which govern neurotransmitters in the brain. These in turn, govern whether a person feels satiated or happy and content versus craving and addicted and out of control. But when you are able to put all of this together, plus address many of the other parts of the total load and detoxify them according to HUMBLE HEALING principles, they can heal as well.

(1)Larson JM, Alcoholism —THE BIOCHEMICAL CONNEC-TION, Villard Books of Random House, NY, 1992
(2)Richardson MA, AMINO ACIDS IN PSYCHIATRIC DIS-EASE, American Psychiatric Press, Inc, 1400 K Street NW, Suite 1101, Washington DC 20005, 1990,
(3)Blum K, ALCOHOL AND THE ADDICTIVE BRAIN, The Free Press, a division of Macmillan Inc, NY, 1991.
(4)Slagel, P, THE WAY UP FROM DOWN,(available from N.E.E.D.S.)

How Do I Start?

Some of the most fun patients are those who have read every-thing we've written, done everything we've suggested, and want to brain storm, see what's new and go to even higher levels of wellness.

On the other end of the spectrum is another type of challenging patient. The person who is suddenly very sick, hates to read and in fact, has never read a thing about nutrition and environ-mental problems, and knows nothing about good health. He does not even know that chlorine and fluoride in city waters damage enzymes and can contribute to cancer. He does not know that silver amalgam fillings in the teeth can mimic any symptom including cancers. He does not know that pesticides are everywhere in our air, food, water, home and office envi-ronments and these two can mimic any symptoms including cancer.

I'll never forget one time when I was telling a well educated, young, engineer to eat whole grains. He innocently asked, "Do you mean like shredded wheat?" And this probably tells us where a lot of people are in terms of their health I.Q. So, if we start simply with one of these impossible types, lets try to build on what might be perhaps the seven most important trade-offs.

The Seven Trade-Offs

(1) First and foremost, you should **get off all sugar** containing products.

This includes honey, maple syrup, yinny rice syrup and any other sweeteners. Sugar can be disguised as corn syrup, dextrose, maltose, glucose, fructose, fruit sugars, and a host of other names. Sugar is the one most important, negative nutrient to avoid if you have any glimmer of hope about getting well regardless, of your condition.

For those wanting mechanisms and references, TIRED OR TOXIC? talks about enzymatic glycosylation which is a chemical reaction that sugars go through in the body whereby they can mimic any and all of the worst chemically induced symptoms you can imagine. Sugar also provides no nutrients, but it uses up many in the process of being metabolized. So, it is a real negative for it makes us less healthy than we were when we ingested it. Worse, sugar (being acid) uses up alkaline buffers that are needed for normal metabolism and healing.

What can you trade off sugar for? Your juicer. **Start juicing** apple juice if you need sweets and then graduate to less sugar with beet, carrot, and/or cabbage juice. You can have these juices whenever you feel the urge for sweets several times a day. Or make the sweet vegetable drink in THE CURE IS IN THE KITCHEN. Regardless, try to get organic vegetables whenever possible. It is worth the extra effort. Try looking at your local farmers' market on Saturday mornings; you may be surprised that people sell 25 lbs. bags of these vegetables for the very purpose of juicing.

So, there you have a good start. All we're doing is getting rid of sugar and replacing it with nutritious vegetable (or fruit) juices that are drunk within 20 minutes of juicing them. If you are having terrible sweet cravings at work, make the sweet vegetable drink (from YOU ARE WHAT YOU ATE) and carry it in a thermos to work.

Merely cook up finely diced squash, cabbage, carrots and onions in 4 times the volume of good water. It's a sweet alternative, high in nutrients. You can even put some sea palm **seaweed** in it for extra minerals; this would make an excellent, nutritious drink for you and it's a cinch to make and should be available at all times. You should eat the seaweeds and MACRO MELLOW has lots of ideas for spreads and breads that you can make from the left over vegetables or you can just eat them or blend them into a soup.

(2) The second trade-off will be to **get rid** of all your bad drinks such as **coffee, tea, alcohol, sodas and yes, even your ciga-rettes**. These also deplete alkaline buffer reserves, and use up more nutrients or flush them out in the urine. As minute examples, each cigarette lowers the vitamin C, and alcohol causes magnesium to be lost in the urine.

What can you trade these for? Good, pure, clean, **spring water,** or if you prefer, your **sweet vegetable drink.** Just imagine, as soon as you ditch coffee, your reduce your load of chlorine and fluoride, both of which damage enzymes. Disease, sickness, chemical sensitivity, cancer, arteriosclerosis, high cholesterol, diabetes, asthma, eczema, arthritis, any malady you can think of is merely the inability of the body to detoxify itself and keep

336

up with the damaging things that are put into it everyday.

Not having coffee also deprives you of your daily dose of aluminum which can contribute to Alzheimer's presenile dementia, for most coffee makers have an aluminum reservoir inside the machine in which the water is brought to boiling. And by not having the coffee, you lower the caffeine dose to your detox system, for caffeine is a drug. If you drank decaffeinated, you miss your dose of cancer-causing dry cleaning fluid, or trichloroethylene, which is commonly used as an extracting solvent to remove some of the caffeine.

Since you are going to be off coffee anyway, you might as well bring your own water and you might as well make it nutritionally superior water i.e., sweet vegetable juice.

Likewise, the sodas deplete minerals like chromium and cause sugar cravings that lead to obesity. If they contain nutrasweet, they interfere with amino acid metabolism in the brain of some, causing headaches, depression, fatigue and other symptoms. Bare minimum, they cause overwork of everyone's detox system, as this chemical has to be detoxified. Also the sodas potentiate osteoporosis, as the phosphates in them compete with calcium for absorption, and win.

(3) The third trade-off is to **get rid of all processed foods**, chips, pizza, anything in a bag, a box, a jar, anything that has conventional salt in it (read THE CURE IS IN THE KITCHEN for the problems that regular salt causes).

Use small amounts of real sea salt in flavoring your cooking. As for the processed foods, if they have a list of ingredients or chemicals or words that do not mean whole, unadulterated foods, you do not want to put them in your healing body. And what do you trade this for? Organically grown foods, many of which can be purchased in your local health food store. These include **whole grains, vegetables, and beans.**

If you need protein, you may have **fish,** but make sure it is not farmed. The benefits of fish are that they are higher in Omega 3 oils. They get these by eating other fish and seaweeds. Unfortunately, farmed fish (and you have to ask at the market) is not grown in the ocean. Real fish eat seaweed and other fish. Farmed fish eat chemicalized, commercial, dog food-type pellets high usually in Omega 6 oils. So, you might as well have a good steak and enjoy it.

When you get off processed foods, you not only lose the chemicalized version of salt, but you get rid of those damaging hydrogenated oils that abound in all the baked goods, especially.

MACRO MELLOW will tell you how to begin to start to cook these types of foods. YOU ARE WHAT YOU ATE then tells you how to get into a more strict level of healing if you need it and THE CURE IS IN THE KITCHEN is the strictest form for those who want to see what maximal health feels like. If you are a carnivore type and need the high meat, fat and oil diet then you should eat that. But again, organic food is the most important. And then there are several stages in between the two extremes, which may actually be where you belong.

Once you start cleaning out by getting rid of the sugars, incorporating juices, getting off coffee, getting rid of the junk food, having clean water and exchanging processed foods for organic, whole foods, you may have some walloping discharges or withdrawal symptoms for a few days. Make sure you have someone with you who is knowledgeable about what you are going through. The coffee enema will shorten its course and severity.

Remember, you can do coffee enemas at any stage if you have bad withdrawal symptoms and want to clean out faster. If you are a little afraid of them, use only a half tbsp. per quart of water to begin with, and work yourself up as tolerated to the prescribed dose. If you are really sick and know you need them, use the Gerson recipe of 2- 3 tbsp. per quart of water boiled for 5 minutes, simmered for 20 minutes and then cool until completely tepid, holding only a comfortable amount (2 cups or less) infused with minimal pressure, by gravity flow, and held for ten minutes. Two or three of these at a session, sometimes two or three times a day, are necessary depending upon the level of toxicity. These would be the maximal levels in general. Anyone doing the enemas should have individual key nutrient levels done once a month the first 3 months, then every other month, to be sure they are not depleting them. And stop them and consult your physician for a nutrient assessment if arrhythmia (irregular heart beat) or any other symptom appears or worsens.

(4) The fourth trade-off is to **stop** breaking down the body with **chemical assaults**, but rather, give it a rest so it can restore itself.

Remember, we are the first generation of man ever exposed to so many chemicals. Everytime we go to the grocery store and breathe one molecule of pesticide, even though we can't perceive the smell, we are using up and loosing nutrients forever.

So, you need to **reduce your chemical overload** as much as is possible for you at this point in time. THE E.I. SYNDROME will go into that in detail, but you can start with a good **air cleaner** in your bedroom and remove any unnecessary cosmetics, dry cleaned clothes, polished shoes, dust catchers, carpet, and any other things that are possible, and especially get rid of any electric blankets or heating pads and pull the bed away

339

from the wall so that you are getting minimal electromagnetic fields. Try to detox your person and **reduce your total load** in general by wearing less scented toiletries and cosmetics. TIRED OR TOXIC? will give you all of the directions as you get more sophisticated and ready to go to higher levels of wellness.

So concentrate on having clean, air, food and water; an air cleaner, organic, whole foods and a water filter will compensate for a host of things gifted to us by the 21st Century. Then you can work on further environmental controls starting with the bedroom. Make sure you awaken feeling great, for if the environment where you spend a third of your life and the majority of your healing time is not conducive to healing, how will you ever get well? Expose a mold plate in there to see how high the mold growth is. This alone can make you awaken exhausted, headachey, congested, and ready to go back to bed.

(5) The fifth phase is to trade your **T.V. time** for **books**, predominantly about your spirituality and about environmental medicine.

Now that your brain is clearer and you are feeling better, you will be amazed at how much you have to learn yet. What occupies your brain all day has as much bearing on your health as what occupies your stomach, and what is in the air you breath, and the what is in the water you drink. There are numerous other entities that can keep a person sick; the total package is crucial just as much so in cancer as in chemical sensitivity. And a great start in guarding against having the toxic level too high is to read and learn about environmental medicine. For like it or not, **you are the sum total of what you eat, breath, drink & think.**

Who would you bet $1,000 of your hard-earned money on to get well faster? Would you lay your money down for a person who watches T.V. filled with brutal killings, rape, high speed chases, foul language, street gangs, drug addicts, and merciless beatings? Or would you prefer someone who reads his BIBLE (or their chosen spiritual material), trying to figure our how to be a better person and studying the word of God to decide what He wants him to do with his life? Also this person would read a great deal about all the techniques in this book as well as references pertaining to how to get himself well, against all odds.

(6) **With the help of your doctor,** your goal should be to get **off as many medications as possible,** and trade them in for **supplements** that must be deficient. For if you are on medications, most likely you have nutrient deficiencies.

This is because (1) medications only cover up or hide the symptoms. But you want to find the causes, if possible, and get rid of it once and for all. For example, is your high blood pressure due to a magnesium or calcium or potassium deficiency (for which there a numerous references in the literature)? Or do you have high cholesterol because you are deficient in chromium, manganese, magnesium, etc.? (2) The second reason for trying to get off as many medications as possible, is that they are a foreign chemical and use up or deplete nutrients in the body's work of metabolizing or detoxifying them.

So, now your goal is to replace everything that is damaging with things that are beneficial so that you may unload the body and allow it to heal. Most medicines do not cure, except antibiotics by killing bugs. Instead, most medications merely mask symptoms. The only thing that heals or cures a body is the body chemistry itself and it must be healthy enough to do so. And the energy to do so comes from food.

In the course of getting off medications, and finding why you

341

needed them in the first place, you will discover deficiencies. You have to. If nothing is found, check to see that the correct rbc levels were done and extend into the total load to find what is awry in your system to have created your symptoms.

A good start would be to do the magnesium loading test and rbc levels: zinc, copper, chromium, molybdenum, manganese, potassium, selenium and rbc folate. Then do an ionized calcium, and vitamins B1, B12, B6, A, C, E, and 1-OH D3.

Then get on a balanced program to correct the deficiencies, check to see what corrected in a few months, and proceed to other assessments if wellness is still elusive. Just whittle through the total load, depending on what seems likely, whether it be amino acids in a chemically sensitive person, or essential fatty acid deficiencies in a depressed person, or burdens of heavy metals, pesticides and other toxicities in someone with odd numbness and tingling and body pains that no one can figure out.

To build the body, start with the primary anti-oxidants, vitamins A, C and E at total daily levels of 10,000-30,000 for A, 2,000-15,000 for ascorbic acid or C and 400-800 for E, plus a good multiple mineral. Of course, there are many other nutrients needed. A multiple B vitamin could be added and the magnesium loading test should be done as quickly as possible. A powerful product called BIO-AE-Mulsion Forte (Biotics, Houston Tx or N.E.E.D.S.) is a special liquid form of vitamin A which is particularly well-absorbed and healing.

(7) Last of all, **assess your life** and **decide** what you are going to trade so that you have time to begin some HUMBLE HEALING. It is your choice, it is your life.

I suggest you start with your doctor with the above omissions(1-6), then continue with your doctor to juicing, then enzymes, the coffee enemas, then the occassional bowel cleanse.

As you have seen, it does not matter what we call anything. It can be chronic fatigue, fibromyalgia, lupus, multiple sclerosis, sarcoidosis, asthma, cancer, the name or label is inconsequential. **The bottom line is how much do you have to do to get your body healthy enough to win, healthy enough to heal itself. Healthy enough to experience wellness, against all odds.**

Obviously, this will also entail changes in your lifestyle and probably even your friends. You may want to join some local support groups of people who are into nutrition and health or spirituality, so that you'll have stimulating friends and ideas to help you get well and stay well.

Then again, you certainly can take your sweet vegetable drink with you to the local smoke-filled bar after work if you want to wear a scuba tank on your back and mask over your eyes and nose so that you don't load up with toxic smoke. It's all up to you. The amount of work and dedication you will need will depend upon your genetics, the severity of your disease and your will to live and be healthy. Obviously not all of this is needed by everyone. But certainly, those with cancers and serious illnesses should use the enzymes to break down cancers, autoimmune antibody complexes, arterial plaque, and fatty tissues harboring foreign chemicals.

Once you use enzymes, you will be commited to coffee enemas, since accelerated breakdown overloads the body with metabolic waste which must be gotten rid of quickly in order for the person to avoid severe toxicity. In cancer patients this toxicity can be fatal. Therefore, skin brushing and coffee enemas are a must if you are going to use enzymes.

343

So an oversimplified start for the 7 trade-offs would be:

Trade	For
1. Sugar	Fresh vegetable juices
2. Processed foods	Organic whole foods
3. Coffee, alcohol, sodas	Filtered spring water
4. Chemical overload	Environmental controls, air cleaner
5. T.V.	Spirituality, reading
6. Medications (physician-assisted)	Nutrient levels and
7. Your choice	HUMBLE HEALING PROGRAM

In other words,
CUT the CRAP out of your life!

C = coffee, cigarettes and chemicals
R = refined sugar & flour products
A = alcohol
P = processed foods as in anything that has passed through a factory and comes in a bag, jar, wrapper or box with a list of chemicals on the label. And once you do all this and start working on the rest of your total load, you should also get to a point where, with the guidance of your doctor, you can shrug many of your **prescription** drugs.

Instead, eat only whole, organic foods, like whole grains, greens, and beans, seeds and weeds, roots and fruits.

HUMBLE HEALING PROGRAM

(1)   Diet, organic and unprocessed as possible. When in doubt, start alkaline (modified vegetarian), 1/3 raw. If you definitely are a carnivore, have your lipids checked once a month for the first 3 months, then every 3-6 months thereafter until you gradually swing into a less carnivorous diet, and into more whole grains, beans, fresh vegetables, seeds and nuts.

(2)   Vegetable juices, chewed

(3)   Fast one day a week, if there is no cancer

(4)   Supplements two weeks on, one week off, or every other day.

(5)   Pancreatin

(6)   Coffee enemas, daily, 3 weeks a month.

(7)   Skin brushing, singing, body work in the form of yoga, exercise, massages, network or other chiropractic, etc.

(8)   Colon cleanse, gallbladder flush on alternative months. Acidophilus to restore flora if stool analysis reveals deficient amounts.

(9)   Consistency and time.

(10)   Spiritual: Tap into universal energy for healing.

(11)   Rectal nutrients versus I.V., if I.V.'s unavailable and person is very ill.

(12)   Accessory measures, like assessing the pH of saliva and urine, taking sodium alginate, etc.

NOTES ON THE INDIVIDUAL ASPECTS OF THE PROGRAM

(1)   As discussed, a trial will tell you which diet is best, and as you heal, you may change. By all means, if you are doing a carnivore diet, have the cholesterol, triglycerides, HDL, LDL, and apoliprotein A1 & B drawn to be sure it is not lipidemic for

you. The modified vegan is the best for the most people, and strict macrobiotic is the most healing for the largest majority with more severe problems.

So if you are a betting man, the odds are in your favor to start with alkaline (modified vegetarian, which includes fish and fowl, or macro). Even for those who later turn out to be carnivores, it is a good cleansing diet and usually gets them off to a good start. For others, they need to start with the carnivore diet while they clear Candida problems, and many cancers of blood-forming tissues, then they can switch to macro.

(2) For juicing, start with carrot if you are able: if not tolerated, try apple, beet and or cabbage and parsley. But try to keep the juice under 2 cups twice a day, especially if you are doing apple juice, as the sugar is undesirable, although a marked improvement from whence you came.

(3) There is a lot to be said for giving the system a rest one day a week. Many find they feel surprisingly well when they fast, which is often a sign of hidden food allergies.

(4) There is no blanket prescription for nutrients, for each person has individual needs. But certainly most can benefit from good levels of vitamins A, C, E,, and a multi- mineral (containing at least copper, potassium, zinc, selenium, manganese, magnesium, vanadium, calcium, molybdenum, chromium), bare minimum. Add appropriate doses of D, B; magnesium (citrate if need alkalinizing), CoQ10, taurine, flaxseed oil, glutathione, other minerals like boron, "accessory" nutrients like choline citrate, glycine, methionine, taurine, carnitine, lipoic acid, L-proline, L-lysine, N-acetyl cysteine, glutathione, etc. after checking at least a few of the more commonly deficient levels (as suggested above) first.

346

A big problem is that you cannot possibly take all the wonderful nutrients in a day that you need (that is, with any powerful amounts). Therefore, I would suggest you see what's broken first, fix that, then assess whether you need to go further in that direction with more sophisticated assessments or can reserve your resources for other areas.

After having seen thousands of self-prescribed and physician-prescribed nutrient programs, I must add a word of caution: although there are no absolutes in medicine, the most common mistake I see is imbalance and overdose of specific nutrients. For example, beyond 10,000 mg of vitamin C, you can start to seriously flush out calcium and other minerals. High doses of zinc can flush out copper, molybdenum, iron, manganese, etc. Likewise, vitamin E has a bell-shaped curve of therapeutic effectivieness. In other words, more is not better, but on the contrary, there is a peak for most people where the optimum dose lies between 400 - 1200 I.U. Beyond that, you start to get diminishing returns and it becomes a drain on the system (and part of the total load), rather than helping it.

Likewise, when essential fatty acids are used (like flax oil to correct the "wrong " fatty acids in the cell membrane that are damaging the potassium pump and causing an rbc potassium deficiency with resultant muscle weakness, fatigue and cramps), there must be a relative increase in vitamin E to aid in the extra biochemical work that is going on in the cell membrane (logical, isn't it, when you now understand the chemistry of how vitamin E sits in the membrane to protect it?).

And when taking supplements, remember that there are only so many mineral transporters to carry minerals across the gut wall. It is as though they all need specific soldiers to bring them over. So it makes sense that you can save money on supplements by having a pocketful that you nibble from throughout the day, rather than slugging down a handful at once. This is particularly useful if you have a particular nutrient that is difficult to correct, like copper. Even if you are not inclined to nibble at the nutrients all day, at least take your most difficult to correct one at a separate time from all the other ones. This maximizes the chance of getting it assimilated, since you are taking it at a time when it has no competition for absorption from other supplements.

(5) Regarding the pancreatic enzyme, the best form of enzyme would be organic glandular pork pancreatin. You may use lamb or beef if you are sensitive to pork. Other pancreatic enzymes are proported by Dr. Kelley (person communication) to contain Bacillus subtilis, an important bacteria which you do not need in your system. I do not know how to determine the validity of this at present, so there are some things I take by faith when I have seen such impressive results.

It is cost prohibitive for many to take 3-8 pancreatin (with no food or supplements 2 hours before or after) 2-5 times a day. But that is the dose many severe cancers or antibody-mediated diseases need. If they are very sick, they may have to cut back, as they simply will not tolerate the flood of cancer breakdown products in their systems. A less expensive necessity may be to have just two doses a day: 4-8 capsules before bed on an empty stomach and 4-8 again on an empty stomach between 2 and 5 a.m. There is a quantity discount available by suppliers, (and I would call and compare prices). This allows the body to have the high doses of the enzyme at the optimal healing time, rather than throughout the day to facilitate food absorption as well. Also recall that a one month trial periodically (once or twice a year) may show you that you took them in the nick of time.

There are other fine enzymes (Tyler and NESS are examples

that quickly come to mind), but I have not observed cancer patients who substituted these and so have no data at present. They are made from Aspergillus, but make fine substitutes for those intolerant of animal-based enzymes.

(6) If you are leary of the coffee enema, start with clean water (not from the tap). Then add only 1 tbs of coffee to the quart, rather than two. If you feel weak after a coffee enema, try drinking 2 tbs. of apple cider vinegar in a glass of water with either a teaspoon of honey or 2 tsp. maple syrup before the next enema. Be sure to rinse your teeth with bicarbonate of soda to prevent dissolving the enamel with the vinegar.

(7) Body work is not emphasized enough in medicine. But you will know when you are doing the right thing when you feel your skin stimulated, tingling, and invigorated, with blood flowing to muscles and tissues you forgot you had, and when you no longer ache or hurt or have any tender "trigger" points. Extra vitamin B3 (called niacin) is also useful for opening clogged or stagnant areas. The dose and procedure needs strict supervision and individualization.

(8) These special parts of the program are obviously for the much more ill individual, and one who will need individual assistance. A good start for many who are not well, however, would be to get a stool analysis for types and amounts of bacteria, fungi, protozoa, and other parasites, plus an indication on how well you are digesting and assimilating food. There are permeability tests for the leaky gut and a D-xylose absorption test to see if you are absorbing well. There are multiple other ways to assess the gut for health and optimal function.

(9) Don't abandon your program just because you are not well the first week ! Natural healing takes time. Only drugs

produce instantaneous results. But always get medical help if you are getting worse. Do not wait just because it is not time to report back yet. Also, be on the constant look-out for how you can improve your dedication to your wellness. And have pre-planned ways to help yourself over the obstacles that are bound to be thrown in your way. For example, if you know the only beverage available when you go to a friend's house is a soda, take your own glass-bottled water.

(10) Don't be afraid to ask God for help, but it must be done with sincere faith. Studying His word helps you gain deeper understanding.

(11) Some people have such poor absorption and marked deficiencies, that rectal instillation, under medical supervision may be worth considering.

(12) In future editions of the newsletter and books, we plan to explore the worthiness of having people check the acidity/alkalinity or pH of their saliva and urine, to determine whether this will be beneficial.

Sodium alginate, for example, is an inexpensive non-prescription product that can mobilize heavy metals. It may be taken as a course of three tablets three times a day for one week a month times three months. It is preferrable to collect urine for heavy metals during that time to determine that indeed it is helping to mobilize and which metals in particular. Sometimes there is more than one heavy metal in the tissues, and they come out in very specific order. There are many procedures that will be learned, and many that are already known but are beyond the scope of a book, but are better dealt with on an individual and highly supervised basis.

Any who have followed us through the years know how

intense our research has been and that there is a steady and continual flow of new ideas. For that reason they check back each year to see what is new that would pertain to their progressive improvement in wellness or that would help solve any problems that have cropped up in the interim.

∗∗∗∗∗∗∗∗∗∗∗∗∗

" I'M OVERWHELMED ! "

"I'm OVERHWELMED!" That is a normal reaction. Don't try to do everything at once. Start easy. If you find yourself saying, "I'd rather be happy than healthy", look at what you have to live for and what you have to be greatful for. As many people often tell us after having spent a day in the testing room with other patients from around the world, "I thought I was sick! My problems are nothing compared with what I heard upstairs."

Begin possibly by looking for simple ways in which you can begin to slowly improve your health. If you are hooked on 3 donuts and 2 cups of coffee for your morning jumpstart, try to cut down to 2 donuts and 1 cup of coffee the first week. Add in brown rice and some veggies to make up the difference. Then the next week cut to one donut and half a cup of coffee. But remember to **always give yourself something more nutritious to make up the difference** in lost calories. Make sure you come out ahead....a winner.

And if you find it utterly impossible to think of going a day without a particular food, then recall that it is the overall proportion that means a great deal. For example, if you are used to guzzling a 6-pack of soda a day, try for 2 or 3, while increasing the greens and whole grains in a form that would be appealing to you. Sure, it may not be perfect, but if it is a step freed from suffering. In a world where the emphasis has

351

up from where you were, you are that much further ahead. **Proportions mean a lot.** If you can increase the more nutritious foods, the smaller amounts of the ones you do not need will not have as deleterious an effect as compared with when they constituted a major part of your diet. And a funny thing often happens. As you make these small nibbles toward a healthier diet, you may find you feel better and do not have as much craving for the old stand-bys. That is because you have begun correcting some of the deficiencies that caused the cravings in the first place.

If you need sugar, make the sweet vegetable drink, or get a whole grain organic bread with fruit juice-sweetened jam. Don't try to overwhelm yourself and be doomed for failure. And if you do fail (we **all** do many times over in the process of learning), **do not put guilt on yourself.** Instead look at what you have learned and accomplished, and start over when you are ready.

By now, you are much smarter than that, anyway. When you need help, don't be afraid to ask. Those of us in this field have all sorts of resources in our offices to help you be successful when you feel you are at an impasse. We'll tailor a diet to your needs and lifestyle, prescribe nutrients to correct your deficiencies, and plough through your total load with you in search of the causes of your symptoms. And don't give up too easily on your doctor. Statistically, he or members of his family will be in need of healing. And there is nothing like personal illness to humble a physician and spark interest. How do you think I got motivated to do all this work?

God has given us all unique gifts. Look at all the important discoveries and reports that permeate the references in this book. So many people with brilliant, inquisitive minds have spent their precious lives researching, so that others could be freed from suffering. In a world where the emphasis has shifted to the material, likewise there has been a shift in medicine to high tech, that in turn supports the material. Much of this is wonderful and has its place. But let us not allow it to totally over-ride or displace the less costly. You have heard some of the evidence.

For man has a unique way of twisting things of the world to his advantage, and sometimes accompanying that is an agenda to destroy anything that conflicts with his agenda and that he has not taken the time to understand. We sometimes cling tenaciously to things we dare not question. But this fear only paralyzes real growth. Fortunately, the preponderance of people have the good of mankind at heart, I feel.

So the next time you hear, "There is nothing more that can be done", just remember what that translates to. It merely means in the limited view of that person, he not only does not know what else to do for you, but he does not know anyone else to send you to. But in view of the vast limitations of some aspects of medicine, being governed by powers that have more of a vested interest in being keepers of the purse and maintaining the ultimate authority, it doesn't mean a great deal. As you have seen, there is a great deal of referenced scientific material that could be inexpensively saving lives right this minute, and it is ignored.

So if you are a **diagnostic puzzle,** or have **exhausted all that medicine has to offer.** Or if you have been told you have to learn to live with it, or your days are numbered; what do you have to lose? Why not hook into some of the means that man has been using to initiate healing for over a century? It is logical, based in scientific research, has a proven track record by many who have done it, and is relatively free of adverse side effects. The only critique I can imagine is that it has no double-blind studies. But double-blind studies are a fabricated standard of drug-oriented medicine and are generally only applicable to the testing of drugs. You cannot double-blind a life-style change. But as you saw with the studies of Carter (JACN 12:3, 1993) and others, the best proof is survival long after everyone else has died.

Basing healing on clean air, food and water, correcting deficiencies that this era has given us, and facilitating detoxification merely returns us to our humble origins, in tune with nature, the universal order of things, the yin and yang or balance of life, and to God. Why not see what a little HUMBLE HEALING can do for you?

With the techniques in this book, there is no question that many of us have healed the impossible. When all else fails, a little humble healing may also allow you to attain **wellness.....against all odds.**

"Small is the gate and narrow the road that leads to life, and only a few find it" (**MATTHEW** 7:14, NIV).

RESOURCES

For an excellent video tape of Dr.Rogers with many patients as well describing their recovery from environmental illness, with diagnosis and treatment, contact

> Robin Kormos Productions
> 149 Avenue A
> NY, NY 10009-8921

This tape is suitable for television, schools, doctors' offices, private individuals, businesses, etc.

Week-long residential seminars are also available at the Kushi Foundation in the Berkshires. These are excellent for patients with end-stage cancers who need a crash course in macrobiotics. For information, write:

> Kushi Foundation Berkshire Center
> Box 7
> Becket, MA 01223
> (413) 623-5741

They also have week-long seminars for physicians which I highly recommend.

For courses for physicians in nutritional biochemistry and for names of physicians (in various stages of learning) near you who may practice some of this form of medicine, write to:

> The American Academy of Environmental Medicine
> P.O. Box 16106
> Denver, CO 80216

Support and informational group for people with E.I., regardless of whether or not they use macrobiotics:

Human Ecology Action League of Central New York
377 Dorthy Drive
Syracuse, NY 13215

For physicians wanting courses on chelation, as well as patients who want to know the location of the nearest chelation physician:

American College for Advancement in Medicine
23121 Verdugo Dr., Ste 204
Laguna Hills CA 92653
ph. 714-583-7666

For books, tapes, and seminars on alternative ways to heal,

Cancer Control Society
2043 N Berendo St.
Los Angeles CA 90027
phone 213-663-7801

The address to our office is:

Northeast Center for Environmental Medicine
Sherry A. Rogers, M.D., Medical Director
2800 W. Genesee St.
Syracuse, NY 13219
(315) 488-2856
but
address correspondances to:
Box 2719
Syracuse NY 13220-2716

356

We also have a quarterly newsletter, called HEALTH LETTER, in which we publish up-to-date findings regarding macrobiotics, nutritional biochemistry (vitamins, minerals, amino acids, essential fatty acids and accessory nutrients) and environmental medicine. There are original and new articles and all is referenced so it is of use for physicians as well. All diseases and aspects of health and medicine as well as politics and insurance items of interest are covered. There is nothing else like it!

Articles from Environmental Medicine column, edited and written by Sherry A Rogers, M.D. Available from INTERNAL MEDICINE WORLD REPORT, 322-D Englishtown Rd.,Old Bridge NJ 08857

1. Rogers SA, Chemical sensitivity: Breaking the paralyzing paradigm. Part I, INT MED WORLD REP, 7:4, pp 1, 15-17, Feb 1- 15, 1992

2. Rogers SA, Chemical sensitivity: Breaking the paralyzing paradigm. Diagnosis and treatment. Part II, INT MED WORLD REP, 7:6, pp 2, 21-31, Mar 1-15, 1992

3. Rogers SA, Chemical sensitivity: Breaking the paralyzing paradigm. How knowledge of chemical sensitivity enhances the treatment of chronic diseases. Part III, 7:8, pp 13-16, 32- 33, 40-41, Apr 15-30. 1992

4. letters to the editor   May 1-15, 1992

5. Rogers SA, When stumped, think environmental medicine, INT MED WORLD REP, 7:10, pp 24-25, May 15-31, 1992

6. Rogers SA, Is it senility or chemical sensitivity?, INT MED WORLD REP, 7:13, p 3, July 1992

7.   Rogers SA, How cost effective is improving the work environment?, INT MED WORLD REP, 7:14, p 48, Aug 1992

8.   Rogers SA, Is it recalcitrant arrhythmia or environmental illness?, INT MED WORLD REP, 7:19, p 28, Nov 1- 14, 1992

9.   Rogers SA, (ed.) Chester AC, Sick building Syndrome and the Nose, INT MED WORLD REP, 8:4, p 25-27, Feb 1993.

****

SCIENTIFIC PUBLICATIONS
OF SHERRY A. ROGERS M.D.
IN PEER REVIEWED MEDICAL JOURNALS

1. Indoor Fungi as Part of the Cause of Recalcitrant Symptoms of the Tight Building Syndrome, **Environment International** 17,4,271-276, 1991.

2. Unrecognized magnesium deficiency masquerades as diverse symptoms, evaluation of an oral magnesium challenge test, **International Clinical Nutrition Reviews**, 11:3, 117-125, July 1991.

3. A practical approach to the person with suspected indoor air quality problems, **International Clinical Nutrition Reviews** 11:3, 126-130, July 1991.

4. Zinc deficiency as a model for developing chemical sensitivity, **International Clinical Nutrition Reviews**, 10:1, 253-259, January, 1990.

5. Diagnosing the Tight Building Syndrome or Diagnosing Chemical Hypersensitivity, **Environment International**, 15,

75- 79, 1989.

6. Diagnosing Chemical Hypersensitivity: Case examples, **Clinical Ecology** 6,4, 129-134, 1989.

7. Provocation-Neutralization of Cough and Wheezing in a Horse, **Clinical Ecology,** 5,4, 185-187, 1987/1988.

8. Resistant Cases, Response to Mold Immunotherapy and Environmental and Dietary Controls, **Clinical Ecology, Archives for Human Ecology in Health and Disease,** 5,3, 115-120, 1987/1988.

9. Diagnosing the Tight Building Syndrome, **Environmental Health Perspectives,** 76, 195-198, 1987.

10. A Thirteen Month Work, Leisure, Sleep Environmental Fungal Survey, **Annals of Allergy,** 52, 338-341, May 1984.

11. A comparison of Commercially Available Mold Survey Services, **Annals of Allergy,** 50, 37-40, January, 1983.

12. In-home Fungal Studies, Methods to Increase the Yield, **Annals of Allergy,** 49,35-37, July, 1982.

13. A Case of Atopy With Inability to Form IgG, **Annals of Allergy,** 43,3, 165-166, September, 1979.

14. Is your cardiologist killing you?, **Journal of Orthomolecular Medicine,** 8:2, 89-97, 1993

SCIENTIFIC ARTICLES BY SHERRY A. ROGERS IN PROCEEDINGS OF INTERNATIONAL SYMPOSIA

1. A Practical Approach to the Person With Suspected Indoor Air Quality Problems, The 5th International Conference on

Indoor Air Quality and Climate, Toronto, Canada, Canada Mortgage and Housing Corporation, Ottawa, Ontario, volume 5, 345-349.

2. Diagnosing the Tight Building Syndrome, an intradermal method to provoke chemically induced symptoms, Man and His Ecosystem, Proceedings of the 8th World Clean Air Congress 1989, Brasser, LJ, Mulder, WC, editors. The Hague, Netherlands, Society for Clean Air in the Netherlands, P.O. Box 186, 2600 AD Delft, The Netherlands. 199-204, volume 1.

3. Case Studies of Indoor Air Fungi Used to Clear Recalcitrant Conditions, Healthy Buildings, '88, CIB conference in Stockholm, Sweden, September, 1988, Swedish Council for Building Research, Stockholm Sweden, Berglund, B, Lindvall, T, Mansson, L-G, editors, 127, 1988.

4. Diagnosing the Tight Building Syndrome, an intradermal method to provoke chemically induced symptoms, IBID, 371.

5. Diagnosing the Tight Building Syndrome, Indoor Air '87, Proceedings of the 4th international conference on indoor air quality and climate, West Berlin, Seifert, B, Esdorn, H, Fischer, M, Ruden, H, Wegner, J, editors, Institute for Water, Soil and Air Hygiene, D 1000 Berlin 33, volume 2, 772- 776.

6. Indoor Air Quality and Environmentally Induced Illness, A technique to revoke chemically induced symptoms in patients. Proceedings of the ASHREA conference, IAQ 86, Managing Indoor Air for Health and Energy conservation, 71-77, ASHRAE, 1791 Tullie Circle, NE, Atlanta, GA 30329.

Also listed in Indoor Air Referenced Bibliography, United States Environmental Protection Agency, Office of Health and Environmental Assessment, Washington, D.C., July, 1990, pg.

C81 and C162.

BOOKS BY S.A. ROGERS, M.D.

1. The E.I. SYNDROME is a 650 page book that is necessary for people with environmental illness. It explains chemical, food, mold and Candida sensitivities, nutritional deficiencies, testing methods and how to do the various environmental controls and diet in order to get well. Many docs buy these by the hundreds and make them mandatory reading for new patients, as it contains many pearls about getting well that are not found anywhere else. In this way it increases the fun of practicing medicine because patients are on a higher educational level and time is more productive for more sophisticated levels of wellness. It covers hundreds of facts that make a difference between E.I. victims versus E.I. conquerors. It helps patients become active partners in their care while avoiding doctor burn-out. It covers the gamut of the diagnosis and treatment of environmentally induced symptoms.

2. TIRED OR TOXIC? is a 400 page book, and the first book that describes the mechanism, diagnosis and treatment of chemical sensitivity, complete with scientific references. It is written for the layman and physician alike and explains the many vitamin, mineral, essential fatty acid and amino acid analyses that may help people detoxify everyday chemicals more efficiently and hence get rid of baffling symptoms. The program shows how to diagnose and treat the majority of everyday symptoms and use molecular medicine techniques. It also gives the biochemical mechanisms of how Candida creates such a diversity of symptoms and how the macrobiotic diet heals "incurable" end stage metastatic cancers. It is the best book of the 4 for the physician.

3. YOU ARE WHAT YOU ATE is a book to show patients how

361

to begin the macrobiotic diet, with which so many universal reactors have lost their food, mold, Candida and chemical sensitivities, as well many other people have healed the impossible with this diet.

4. **THE CURE IS IN THE KITCHEN** is the first book to ever spell out in detail what all those people ate day to day who cleared their incurable diseases, undiagnosable symptoms, relentless chemical, food, Candida, and electromagnetic sensitivities, as well as terminal cancers. Dr. Rogers flew to Boston each month to work side by side with Mr. Michio Kushi, as he counseled people at the end of their medical ropes, as their remarkable case histories will show you. If you cannot afford a $500 consultation, and you chose not to accept your death sentence, why not learn first hand what these people did and how you, too, may improve your health.

5. **MACRO MELLOW** is a book designed for 4 types of people:
(1) For the person who doesn't know a thing about macrobiotics, but just plain wants to feel better, in spite of the 21st century.
(2) It solves the high cholesterol/triglycerides problem without drugs and is the perfect diet for heart disease patients.
(3) It is the perfect transition diet for those not ready for macro, but needing to get out of the chronic illness rut.
(4) It spells out how to feed the rest of the family who hates macro, while another family member must eat it to clear their "incurable" symptoms.

The delicious low-fat whole food meals designed by Shirley Gallinger, a veteran nurse who has worked with Dr. Rogers for over a decade, use macro ingredients without the rest of the family even knowing. It is the first book to dove-tail creative meal planning, menus, recipes and even gardening so the cook isn't driven crazy.

362

PRESTIGE PUBLISHING
P.O. BOX 3161
Syracuse, NY 13220
(800) 846-ONUS
(315) 455-7862

Please send the following books: Quantity Sub-total

The E.I. Syndrome...................$ 14.95   _____ _____
You Are What You Ate........... 9.95   _____ _____
Tired or Toxic?........................... 17.95 _____ _____
Macro Mellow........................... 13.95   _____ _____
The Cure Is In The Kitchen..... 14.95   _____ _____
Wellness Against All Odds......17.95   _____ _____

Health Letter(quarterly)newsletter..30/yr _____

Mold Plates (one room)...........25.00   _____ _____

Formaldehyde Spot Test.........40.00   _____ _____
      (over 50 tests)
                                      Sub-total   _____

                    *Quantity discount   _____
            NY State residents add 7% sales tax   _____
**Shipping/handling $3 each item......................   _____

Total enclosed.......................................   _____

*Discounts available on ten or more books.
**Ship/hand $3.00 each item in the continental U.S., $6.00 each
elsewhere.

INITIAL SUBSCRIPTION
OR
— RENEWAL—
NORTHEAST CENTER FOR ENVIRONMENTAL MEDICINE
HEALTH LETTER
P.O. Box 3161, Syracuse, NY 13220
(315) 455-7863
1-800-846-ONUS

_____Please start my subscription for _____years.

_____Please renew my subscription for _____years.

Subscription rates: (United States) One year, $30.00
Two years, $60.00

(International) One year, $40.00 (U.S.)
Two years, $80.00 (U.S.)

_____Charge to:_____VISA_____MasterCard

#_____Exp._____

Signature:_____

Name_____

Address_____

City_____State_____Zip_____

Telephone _____

Northeast Center For Environmental Medicine Health Letter is published quarterly by Prestige Publishing, P.O. Box 3161, Syracuse, NY 13220.

Index

(abbreviated)

A

abdominal pain   240, 243
acid-loving   54, 73
acne   22
acute pain   232
ADDICTION   121
adrenal   115
aggitation   201, 202, 292
AIDS   103, 116, 120, 131, 139, 163
alcohol   51, 62, 67, 74, 196
ALCOHOLISM   327, 333, 334
alcoholism   139
alkaline-loving   56
Aluminum   103, 225, 239, 243, 245, 246, 253, 329, 337
Amalgam   243
amalgam   240, 243, 334
AMINO ACID   334
Amino acid   110, 145, 147, 158, 160, 162, 202, 242, 250, 303, 308, 322, 326, 334, 337, 342
amino acid   93, 357, 361
Amino aciduria   242
anergy   115
ankylosing spondylitis   237, 251, 291
antagonist   175
Antibodies   121, 237
antibodies   120, 136, 138, 236, 237, 250, 251, 305
antibody   85, 86
Antihistamine   179
antihistamine   175, 305, 307
anxiety   201, 207, 292, 293

apoliprotein A1 & B   346
area of weakness or previous damage   232
arrhythmia   154, 155, 171, 197, 198, 222, 234, 288, 289, 322, 328, 339, 358
Arsenic   240, 242, 245, 246
arteriosclerosis 112, 118, 151, 152,
154, 162, 163, 168, 193,
199, 207, 208, 213, 218,
229, 284, 290, 294, 299, 304
arthritic spurs   231
ARTHRITIS   220
Arthritis   9, 23, 81, 84, 85, 86, 102, 112, 116, 118,
136, 138, 139, 140, 142, 143, 153, 215
asthma   2, 29, 33, 48
ataxia   240, 243
atherosclerotic plaque   192
Atrial fibrillation   222
atrial fibrillation   222
attention deficit disorder   242, 327
auto-immune   249
autoimmune   112, 116, 118
automatic nervous system   290
autonomic nervous system   290

B

B vitamins   135
B12   253, 309, 342
BALANCE   64
balance   62, 65, 68, 69
Beans   5, 50, 55, 64, 74, 107, 211
bell-shaped curve   161, 347
Beta-carotene   122, 162, 189, 191, 206
Beverages   28, 45
Bio Tech   144
biochemical blunders   207, 294

bizarre palsies   240
bizarre tremors   243
bladder spasms   171
bleached white rice   196, 287
Blood pressure   171
blood pressure   92, 150, 151, 152,
156, 170, 179, 180, 182, 193, 217, 229, 231,
239, 284, 303, 290, 327, 341
body pains   240, 342
bone calcification   210, 297
brain fog   84, 102
breast cancinoma   190
BRUSHING   110, 132, 141
buffers   127
burdock weed   67

C

c   81, 100
CACHEXIA   106
Cadmium   239, 241, 242, 245
caffeine   90, 94, 100, 102, 337
Cal amo   129, 130, 132
cal amo   143
CALCIUM   221
Calcium   34, 127, 129, 130, 143, 156, 172,
197, 198, 202, 206, 210, 212, 214, 215, 216, 229,
231, 288, 289, 293, 296, 297, 298, 301, 302
calcium   28, 33, 34, 40, 45
Calcium channel blocker   198, 288, 289
Calcium pump   198, 288
CANCER   107, 108, 109, 113, 114, 115,
131, 142, 202, 204, 215, 220, 224
Cancer   167, 203, 230, 255
cancer   81, 82, 83, 84, 88, 92, 93, 95,
105, 106, 108, 109, 110, 111, 112, 113,

114, 115, 116, 118, 119, 120, 122, 131, 133, 137, 140, 141,
142, 145, 146, 149, 150, 159, 160, 162, 163, 164,
166, 167, 202, 203, 204, 208, 218, 223, 224,
228, 229, 230, 239, 240,
242, 249, 251, 253, 254, 255
Cancer of the prostate   327
cancer of the prostate   242
cancerous conditions   186
CANCERS   145, 149, 150, 163, 164, 166,
167, 175, 176, 177, 184, 185, 186,
188, 202, 224, 229, 254, 255, 299, 303, 306,
326, 327, 331, 334, 343, 346, 348
cancers   355, 361, 362
CANDIDA   134, 135, 137, 140, 203, 253, 254, 305
Candida   2, 3, 46, 50, 52, 62, 71
carcinogenesis   190, 202
cardiac arrhythmia   155, 171, 197, 198, 288, 289
cardiac disease   213, 217, 242, 299, 303
cardiac myopathy   207, 294
cardiologists   181, 194, 285, 328
carnitine   61
CARNIVORE   20, 21, 47
Carnivore   16, 18, 19, 37, 39, 40,
41, 46, 47, 49, 50, 51, 52, 54, 5
5, 56, 69, 70, 72, 73, 74, 176,
179, 248, 252, 338, 345, 346
Carotenoids   187, 190, 191
carpets   81
Castor Oil Compresses   134
catecholamine induction   201, 292
cause of nutrient loss   149
cbc   152
celiac disease   120
Charles Coleson   288
chelate   244

chelators   244
chemically sensitive   95
chemicals   81, 82, 87, 91, 100, 105
Chemicals deplete vitamin A   186
chemotherapy   150, 161, 186, 187, 202, 205, 299, 300, 302, 306, 321, 326, 332
CHLORINATED WATER   226, 228, 229
Chlorination   230
Chlorine   228, 229
chlorine   95, 105, 228, 229, 230, 334, 337
Cholesterol   56
cholesterol   9, 55, 56, 65, 71
cholinate citrate   347
chromium   52, 61, 65
CHROMIUM CYCLE   169
CHROMIUM DEFICIENCY   155, 167, 168, 169, 207, 218, 294, 304
CHRONIC BACK PAIN   231, 237
chronic cystitis   250
chronic dermatoses   242
chronic fatigue   152, 154, 201, 213, 234, 242, 250, 291, 299, 303, 331, 343
chronic low back pain   154, 236
chronic shoulder   2
chronic sinusitis   2
chronic upper respiratory infections   242
chymotrypsin   113
citric acid cycle   50
CLEANSING   110, 123, 124, 126, 128, 137, 143
coagulation   173, 174
coenzyme A   50
COFFEE ENEMA   82, 90, 95
Coffee enema   88, 103, 105
coffee enema   81, 82, 83, 84, 85, 86, 88, 90, 91, 92, 93, 94, 98, 99,

100, 101, 102, 103, 106, 110, 112, 113, 121, 125, 129, 204
COLON CLEANSE   100, 123, 124, 126, 128, 137
colon problems   136
COMMON COLD   91
confusion   240
Consistency   249, 345
consistency   248, 249
Copper   65, 67
copper   94
CoQ10   347
coronary heart disease   56, 57, 214, 216
CRAVING CYCLE   167
cravings   51, 61, 62, 63, 66, 67
cravings for sweets   168
CUT the CRAP   344
cyclooxygenase   176

D

D-alpha tocopherol   164
D-XYLOSE TEST   254
Dairy Products   33, 41, 42
Darvon deficiency   63, 68
deficiencies   52, 53, 54, 56, 61, 64, 65, 73, 284, 285, 303
degenerative diseases   151
dementia   193, 284, 337
depression   81, 139, 152, 162, 169,
171, 201, 239, 240, 250, 251, 292
detox   48, 49, 50, 52, 54, 71, 72, 73
DETOXIFICATION   133, 142
Detoxification   108
detoxification   87, 89, 91, 103, 104, 110, 129,
131, 135, 137, 149, 162, 202, 244, 246
detoxify   83, 89, 90, 100, 105, 122, 133, 145,
146, 149, 152, 156, 198, 206, 234
DIABETES   216, 302

Diabetes   303
diabetes   52, 62, 137, 168, 209, 213,
220, 296, 299, 306, 303, 337
diagnostic puzzle   353
diarrhea   240, 243
difficulty walking   240
dissolve arterial obstructions   119
diuretic   197, 198, 209, 220, 288, 289, 296, 306
DNA   174, 286, 303
Dr. Bernie Siegel   294
Dr. Delores Krieger   295
Dr. John Beard   111
Dr. Joseph Gold   106
Dr. Kelley   348
Dr. Linus Pauling   163, 203
Dr. Vivien Newbold   326
Dr. William Rea   53
drug   1, 9
dysbiosis   117, 136, 137, 144, 254

E

E.I.   2, 6, 11, 28, 53, 91, 135, 186
eczema   2
EDTA   149
EMF   81
endocrinologists   330
ENEMA   82, 90, 95, 96
enema   81, 82, 83, 84, 85, 86, 88, 90, 91, 92,
93, 94, 95, 96, 97, 98, 99, 100, 101, 102, 103,
104, 105, 106, 110, 112, 113, 119, 121, 125,
129, 174, 177, 185, 332, 339, 343, 344, 345, 349
energy   49, 50, 52, 87, 135, 153, 162
entero-hepatic circulation   90
ENVIRONMENTAL MEDICINE   231, 232, 236,
253, 255, 305, 327, 329, 340, 355, 356, 357, 364, 365

ENZYMES 83, 93, 100, 110, 111, 112, 113, 115,
116, 117, 118, 119, 120, 121, 122, 137, 142, 143, 152,
153, 154, 158, 159, 165, 177, 185, 228, 230,
236, 240, 243, 246, 247, 334, 337, 343, 344, 348, 349
ESENTIAL FATTY ACIDS 77
esential fatty acids ˙74

F

Faid 287, 317
FAITH FACTOR 284, 316
farmed ocean fish 211, 297
FASTING 77
Fatigue 240
fatigue 81, 84, 100, 135, 139, 140, 234, 242, 250, 251
Fatty acids 186
fatty acids 81, 93, 110, 145, 147,
158, 160, 165, 179, 180, 181,
183, 192, 194, 195, 215, 229, 250, 285, 286, 301, 347, 357
fellowship groups 288
flaxseed 26, 36, 44, 347
FLUSHING 93, 110, 127
FOOD ALLERGY 237, 249, 303
Food allergy 249, 250
Food antigens 139
food antigens 138, 139, 141
foot drop 242
French catheter 95

G

gall stones 128
Gallbladder flush 127, 131
gallbladder flush 127
gamma linolenic acid 192
GARLIC 71
Garlic 71

garlic   71, 72, 74
gas heat   235
gastroenterologist   89
gastroenterologists   329
Gerson   6, 7, 11, 12, 13, 19, 25, 35, 42, 57,
58, 75, 79, 80, 83, 122, 179, 223, 333, 339
gingivitis   243
glands   115, 330
glutamic acid   72, 73
glutathione   87, 91, 100, 107, 108, 109, 149, 347
glutathione-S-transferace   91, 100, 107, 108
GLUTEN   249, 250, 251
Gluten   250
gluten   250, 251, 252, 254, 255
gluten enteropathy   120, 251, 254
GLUTEN-SENSITIVITY   249, 250
glycine   347
glycosylation   52, 53
God-given symptom   63
Grains   5, 13, 18, 19, 21, 25, 26, 27, 29, 30, 32,
42, 46, 49, 50, 51, 56, 64, 74, 211, 226, 250, 332, 335, 338, 345
Great Smokies Laboratory   144
grocery store cooking oils   193
GUILT   61, 62, 66
gynecologists   330

H

HDL   346
headache   83, 84, 102, 132, 134, 168,
204, 240, 243, 321, 337, 340
HEAL   3, 5, 6, 9, 10
heart attacks   193
HEAVY METAL TOXICITY   239, 240, 241, 243,
244, 245, 253
high blood pressure   193, 229, 239, 284, 327, 341

homeostasis   156, 169
hospital dieticians   181
HUMBLE HEALING   321, 334, 343, 344, 345, 354
Humble Healing   311, 332, 354
HYDRAZINE SULFATE   106, 108, 109
hydrocephalus   161, 162
hydrogenated   193, 211
hydrogenated oils   54, 57, 211, 297, 329, 338
hyperactivity   242, 250, 308
hypercholesterolemia   152, 155
hyperlipidemia   187
hyperpermeable   94, 138, 140, 236, 251
HYPERTENSION   229, 230, 231
Hypertension   171, 172
hypertension   150, 170, 171, 173, 180,
197, 198, 212, 215, 217, 219, 229, 230, 231, 238, 251, 288,
289, 298, 301, 303, 305
hypocalcemia   199, 220, 290, 306
hypoglycemia   168, 169, 187, 207, 212, 294, 298, 314
hypokalemia   180, 197, 199, 200, 220, 288, 290, 291, 306
Hypomagnesaemia   214, 301
Hypomagnesemia   214, 300
hypomagnesemia   198, 199, 220, 222, 289, 290, 306
hyponatremia   220, 306
hypophosphatemia   199, 220, 290, 306

I

IgA   93, 94, 135, 204, 239, 240, 242, 243
immune system damage   240
impotence   193
incinerators   242
infertility   201, 292, 307
insomnia   171, 207, 293, 308, 333
insulin resistance   168
internists   328

Intestinal spasms   201, 291
intravenous magnesium   199, 222, 290
IRON   190, 195, 231, 238, 239, 286, 364
Iron   125
iron   100, 120, 139, 147, 149, 150, 153, 176, 181, 186, 201, 202,
204, 206, 208, 209, 211, 217, 223, 224, 226, 232, 236, 240, 241, 244,
246, 247, 253, 255, 292, 293, 294, 295, 296, 297, 303,
297, 300, 305, 310, 311, 312, 323, 327, 329, 330,
331, 334, 335, 340, 344, 347,
355, 356, 357, 358, 359, 360, 361, 365
irritability   201, 202, 292
irritable bowel   140, 251

J

jitteriness   104
JUICING   93, 100, 110, 122, 142, 299
juvenile chronic myelogenous leukemia   185

K

Kelley Program   7, 112
kidney damage   239, 240
Klaire Laboratories   143
Klebsiella   237, 251
kudzu   67

L

Labelitis   321
labelitis   255, 321
lactase   252
LDL   346
lead poisoning   239
LEAKY CELL MEMBRANES   54
LEAKY GUT   249
leaky gut   249, 350
LEAKY GUT SYNDROME   94, 117, 134, 138,

139, 141, 144, 249
learning disabilities   139
learning disorder   250
LeShan   226, 294
leukemia   5, 6, 150, 161
lipid metabolism   198, 217, 289, 303
lipoic acid   347
liver   11, 12, 15, 35, 36, 39, 42, 45
liver flush   130, 131
loss of amino acids   242
low blood sugar   187
lupus   116

M

Macrobiotics   2, 3, 4, 46, 64, 75
magnesium   83, 86, 89, 90, 94, 99
MAGNESIUM CYCLE   169, 170
Magnesium deficiency   154
magnesium deficiency   89, 90, 99, 150, 155, 170, 171
magnesium loading test   94
magnesium sulfate   219, 222, 305
maillard   52
malabsorption   254
Malnutrit;insulin response   219, 305
Malnutrition among hospitalized patients   218, 304
manganese   52, 61, 148, 152, 153, 158, 159, 169, 206, 232, 234, 240, 293, 329, 333, 341, 342, 346, 347
Margarines   194
margarines   193, 194, 195, 211
Mercury   240, 243, 245
metabolize cholesterol   155, 329
metastatic cancer   112, 361
methionine   347
microcytic anemia   153
migraine   201, 250, 291, 327, 330

migraines 2
mineral 2, 3, 18, 19, 24, 25, 27, 28, 30, 31, 32, 33, 34, 35, 37, 39, 43, 45, 57, 64, 65, 68, 72
mineral deficiency 101
mineral deficiencies 116, 148, 151, 169, 323
mineral transporters 153, 348
molasses 95, 96, 98, 103
molybdenum 244, 342, 346, 347
mood swings 139, 168, 169, 250
MSG 233, 252
muscle contraction or spasm 197, 288
muscle relaxation 197, 288
Mustard Foot Soaks 134

N

N-acetyl cysteine 347
N.E.E.D.S. 95, 109, 118, 124, 143, 225, 334, 342
Natrens Inc, 144
natural hygiene 83
Navy SEAL trainees 151
neoplasia 190
nerve disorders 240
neurologists 330
niacin 102, 162, 349
nightshades 232, 233
nitroglycerine 104
non-chlorinated water 226
non-steroidal anti-inflammatory drugs 89
numbness 240, 251, 342
Nutricology, dba Allergy Research Group 143

O

obesity 169, 337
OILS 77
Oils 54, 57, 82, 133, 165, 193, 194, 195, 211

Omega-3 oil   176
oncologists   287, 300, 330
OPPOSITES   73
Opposites   73
ORNISH   57
Ornish   57
orthopedists   330
osteoporosis   154, 156, 210, 212, 229, 230, 296, 298, 337
ovary   115
OVERWHELMED   351
oxidation   153, 167, 303
oxidized form   163
ozonation   229

P

pancreas   83, 111, 114, 116, 117, 167, 229, 230
panic   201, 202, 240, 292, 290
panic attacks   201, 292
parasympathetic   290, 291
paresthesias   240, 251
Pat Robertson   293, 325
pediatricians   328
peripheral neuropathies   242
peripheral neuropathy   242
pesticides   117, 312, 334, 342
phosphorous   127
phosphorous acid   127
pituitary   115
placenta   111, 114
PMS   171
poor digestion   169
poor I.Q.   240
postviral fatigue syndrome   192
POTASSIUM   55, 56, 57, 58, 59, 60,
79, 93, 99, 100, 103, 107

pregnancy   201, 292, 322
premature aging   152, 167, 193, 284
Processed foods   344
processed foods   54, 60, 62, 74, 145, 146, 148,
165, 181, 186, 195, 196, 210,
211, 226, 286, 287, 296, 297, 308, 309,
313, 329, 337, 338, 339, 344
prostate cancer   167, 191, 192
psychoneuroimmunology   295
Psyllium   125, 126
psyllium   123, 124, 125, 126
PURGE   92, 131, 132
putrescene   66

R

radiation   202, 204, 254, 300, 312, 321, 326
radon   81, 82
Rapp DJ   313
rbc chromium   94
rbc copper   94
rbc manganese   94
rbc zinc   94
reasonable and customary   155, 199, 290
recalcitrant cardiac arrhythmia   197, 288
Remission   189
remission   184, 185, 189
RETINOIC ACID SYNDROME   92
Retinoids   182, 187, 188, 190
retinoids   190, 192
retinol   190, 192
rheumatologists   329
Robertson   293, 318, 325

S

S.O.D.   159

Salt and Soda Baths   133
SCHIZOPHRENIA   121
schizophrenia   120, 121, 139
see your test results   159
Seeds   18, 21, 26, 29, 30, 31, 32, 37
selenium   342, 346
serum magnesium   155, 156, 157, 158, 197,
198, 219, 222, 234, 288, 289, 305
Shirley Gallinger   64
sick feeling   84
SICK GET SICKER   193, 198, 202, 208, 210, 211, 236,
247, 251, 284, 289, 292, 294, 296, 297, 309
sigmoid colon   90, 97
Sodium pump   172
sodium pump   170, 197, 213, 288, 299
spiral mechanism   202, 292
SPIRITUALITY   228, 284, 285, 289, 290, 291, 292,
294, 295, 296, 297, 301, 340, 343, 344
spreading phenomenon   247, 289
squamous cell   185
stagnation   173
standard American diet (SAD)   148
STEAMING   22, 59
Stress   296
stress   196, 201, 224, 235, 287, 292, 291, 296, 313
strokes   193, 200, 284, 291
sucrase   253
Sudden death   198, 289
sudden death   154, 171, 197, 198, 209, 215, 219,
229, 234, 239, 288, 289, 296, 301, 305
sugar metabolism   168
Sugars   135
sugars   22, 38, 44, 52, 117, 119, 135, 335, 338
superoxide dismutase   146, 159
surgeons   329

surgery 202, 204, 214, 226, 232, 237, 300, 326, 329, 331, 332

sweats 168

sweets 51, 210

sympathetic nervous system 231, 290

symptoms 84, 89, 92, 94, 99, 102, 105, 113, 119, 127, 132, 134, 135, 139, 140, 147, 148, 149, 151, 152, 156, 157, 170, 171, 195, 197, 198, 200, 201, 207, 208, 211, 214, 230, 232, 233, 234, 235, 236, 237, 238, 239, 240, 241, 242, 243, 245, 246, 250, 252, 253

T

tamoxifen 306

target organ 232, 233, 234, 236, 250, 294, 284, 331

target organ age 232, 233, 234, 236, 250, 284, 331

taurine 347

The 4-PC 81

thiaminase 50

thiamine 50

thymus 115

THYROID 300

Thyroid 136

thyroid 115, 116, 136, 153, 175, 176, 249

thyroiditis 116, 249

TIA 193, 196, 198, 200, 201, 209, 210, 211, 217, 218, 220, 229, 231, 239, 243, 246, 250, 284, 287, 289, 291, 292, 295, 296, 297, 303, 304, 287, 288, 291, 292, 293, 300, 302, 303, 306, 308, 311, 313, 316, 317, 318, 319, 324, 332, 334, 337, 342, 343, 347, 353, 355, 357, 361, 364

Tilden 89

tingling 240, 251, 342, 349

TIRED OR TOXIC? 92, 110, 147, 157, 158, 160, 165, 166, 183, 218, 304, 307, 328, 335, 340, 361

Tired or Toxic? 363

tongue 84

TOTAL LOAD 223

total load 208, 210, 223, 224, 235,

239, 247, 248, 249, 254,
255, 294, 295, 296, 291, 294, 328, 334, 340, 342, 344, 347, 352
Tourette's 139
TOXEMIA 87, 89
toxemia 87
toxic brain syndrome 242
toxins 51, 66, 84, 88, 90, 94, 100, 103
Trade-offs 335
trade-offs 335, 344
trans fatty acids 194, 195, 229, 285, 286
triglycerides 156, 168, 170, 187, 346, 362
trophoblast 111, 114, 141, 142
tryptophan 308
tumors 66, 67, 80
Tyler Encapsulations 143

U

ulcerative colitis 250
ulcers 243
UNIVERSAL HEALING POWER 295
urologists 330

V

vaginitis 250
vanadium 346
vascular calcifications 210, 297
vascular spasms 201, 291
vegan 48, 50, 56
Vegetables 7, 55, 56, 57, 58, 59, 60,
64, 68, 69, 72, 122, 123, 202, 211
ventricles 161
villi 136, 137, 250
visual disturbances 243
VITAMIN 114, 184, 187, 224
Vitamin 72, 163, 164, 165, 184, 186, 202, 207, 294

vitamin 2, 3, 11, 19, 22, 24, 27,
28, 30, 31, 32, 38, 39, 43, 44, 50, 65, 68, 70, 72,
74, 83, 90, 92, 93, 102, 110,
124, 135, 145, 147, 148, 149, 150, 155,
157, 158, 160, 161, 162, 163, 164, 165, 166, 173, 174, 175,
177, 181, 182, 184, 185, 186, 187, 188, 189, 191, 192, 193, 202,
203, 205, 206, 207, 208, 209, 214, 215, 241, 250, 252, 253, 284,
294, 295, 300, 308, 330, 336, 342, 346, 347, 348, 349, 357, 361
vitamin A   92
vitamin A analogs   185
vitamin B3   102, 349
vitamin B6   149, 173, 174
vitamin D   70
Vitamin E   207, 294
vitamin E   202, 205, 206, 207, 208, 209,
214, 215, 294, 295, 300, 347, 348
Vitamin K   72
vitamin K   72

W

wasting away   106
weakness   168, 232, 347
white flour   74, 170, 196, 226, 287
Whole grain cereals   42
wrist drop   242

X

Xenobiotic   247
xenobiotic   108, 147, 149, 208, 234, 235, 236, 294, 296, 328

Z

zinc   94
Zinc deficiency   154, 358
zinc deficiency   154